recommend this book. Thanks, Samantha Craft, for putting this good thing into the world."

~ Jeanette Purkis, Autistic Advocate, Artist, and Author of *Finding a Different Kind of Normal* and *The Wonderful World of Work* and Coauthor of *The Guide to Good Mental Health on the Autism Spectrum*

"*Everyday Aspergers*, the new book, as much as the blog, is a valuable resource for anyone in any way touched by ASD, as well as an honest insight for anyone else into the workings of Samantha Craft's wonderfully poetic brain. To try and explain in what way her writings have improved my life, my marriage, and my relationship to friends and family would be to write a whole other book. She is a kind and incredibly insightful human being, whose experiences resonate with many people on the autism spectrum, male and female alike. I particularly appreciate her wonderfully elaborate 'Ten Traits (Females with Aspergers)' list. *Everyday Aspergers* will—no shimmer of doubt in my mind—help generations of people in need of a familiar voice."

~ Jasmin Egner, Autistic Actress, Autism and Mental Health Advocate

"'The Encyclopedia of Aspergers'—written by someone who lives it every day. Funny, honest, touching, and real, *Everyday Aspergers* is a book that can be turned to again and again—for reference, support, and for reassurance. I recommend it highly."

~ Rachael Lucas, Author of *Sealed with a Kiss* and *Wildflower Bay*

"There has never been another book like *Everyday Aspergers*. In prose that is alternatingly playful, witty, brave, heartbreaking, and encouraging, Samantha Craft explores her experience of life on the spectrum in meticulous and comprehensive detail. Many parts of the book—including '116 Reasons I Know I Have Asperger's Syndrome' and her description of her journey to 'Planet Aspie' and return to Earth—are classic, stand-alone set pieces that rank with the very best writing from autistic self-advocates. This book is a gift for autistic people in general, for autistic women in specific, and for neurotypical readers who want to become more effective allies. By exploring her autism, Craft teaches us all how to be more compassionate and alive human beings."

~ Steve Silberman, Author of
NeuroTribes: The Legacy of Autism and the Future of Neurodiversity

"This book is stunning, beautifully written with a raw and arresting honesty that illuminates the details of living and being autistic/Aspie. Dip in and out or read right through, you will find something that resonates with you as being autistic is being human."

~ Emma Goodall, PhD, Author of
Understanding and Facilitating the Achievement of Autistic Potential
and *The Autism Spectrum Guide to Sexuality and Relationships*
and Coauthor of *The Guide to Good Mental Health on the Autism Spectrum*

"*Everyday Aspergers* is a fun, poignant series of snapshots into the mind of a wife, mother, educator-turned-therapist during the days she spent processing her own late diagnosis. Each vignette is a sweet morsel of insight and generosity of spirit as she lays raw her very personal journey. Finally something for families and especially women to read a day at a time—as it was written— as they also take their own small steps to self-awareness and insight."

~ Dena L. Gassner, PhD Student
in Social Welfare at Adelphi University; National Board Member Arc US
and GRASP; Director of the Center for Understanding

"Samantha Craft has put together a series of personal stories which offer an amazing insight for Aspergirls specifically. Her journey of acceptance, inclusion, and understanding of her own identity is inspirational and I will share this book with all of my clients on the spectrum. I am beyond impressed with her journey and her commitment to sharing her personal life with other people on the spectrum. Amazing work!"

~ Frank Gaskill, PhD, Author of the graphic novel *Max Gamer*,
a Contributing Author to *The Walking Dead Psychology*,
and *Star Wars Psychology: The Dark Side of the Mind*.
He is also the host of the "Dr. G. Aspie Show."

"Craft is a positive and professional strengths-based role model with many gifts. Her insightful story illuminates the multiple attributes I've observed in the hundreds of females I've assessed and diagnosed on the autism spectrum. The information is current and prolific. Her self-reflection, intelligence, humor, and faith are refreshing. This is one book that I'll be recommending in my 'what next' sections with my clients. *Everyday Aspergers* will no doubt serve as a helpful resource to many."

~ Tania Marshall, MS, Psychologist and
Gold-Winning Author of
I Am AspienWoman and *I Am AspienGirl*

"*Everyday Aspergers* is easy to read, accessible, and incredibly relatable. As an autistic woman myself, I found countless points of commonality with Craft's experiences and thoughts about life. The book is passionate—a great work of advocacy, as well as an honest and heartfelt personal account of the author's life. The book presents a life lived with challenges but also with great strengths and quiet wisdom. Craft shatters a number of myths around things like autism and empathy, creativity and love. It was moving and meaningful on many levels. If you are on the autism spectrum yourself, or know, love, or care for someone who is, I strongly

EVERYDAY ASPERGERS

EVERYDAY ASPERGERS

SAMANTHA CRAFT

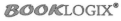**BOOK**LOGIX®
Alpharetta, GA

Some names and identifying details have been changed to protect the privacy of individuals.

The author has tried to recreate events, locations, and conversations from his/her memories of them. In some instances, in order to maintain their anonymity, the author has changed the names of individuals and places. He/she may also have changed some identifying characteristics and details such as physical attributes, occupations, and places of residence.

The information provided in the book *Everyday Aspergers* is for informational purposes only and is not intended as a substitute for advice from a physician or other health care professional. The information in this book is not intended for diagnosis or treatment of any medical condition. It is not advisable to stop taking any medication without consulting a medical physician. Stopping psychiatric medications without medical supervision can be extremely dangerous.

ISBN: 978-1-61005-805-6
Library of Congress Control Number: 2016909542

10 9 8 7 6 5 4 3 2   0 6 3 0 1 6

Printed in the United States of America

∞This paper meets the requirements of ANSI/NISO Z39.48-1992 (Permanence of Paper)

To Bob and my three beautiful sons

"I believe the greatest gift I can conceive of having from anyone is to be seen, heard, understood and touched by them. The greatest gift I can give is to see, hear, understand and touch another person. When this is done, I feel contact has been made."

—Virginia Satir

CONTENTS

ACKNOWLEDGMENTS

Thanks go out to Bob, my former husband, who remains a dear friend and supporter in my life and a loving father to our three teenage sons; thank you for our nineteen years together and for all the times you repeatedly listened to my writings. Thank you for your continued assistance with my vocational endeavors; I am fortunate to know you. Further thanks to my three handsome sons; thank you for accepting me with all my quirks and loving me regardless, for your contributions to my writings through your own life happenings, and for being the cool dudes you are—intelligent, open-minded, considerate, and patient. An additional thank-you to my partner, Ryan—your unyielding emotional support, unconditional love, and understanding of my autism got me through the editing process and much more. My utmost appreciation goes out to Steve Silberman, Tania Marshall, Dena Gassner, Emma Goodall, Jeanette Purkis, Jasmin Egner, Frank Gaskill, and Rachael Lucas; thank you, with countless gratitude, for kindly fitting in time to review my manuscript and more importantly for all you do to support individuals on the autism spectrum. In addition, I am sending out a huge cloud of fluffy thank-yous to the readers of my online writings that made *Everyday Aspergers* possible—without you, I would have not had the strength or encouragement to turn my writings into a book. And a big thanks to the kind members of the *Everyday Aspergers* Book Group who helped with final revisions and editing. And let me not forget to acknowledge the patience and expertise of the members of the BookLogix team. A huge hug of thanks to all my friends through the years who stuck with me, including Patricia P., Lynn H., Lisa L., Mary K., Alyce A., Steffanie K., Lisa G., Aileen K., David W., Jodie C., Anna Marie C., Sue S., Cynthia B., Shawna H., Fran, Jill, and Wati. I am blessed beyond measure to have you all in my life. A big thank-you and love to Lisa (my lifelong friend) and Anthony (my high school sweetheart); you both made high school life bearable. Much love as well to my extended family, including Grandma Evy and all my cousins, aunts, and uncles. You are a hoot to know and a joy to cherish! A blessing goes to my namesake Aunt Marcelle, and to Aunt Kathleen, Aunt Cathy, and my intelligent and generous parents. A wave and kiss toward the heavens to Grandpa Mac, Louise, Nano, Nana, Aunt Francesca, Andrea, Mrs. Silva, Uncle Paul, Helen, Charles, "Drake," "Ben," and Mrs. Craft. Lastly, I'd like to thank my childhood dog Justice for being my constant companion.

INTRODUCTION

I remember the exact day my middle son was diagnosed with Asperger's Syndrome: January 13, 2005. He was five years old. His long-awaited appointment at the UC Davis Mind Institute just so happened to be on the same day as my youngest son's birthday and the day right after my minivan was rear-ended in a highway accident. I recall too well the previous months leading up to the appointment and still feel a tiny quiver of unease when I think back to the years before my son's diagnosis. Particularly poignant was the afternoon I gently pulled my little man (who was screaming and slithering on the floor) across the waiting room and into the family doctor's office. That practitioner's advice: "I suggest you take a look at your parenting skills." I remember, too, the time period shortly following my son's diagnosis—how the behavioral specialist and child psychologist that visited our home basically gave up on assisting. I can still see the behaviorist's hands up in the air and hear him whispering, "I honestly don't think there is anything I can do." I remember crying and feeling extremely isolated. And I remember slowly pulling myself up and doing what I had to do to be my child's supporter.

Overall, the ramification of my son's diagnosis of Asperger's Syndrome caused a spiral effect; it spun out like a top, colliding and stirring every aspect of our family's life. My diagnosis fallout was different. By the time I was in my early forties, my middle guy was content and, for the most part, functioning at a high level of independence. Our family unit was also functioning well. I had long since retired from teaching and advocating for children with special needs and was at home taking care of my three boys. I was content with my husband. Life in general felt easy. Everything seemed in its place: our marriage, our home, our children's education, our vocations. Everything was satisfactory. I had just started in on a new career path and was attending a local university to attain a degree in mental health counseling, something I'd originally started prior to the birth of our first son. It was at this time that I sought out a private practice therapist as part of the counseling program's requirements. The therapist I saw was quick to diagnose me with Asperger's Syndrome. About thirteen months later, a licensed psychologist "officially" confirmed my diagnosis; however, by that time I was already floating aimlessly in the autism matrix, bewildered by the complexities of my own thought processes in regard to the "syndrome."

Unlike the diagnostic journey with my son—in which my own logic and skills took over and I circumvented the grief and challenges with solution after solution—here, I found myself trapped inside my mind with no rescue in sight. This is where my writings began, with me in this internal spinning state.

Each account in this book represents a numbered journal entry that I selected, refined, and polished from well over twelve hundred pages of my online writings. The majority of the posts are in the same chronological order as when they were originally scribed. The journal entries are intermingled with vignettes—short stories that I completed approximately a decade ago when I was first called to share my journey. These vignettes, inspired by true events, were completed long before I knew I was autistic. Today, I find it interesting to observe the nuances of Aspergers bulging through the pages of these older tales.

In considering the language use in this memoir, it is important to point out that the selections in *Everyday Aspergers* were originally composed when Asperger's Syndrome was a stand-alone diagnosis. At that time, not much was written or discussed about females on the autism spectrum, particularly not the rules of semantics to utilize when referring to other autistic women. In the four years since my online writings began, much to do about semantics in relation to autism spectrum disorders has emerged. Even the word "disorder" is a trigger word for some, myself included. Today, I prefer to write and say, "I am autistic," or "I am Aspie," when referring to myself, versus "a person with autism/Aspergers." Primarily because I don't *have* Aspergers—rather, I *am* Aspie. Aspergers is innately who I am as an individual and not some tagline—like a disease (people first versus condition/diagnosis first). With that said, while I am sensitive to the ongoing terminology debate and the growing trend (and need) to move beyond identifying one's self with a "disorder," in order to keep the authenticity and voice of the original works, including accurately reflecting how I experienced life and trends in the societal and psychological fields at the time, I chose to not make any specific broad-based terminology alterations. This same line of reasoning applies to my decision not to use non-gender-specific pronouns.

It is also important to point out that the writings presented in *Everyday Aspergers* reflect my life experience. The conclusions, theories, observations, and so forth are uniquely mine in the sense that I created my literature "art" by drawing from my own knowledge base and from there expanding and scaffolding off of the old to bring into light the new. My portrayed journey is not meant to depict autism or Aspergers in its entirety and in no way endeavors to do so. If anything my tale is a velvety, cornflower-blue sliver of a sapphire—a fragmented portion of a greater, sparkling whole. This is my story and my story alone, tainted by the limitations of my individualized and biased perceptions and the totality of scarred memories. Nonetheless, I have rendered to the best of my ability the twinkling whole of my truth. And in that, in setting my point of intention on the quest to be authentic, I have done my best.

I have traveled through the words you are about to enter a thousand times over—in memory, in reflection, in prayer, and in reading. In them is my life song, my hopes, my life. It is with great love I pass on this interwoven journey to you. And it is my sincerest wish that the words serve a purpose in some way, feasibly to provide a substantial view of the mind of a woman with Aspergers and, furthermore, to shine an incandescent light for those of us living inside the spectrum.

1. EYES

We each view life differently. Our understanding of this life experience is primarily based on our individual genetic makeup, societal influences, family environment and dynamics, adopted belief systems, and the limitation of the five senses. Some would go further and postulate that our experience of this life is based on a collective spiritual journey, perhaps even an ancestral journey, and/or that we are living a life already preordained and set out in an exact blueprint. There is the concept of emptiness. There is the idea of heaven—the thought of the collective unconscious, the faith of a higher power. Some even hold true to the fact that we are living in multiple dimensions, creating infinite destinies with each and every decision, each and every breath. Others believe this life is finite and that the real reward rests beyond. Each of us holds something to be true about our experience of the world—even if that truth is that of simply believing there is no truth. I'm not here to conjecture the theory of my existence, and definitely not your existence. Nor am I writing to make some claim that I know the workings of the vast mechanisms of our minds—the place (perhaps) where existence is manifested. I'm here only to examine the workings of my mind and spirit, and how, in this present moment, life appears through the eyes of a woman with Aspergers.

2. Brain Blizzard

As of late, much of my processing has been focused around my recent understanding of Asperger's Syndrome. While I knew I had some Aspergers traits and had profusely studied the subject matter, I'd yet to truly come to terms with the diagnosis for myself. I was actually quite surprised at the reaction I had after my mental health counselor said something to the effect of "You? Yes, you definitely have it." Beyond the major aha that lit up every cavern of my brain, what surprised me the most upon hearing her opinion were my thoughts and behaviors that followed. Within minutes after my therapy appointment, I entered a precarious tailspin of depression accompanied by rapid thinking. I wrote and wrote, journaling out all of my feelings. And then I charged forward to the next step—something I always do, this charging. For instance, I'll feel anxiety about some sort of news or realization, and then move quickly from a state of anxiety to one of organizing and fixing. With this Aspergers discovery, I went from an emotional state of depression to the act of barging straight into the logical: *What do I do with this information?* I have this irresistible urge to put things in order, whether in the physical sense (e.g., books, DVDs, furniture) or in the mental sense. My head started whirling with possibilities—perhaps I could run support groups, perhaps I could query a literary agent and write a book, perhaps I could be a subject in a psychological study, perhaps I could get my doctorate and ultimately change the prognosis for females with Aspergers, maybe I could . . . You see the point. And truth be told, in my mind all the *coulds* that I listed were loud *shoulds*. I'm trying to paint a picture here. Trying to explain that beneath this lump of Asperger's Syndrome that literally feels like an enormous sandbag on my chest, I'm pushing up and out and searching for ways to make sense of it all, while at the same instant, I'm stepping back and watching my silly self recognize that the reason I'm trying to make sense of it all, at such high-speed and in direct measures, is likely a result of having this condition to begin with. I'm trapped in those mirrors, the type that face one another so the viewer sees herself multiplied into infinity. Except I am the viewer examining the viewer examining the viewer. It's a blizzard in my brain.

3. IDENTITY

This journey is all about my identity. I'm trying to figure out how Aspergers defines who I am as an individual. It's all about ego, a Tibetan monk might inform. Yet for me it's all about settling my brain. I'm currently compartmentalizing my traits and attributes in a similar way to how I box up everything else in my life. The human brain instinctively categorizes and organizes in an attempt to classify and understand what it is taking in. My brain, an Aspie brain on overdrive, is likewise trying to categorize and organize by scaffolding off of past experiences and my collective knowledge base. Though during the process, my brain gets stuck and doesn't know where to store all of this new information. I've run out of boxes, or they've been misplaced or mislabeled, something to that degree. What it comes down to is that I'm not sure how to classify this condition and therefore not sure how to classify my identity. I'm not sure of the effects, the consequences, the outcomes, not sure at all about where to place this on the shelves of my subconscious. I've tried to figure Aspergers out repeatedly, tried to connect the feasible diagnosis with something similar in another's life. Is this like finding out you have diabetes? (No.) How about that your father was another ethnicity than what you first thought? (No, but closer.) What about someone telling you that the whole entire way you understood and processed your life, which you believed to be typical, was in fact entirely different than much of the mainstream population? That in truth your brain was wired differently? (Oh, much closer but not quite there.) Okay, then what if someone said, "You are an alien dropped down from another planet trying to figure out the ways of the world with a brain that doesn't work the same way as most people around you?" (Now that, the alien business, makes the most sense.) Today, with this Aspergers gig, I wonder if I'm clinging on to the Aspergers role—my new identity, so to speak—and then trying my best to play the part. To be the best Aspie Alien out there. And if so, am I driving myself to extremes of the condition in the process?

4. DOOR THREE

Someone once told me that there are three doors to self: One door you willingly open and show the world, a second door you open to some, and a third door that usually remains closed—a place where you hold the deepest hurts—secrets that if exposed could make you crumble.

I recently "came out" with my Asperger's Syndrome at the local university that I am attending to obtain a degree in mental health counseling. Suffice to say, it didn't go over very well. In fact, in doing so (in spilling the beans, so to speak), I not only opened door number three but also left it ajar and permanently wedged open. And so it is, after completing such a phenomenal feat, I am feeling the repercussions.

To tell you the truth, before yesterday, I didn't even think to consider the topic of my Aspergers diagnosis a door number three—not in the least. I didn't know Aspergers was something I was supposed to keep to myself and feasibly be ashamed about. Or worse, something I ought to fear telling people. I also didn't realize that there's this huge stigma around the word. But based on my professors' reactions, I guess there is a scarlet-letter aura associated with the term. I also thought I understood the three-doors analogy fairly well. It's not rocket science. I presumed that door number one was the no-big-deal stuff in life, like lighthearted jargon regurgitated at cocktail parties. And I reckoned the fictitious door two was stuff that was a little more sensitive, such as personal things you've dealt with, maybe in therapy or another form of processing. And I sort of assumed door three was the deep, deep wounded junk—the place where your scars get ripped open and you bleed all over the place. However, I didn't grasp the notion that the act of sharing the fact that I had Asperger's Syndrome was a door number three in any way whatsoever! I still don't. Regardless, I opened the dang door and feasibly broke it.

5. She Strikes Again

I truly tried to do right. I know enough from life that before I share I ought to first evaluate the situation. I'm referring to the safety of the place and person. I'm *way* overtrusting. I figure that everyone will support everyone, tell the truth, be there when needed, and won't backstab you or let you down intentionally. That's one of the qualities I think is super fabulous about me. I'm not only super trusting but you can trust me. It works both ways, you know? I'm still learning the whole *thingamajig* (Hey, that's a real word and I spelled it right!) associated around building trust. For the most part, in my later adult years, I've been very fortunate in regard to forming long-lasting friendships and working with professionals who are trustworthy. I believe as a general rule that you reap what you sow and that you attract what you put out there. Basically, if you act like a boob, don't be surprised when there are a bunch of boobs around you. And no, I don't mean that literally.

Speaking of *boobs*, lately it's been all boobs at the local university. Seriously, this university, to which I'm paying the equivalent of my entire retirement savings to attend, sure is surprising me. Of all the places on the planet, a counseling program taught by practicing mental health therapists should be the ideal place to be vulnerable—to be myself, to show all my cards. No! Nada! No way in H-E-double-hockey-sticks. Gosh darn it! She strikes again! Without going into obnoxious, overly revealing details, my experience in sharing that my therapist diagnosed me with Asperger's Syndrome went over about as well as yelling "timber" at the top of my lungs at a depth hoar. (A very dangerous snow condition that leads to avalanches. And you thought you weren't going to learn anything.) As it happened, when I told my college instructor about my recent diagnosis (something my personal therapist had advised me to do), my white-bearded professor sideswiped me with a full-on retaliation, explaining, rather irately, that under the umbrella of family system theory, my son and I would be classified as having "broken brains" created by our family dynamics. This wasn't said all in one breath but dragged on and on in the longest ten minutes of my life.

Me? I did what I do when I feel assaulted—I fumbled for words trying to defend myself. The story doesn't end well. Let's just say that after I left in shock, I experienced a lot of tears and way too much verbal processing, letter writing, and editing. Then the topper was a few days following: a confrontational meeting (guised as a mediation) at the university with that same professor, his subordinate, teary-eyed me, and a "witness" who suddenly couldn't remember anything. End result, I dropped the professor's class, agreed to disagree about how we saw the discussion (attack), and ended up spending a few days questioning my place in this entire world!

6. 116 REASONS I KNOW I HAVE ASPERGER'S SYNDROME

1. Writing this list.
2. Enjoying writing this list.
3. Love, love, love animals and bugs.
4. Do I have to leave the house?
5. Nature is heavenly as long as I can stay clean.
6. Collector.
7. Toys are objects to be organized, stacked, categorized, or cleaned.
8. Friday the 13th in 3-D three times because I think the number three is awesome!
9. Red fluffy socks with high heels.
10. Sweater on inside out, again.
11. Memorized how to spell and sing supercalifragilisticexpialidocious in an attempt to qualify for speech class.
12. I was Jacqueline Smith, never Farah.
13. Every stuffed animal named, categorized by birth, and kept until after college.
14. Snoopy in a chair looking out the back of the window of my first car.
15. Seven days straight perfecting my penmanship before I began teaching.
16. Clever Clyde was a famous humanistic caterpillar in the stories I wrote.
17. Buddy One was my imaginary ghost friend.
18. Entering poetry (scam) contests.
19. Hamsters aren't stuffed animals.
20. Goldfish do die when left under the hot sun in a small bowl of water.

21. Childhood friends were students, the members of my club, customers, or placed in another subordinate position.
22. Backgammon pro by age nine. Cribbage pro by age fifteen.
23. Perfected Pac-Man and Space Invaders while watching every episode of *Three's Company*.
24. Called dumb blond, in regard to not getting jokes. I'm a brunette.
25. You do not sit with your legs spread while wearing a cheerleading skirt.
26. If I'm her best friend, why does she need more friends than me?
27. I have a confession to make—I was thinking about lying, but I didn't.
28. Naïve, sweet, gullible, unique, hyper, interesting, odd . . .
29. I have 120 flaws; should I list them?
30. Don't answer the phone!!!
31. Note to self: Read the birthday card before grabbing the money and jumping up and down.
32. Hello? Your toenails do need to be cleaned occasionally.
33. "Snob! You always look away."
34. Victim, with her head down.
35. Statistically speaking, your chances of dying from that are slim. I researched it for five days.
36. Website built, 100 pages total, in five weeks. Go baby.
37. Months and months on freebie websites equals toothbrushes, baskets, lotions, and much more.
38. I had the coolest property on Farmville.
39. Why do fantastic ideas from the night before not seem so fantastic in the morning?
40. Don't answer the door!
41. I don't want to go . . . It's too much work for me to put on a bra.
42. Monopolize a conversation? Who me?
43. Depression, Anxiety, blah . . . blah . . . blah.
44. Verbal processing.
45. Can you say *manuscript?*

46. What exactly is a guilty pleasure? And why would people do something that makes them feel guilty?
47. I don't understand—it's old wives' tales? Not old wise tales?
48. Just Relax. Not comprehending. What does it feel like to relax?
49. Nonfiction galore.
50. Twitching and jumping because it's museum time!
51. Oh no! You did not just change the plan.
52. Carpet, dirt, germs, clutter, blemishes, lips, breath . . . Yuck!
53. Don't hug me right now.
54. Okay, you can hug me, but not too tight, that hurts.
55. Are my shoes on the right feet?
56. I wish I hadn't sent them that garage sale crystal for their wedding present; what was I thinking?
57. Do you think she'll like these earrings I never wore or a gift certificate?
58. What do you mean this letter might offend my professor?
59. Here's a bruise, and another one. Look at this one.
60. Let's drive around the block again and look for a spot. I can't parallel park.
61. Group sports? Swinging a bat? Dressing for PE? Run in fear!
62. All the fun is in the planning. The party itself is terrifying.
63. Why do people bully and tease?
64. Give me a role or a part, and I'll perfect it.
65. Should I dress like my best friend, my spiritual counselor, or the lady on my favorite soap opera?
66. I love having friends my mom's age.
67. Monthly Bunco with the Episcopalian Retirement Group? Why not?
68. Post-social-event debrief time: When I said this, do you think it was offensive? Why did she look at me that way? Should I have kept my mouth closed? Was that appropriate? I'm quitting Bunco; it's too stressful.
69. My only friends in second grade—two twin boys, Chris and Jimmy.

70. My only friend in kindergarten, Keith. He moved to Hawaii.

71. Sure, I can write for ten hours straight. Can't you?

72. Doesn't everyone have a voice reminding them what to do during a conversation: make more eye contact, step closer, nod your head, smile—but not too big—insert giggle, let them talk more.

73. Give me a passion and give me a week to learn everything there is to know about it.

74. Hypochondriac.

75. Stop talking . . . you're hurting my ears.

76. You smell funny.

77. Is that your natural hair color and how old are you?

78. Camping sucks.

79. Criteria for boyfriends? Criteria for friends? What?

80. Name an object. I can tell you 100 uses for it.

81. Let me fix the situation.

82. Just because the thought is in my head doesn't mean it needs to get out. Or does it?

83. Crossing the street so I don't have to pass the stranger on the sidewalk.

84. How do you turn around at the halfway point of a walk without looking silly?

85. No events in college. One friend in college—before she stopped answering my calls.

86. ADHD, PTSD . . . blah, blah, blah.

87. Therapists, psychologists, priests, reverends, psychiatrists, hypnotists, and the like are kind of clueless about recognizing Aspergers in females.

88. I'll just hang out in this closet until the party is over.

89. I'll be in the back room writing until the party is over.

90. I'll be reading in the bathroom until the party is over.

91. Why do you ask me how I am when you don't want to hear the answer?

92. IBS.

93. Funerals are confusing.

94. Let's practice small talk; the ritual is intriguing.
95. Queen of evaluation.
96. Stopped eating lamb at age four, pork at age eleven.
97. Words are beautiful or painful.
98. Fixations, obsessions . . . blah, blah, blah.
99. Let me organize your pantry.
100. I should have asked before buying a puppy?
101. What can I eat that doesn't have pesticides, hormones, mutations, cancer-causing ingredients, sugar, sugar substitutes, dairy, preservatives, chemicals, bleach . . . I'm watching too many documentaries.
102. Time for another organic juice fast. Time for more organic chocolate.
103. Either no one has ever flirted with me in my entire life or I don't recognize flirting.
104. Give me a visual, a guideline, a rule, and stop all the jabber.
105. I can tell you exactly where anything is on my kitchen shelves, but don't ask me where my keys are.
106. Imaginary play is confusing unless there is a script.
107. I like to analyze the sentence structure and grammar in fictional books.
108. It's hard to recognize faces.
109. Do you want to hear this record for the fiftieth time?
110. I'm the one reading the Buddhist book at my son's baseball game.
111. Listen to what I wrote. I edited it.
112. Grown-ups shouldn't lie about Santa or that the government is looking out for our best interest.
113. I trust you.
114. I overshare.
115. I would be happy to eat the same meal every day.
116. That fixation to write this list is gone. I don't know why; it just is. (It really bugs me this isn't number 113.)

7. VIGNETTE, INVISIBLE, AGE 16

For the red-bearded psychologist, there were no readily available reasons for my inferiority. I was an intriguing case indeed—a pretty girl, somewhat charming, and well accomplished. Sitting there in his stately office that gave off an awful stench of new carpet and furniture polish, I began to wonder why I had insisted on seeing someone in the first place. In all honesty, I knew what this man was thinking. He was seeing what they all had seen, the only difference being he was receiving payment. This stranger behind the walnut desk was no different than the rest. He was easy to fool. He hadn't the slightest idea of where to begin looking or what to uncover, and I knew just the right words and phrases to lead him in the wrong direction. He would notice my nice clothes, my youthful face. He would note my kind mannerisms and make a list of all my accomplishments. He'd probably highlight a few catchphrases. And then he'd be done with me; done like the rest, having seen only what he had wanted to see and not trying to see any more. He looked at me in the same quizzical, doubting manner that my girlfriend's therapist had years ago. Though his expression was well-masked, I saw the essence of a smirk behind his steady, pale eyes. And in the same way, I recognized—by the way he nervously fidgeted with his ballpoint pen and wheeled round his chair—he hadn't found the answers he'd been seeking. Perhaps he was aware of my time limitations, the lack of funds, and the urgency of my situation. Seeing how Mother worked just across the street from him and had more than likely had a lunch date once or twice with this man, he was bound to know some of the happenings, or at least Mother's view of it. Quick and easy is how I saw the entire therapeutic experience. Roll her in, figure it out, and roll her back out—even if she's still broken. With my new diagnosis in hand, granted after a brief multiple-choice test and short interview, I now believed my emotional issues rested in my own *inferiority complex* and resulting inability to love myself. However, stepping out on my own, beyond the psychologist's office, one vital question remained: If I was somehow internally flawed by a faulty infrastructure, then how could I feasibly begin to rebuild myself?

8. Oh Crap! Dyspraxia!

I crave writing. When I find a healthy and stimulating venue to pour out my thoughts, I long to return to that place. This is nothing new. I've been processing through writing since I first learned to hold a writing utensil. My favorites were the fat, scented markers. Writing combined with sweet, surprising smells—now that was magical. Today, as an anxiety-ridden adult (living in a fear-based society), I'd probably worry about the toxins in the ink. Go figure. I miss the innocence of my youth, when I truly believed, without an inkling of a doubt (no pun intended), that the world was a safe place. In committing to write every day for a year (and sometimes two times a day—God love me), I've found some added comfort in scanning through other authors' writings about Asperger's Syndrome. This morning, in scanning an article, I came across the word *dyspraxia*. This word isn't new to me. As a teacher, and as an individual with dyslexia, I've come across the term a time or two. All the same, I never took the time to stop and understand what dyspraxia meant. I figured it was something to do with word order. Now, after grueling detective work (just kidding . . . the process took thirty seconds), I'm forced to spill out and spit out of my mind the fact that yes indeed I do appear to have dyspraxia. Pin the ribbon on me!

I now know dyspraxia is a neurologically based developmental disorder affecting fine and/or gross motor planning and coordination, including cognitive tasks, and that the coordination difficulties can affect participation and functioning levels of everyday life skills. If you had been nearby when I scanned down to the "whole body movement, coordination, and body image" section, you would have heard my young voice shout, "Oh, crap!"

Without risking the act of plagiarizing Wikipedia, let me say, in relation to dyspraxia markers, that my timing sucks, my balance sucks—yes, I trip over my own feet—I suck at sequencing movements, and my spatial awareness sucks. I drop things all the time, I knock into people, I can't tell the difference between left and right, and I have trouble determining the distance between objects. If you suck at these things too, then congratulations—you might have dyspraxia! Oh! And in reading on, let me also point out the problems associated with short-term memory, increased propensity to lose things, difficulty following sequences, and sensory-processing disorder. Oh boy! I'm actually very happy at the moment. In my vivid imagination, I'm dancing around on stage, pumping my arms up and down with my palms facing the ceiling, and doing a happy dance. (And I'm twenty pounds lighter.) Why? Because despite these challenges, I taught myself to write, I completed college with honors, and I continue to achieve my goals. I rock! Now the funny thing is (in an odd, remarkable, and sad kind of way), I was a high school cheerleader, and I never could figure out how everyone picked up the moves for the cheer routines so swiftly and effortlessly, while I had to practice for hours on end, and even after that was still typically going the wrong direction.

9. TEN TRAITS
(FEMALES WITH ASPERGERS)

1) We are deep philosophical thinkers and writers, gifted in the sense of our level of thinking—perhaps poets, professors, authors, or avid readers of nonfictional genre. I don't believe you can have Aspergers without being highly intelligent by mainstream standards. Perhaps that is part of the issue at hand, the extreme intelligence leading to an overactive mind and high anxiety. We see things at multiple levels, including our own place in the world and our own thinking processes. We analyze our existence, the meaning of life, the meaning of everything, continually. We are serious and matter of fact. Nothing is taken for granted, simplified, or easy. Everything is complex.

2) We are innocent, naive, and honest. Do we lie? Yes. Do we like to lie? No. Things that are hard for us to understand: manipulation, disloyalty, vindictive behavior, and retaliation. Are we easily fooled and conned, particularly before we grow wiser to the ways of the world? Absolutely, yes. Confusion and feeling misplaced, isolated, overwhelmed, and simply plopped down on the wrong universe are all parts of the Aspie experience. Can we learn to adapt? Yes. Is it always hard to fit in at some level? Yes. Can we out grow our character traits? No.

3) We are escape artists. We know how to escape. It's how we survive this place. We escape through our fixations, our passions, our imaginings, and even our made-up realities. We escape and make sense of our world through mental processing, in spoken or written form. We escape in the rhythm of words. We escape in our philosophizing. As children, we had imaginary friends or animals, maybe witches or spirit friends, even extraterrestrial buddies. We escaped in our play, imitating what we'd seen on television or in walking life, taking on the role of a teacher, an actress in a play, a movie star. If we had friends, we made friendship another means of escape—through control, planning, or perhaps hiding behind them. We were either their instructor or boss, telling them what to do, where to stand, and how to talk, or we were the "baby," blindly following our friends wherever they went. We escaped our own identity by taking on one

friend's identity. We dressed like her, spoke like her, adapted our own self to her (or his) likes and dislikes. We became masters at imitation, without recognizing what we were doing. We escaped through music. Through the repeated lyrics or rhythm of a song—through everything that song stirred in us. We escaped into fantasies, what could be, projections, dreams, and fairy-tale endings. We obsessed over collecting objects (maybe stickers, mystical unicorns, or books). We may have escaped through a relationship with a lover. We delved into an alternate state of mind, so we could breathe, maybe momentarily taking on another dialect, personality, or view of the world. Numbers brought ease, as did counting, categorizing, organizing, and rearranging. At parties, if we went, we might have escaped into a closet, the outskirts, outdoors, or at the side of our best friend. We may have escaped through substance abuse, including food, or through hiding in our homes. When we resurfaced, we became confused. What had we missed? What had we left behind? What would we escape through next?

4) We have coexisting attributes of other syndromes/disorders/conditions. We often have OCD (obsessive compulsive disorder) tendencies, sensory issues (with sight, sound, texture, smells, taste), generalized anxiety and/or a sense we are always unsafe or in pending danger, particularly in crowded public places. We may have been labeled with seemingly polar extremes: depressed/overjoyed, lazy/overactive, inconsiderate/oversensitive, lacking awareness/attention to detail, low focus/high focus. We may have poor muscle tone, be "double-jointed," or lack motor skills. We may hold our pencil "incorrectly." We may have eating disorders, food obsessions, and struggles with diet. We may have irritable bowel syndrome, fibromyalgia, chronic fatigue, and other immune challenges. We may have sought out answers to why we seemed to see the world differently than others we knew, only to be told we were attention seekers, paranoid, hypochondriacs, or too focused on diagnoses and labels. Our personhood was challenged on the sole basis that we "knew" we were different but couldn't prove it to the world, and/or our personhood was oppressed, as we attempted to be and act like someone we were not. We still question our place in the world, who we are, who we are expected to be, searching for the "rights" and "wrongs."

5) We learn that to fit in we have to "fake" it. Through trial and error, we lost friends. We overshared, spilling out intimate details to strangers; we raised

our hands too much in class or didn't raise our hands at all; we had little impulse control with our speaking, monopolizing conversations and bringing the subject back to ourselves. Not because we are narcissistic and controlling, but because that is how we make sense of our world; that is how we believe we connect. We hold a lot inside. A lot of what we see going on about us, a lot of what our bodies feel, what our minds conjecture. We push back the conversational difficulties we experience, e.g., the concepts of acceptable and accurate eye contact, tone of voice, proximity of body, stance, posture—push it all back, and try to focus on what someone is saying with all the dos and don'ts hammering in our mind. We come out of a conversation exhausted, questioning if we "acted" the socially acceptable way, wondering if we have offended, contradicted, hurt, or embarrassed others or ourselves. We learn that people aren't as open or trusting as we are. That others hold back and filter their thoughts. We learn that our brains are different. We learn to survive means we must pretend.

6) We seek refuge at home or at a safe place. The days we know we don't have to be anywhere, talk to anyone, answer any calls, or leave the house, are the days we take a deep breath and relax. If one person will be visiting, we perceive the visit as a threat; knowing logically the threat isn't real doesn't relieve a drop of the anxiety. We have feelings of dread about even one event on the calendar. Even something as simple as a self-imposed obligation, such as leaving the house to walk the dog, can cause extreme anxiety. It's more than going out into society, it's all the steps that are involved in leaving—all the rules, routines, and norms. Choices can be overwhelming: what to wear, to shower or not, what to eat, what time to be back, how to organize time, how to act outside the house . . . all these thoughts can pop up. Sensory processing can go into overload—the shirt might be scratchy, the bra pokey, the shoes too tight. Even the steps to getting ready can seem boggled with choices—*should I brush my teeth or shower first? Should I finish that email? Should I call her back now, or when I return? Should I go at all?* Maybe staying home feels better, but by adulthood we know it is socially "healthier" to get out of the house, to interact, to take in fresh air, to exercise, to share. But going out doesn't feel healthy to us, because it doesn't feel safe. For those of us who have tried CBT (Cognitive Behavior Therapy), we try to tell ourselves all the "right" words, to convince ourselves our thought patterns are simply wired

differently, to reassure ourselves we are safe . . . the problem then becomes this other layer of rules we should apply, that of the cognitive-behavior set of rules. So even the supposed therapeutic self-talk becomes yet another set of hoops to jump through before stepping foot out of the house. To curl up on the couch with a clean pet, a cotton blanket, a warm cup of tea, and a movie or good book may become our refuge. At least for the moment, we can stop the thoughts associated with having to make decisions and having to face the world. A simple task has simple rules.

7) We are sensitive. We are sensitive when we sleep, maybe needing a certain mattress, pillow, earplugs, or particularly comfortable clothing. Some need long sleeves, some short. Temperature needs to be just so. No air blowing from the heater vent, no traffic noise, no noise, period. We are sensitive even in our dream state, perhaps having intense and colorful dreams, anxiety-ridden dreams, or maybe precognitive dreams. Our sensitivity might expand to being highly intuitive of others' feelings, which is a paradox, considering the limitations of our social communication skills. We seek out verbal information in written or spoken form, sometimes overthinking something someone said and reliving the ways we ought to have responded. We take criticism to heart, not necessarily longing for perfection, but for the opportunity to be understood and accepted. It seems we have inferiority complexes; yet with careful analysis, we don't feel inferior, but rather unseen, unheard, and misunderstood. If someone tells us this or that, we may adapt our view of life accordingly, continually in search of the "right" and "correct" way. We may jump from one religious realm to another, in search of the "right" path or may run away from aspects of religion because of all the questions that arise in theorizing. When others question our works, we may become hurt, as we perceive our works as an extension of ourselves. Sometimes we stop sharing our work in hopes of avoiding opinions, criticism, and judgment. We dislike words and events that hurt others and hurt animals. We may have collected insects, saved a fallen bird, or rescued pets. We have a huge compassion for suffering, for we have experienced deep levels of suffering. We are very sensitive to substances, such as foods, caffeine, alcohol, medications, environmental toxins, and perfumes. A little amount of one substance can have extreme effects on our emotional and/or physical state.

8) We are ourselves and we aren't ourselves. Between imitating others and copying the ways of the world, and trying to be honest, and having no choice but to be "real," we find ourselves trapped between pretending to be normal and showing all our cards. It's a difficult state. Sometimes we don't realize when we are imitating someone else or taking on another's interests, or when we are suppressing our true wishes in order to avoid ridicule. We have an odd sense of self. We know we are an individual with unique traits and attributes, but at the same time we recognize we so desperately want to fit in that we might have adapted or conformed many aspects about ourselves. Some of us might reject societal norms and expectations all together, only to find ourselves extremely isolated. There is an in-between place where an Aspie girl can be herself and fit in, but finding that place and staying in that place takes a lot of work and processing. Some of us even have a hard time understanding what we physically look like. We might switch our preference in hairstyles, clothes, interests, and hobbies, frequently, as we attempt to manage and keep up with our changing sense of self and our place in the world. We can gain the ability to love ourselves, accept ourselves, and be happy with our lives; however, this usually takes much inner work and self-analysis. Part of self-acceptance comes with the recognition that everyone is unique, everyone has challenges, and everyone is struggling to find this invented norm. When we recognize there are no rules, and no guide map to life, we may be able to breathe easier, and finally explore what makes us happy.

9) Feelings and other people's actions are confusing. Others' feelings and our own feelings are confusing to the extent there are no set rules to feelings. We think logically, and even though we are (despite what others think) sensitive, compassionate, intuitive, and understanding, many emotions remain illogical and unpredictable. We may expect that by acting a certain way we can achieve a certain result, but in dealing with emotions we find the intended results don't manifest. We speak frankly and literally. In our youth, jokes go over our heads; we are the last to laugh, if we laugh at all, and sometimes ourselves the subject of the joke. We are confused when others make fun of us, ostracize us, decide they don't want to be our friend, shun us, belittle us, trick us, and especially betray us. We may have trouble identifying feelings, unless they are extremes. We might have trouble with the emotions of hate and dislike. We may hold grudges and

feel pain from a situation years later, yet at the same time find it easier to forgive than to hold a grudge. We might feel sorry for someone who has persecuted or hurt us. Personal feelings of anger, outrage, deep love, fear, giddiness, and anticipation seem to be easier to identify than emotions of joy, satisfaction, calmness, and serenity. Sometimes situations, conversations, or events are perceived as black or white, one way or another, and the middle spectrum is overlooked or misunderstood. A small fight might signal the end of a relationship and collapse of one's world, whereas a small compliment might boost us into a state of bliss.

10) We have difficulty with executive functioning. The way we process the world is different. Simple tasks can cause us extreme hardship. Learning to drive a car, to tuck in the bed sheets, to even round the hallway corner, can be troublesome. New places offer their own set of challenges. Escalators, turning on and off faucets, unlocking doors, finding our car in a parking lot (even our keys in our purse) and managing computers, electronic devices, or anything that requires a reasonable amount of steps, dexterity, or know-how, can rouse in us a sense of panic. While we might be grand organizers, as organizing brings us a sense of comfort, the thought of repairing, fixing, or locating something causes distress. Doing the bills, cleaning the house, sorting through papers, scheduling appointments, keeping track of times on the calendar, and preparing for a party can cause anxiety. Tasks may be avoided. Cleaning may seem insurmountable. *Where to begin? How long should I do something? Is this the right way?* These are all questions that might come to mind. Sometimes we imagine a stranger entering our home, and question what they would do if they were in our shoes. We reach out to others' rules of what is right, even to do the simplest of things. Sometimes we reorganize in an attempt to make things right or to make things easier, only life doesn't seem to get easier. Some of us are affected in the way we calculate numbers or in reading. We may have dyslexia or other learning disabilities. We may solve problems and sort out situations much differently than most. We like to categorize and find patterns, and when ideas don't fit, we don't know where to put them. Putting on shoes, zipping or buttoning clothes, carrying or packing groceries, all of these actions can pose trouble. We might leave the house with mismatched socks, our shirt buttoned incorrectly, and our sweater inside out.

10. To See a Dog and Nothing More

I think Scooby is dying. He's not moving. Our Goldendoodle is very, very sick. I don't know if he will make it this time. In early October he was also ill. He had lost fifteen pounds from an internal staph infection in the neck region. He wouldn't eat, wouldn't get out of his designated chair, and was very despondent. Today is a little different—the weight is still on him, but he appears boney, as if a part of him, a part I can't readily see, has been chiseled away. He can barely stand. He has a fever of 103.8 and black, tarry stools keep appearing from the internal bleeding. I can't stand it when a living being is in pain, especially an animal. It tears me up inside and I can't focus. I wonder if he knows that when we took him to the vet yesterday, and he had all those tests and the emergency shots, that we were trying to help him. I wonder if he can feel my own worry. I question if he understands this concept of mortality and the afterlife. I feel guilty, too, because I haven't been the best master. I could have taken him on more walks. There is an agonizing twist in my stomach—the recognition of potential loss— this black wisp of nothingness that reaches up from the depths of me, beneath the physical layer, from some oblique existence, and nips at the tender parts of my being. In the pain I am reminded of all the losses before, all the pets that were once here and now gone, all the people who were part of my life and slipped away.

11. Vignette, Ten Stitches, Age 3

I'd fallen—tumbled backward off my babysitter's shoulders, crashing headfirst onto the unforgiving concrete patio. Through my tears, I saw our Labrador Sugar panting and pacing, and whining some. My small hand met the warm, oozing blood at the back of my head. So much blood.

I awoke, wet and hot, to discover myself trapped beneath a heavy blanket in an unfamiliar place. I turned quickly and tried to rise up, but some force pushed down. I was inside a nightmare. A pungent odor came, a smell similar to Mother's nail-polish remover. Two strangers garbed in white tugged. I felt what had to have been a swimmer's cap of sharp sewing needles being driven into my head. The keening of the pain intensified. My hands closed into tight fists—tiny fingernails indenting the flesh of palms. "Mommy!" I screamed. "Mommy!" My eyes leapt about the four blank walls, darting. I felt carsick. Again, the needling pain. High in the white, a dark-skinned maiden swept my bangs, just like Mother did after a terrible dream. I drifted, leaving behind the nightmare.

In the late-day hour I awoke to find Father, his golden-hazel eyes lowered to the floor and most of his auburn curls combed back. "Hello," Father offered, his voice filling the still of the room. "You're a lucky little girl. You took a bad fall. But they stitched you all up. Ten stitches." I pulled down the blanket and sat up, my dark eyes wide, picturing how Father had recently stitched the red yarn onto the bald head of my plush Raggedy Ann doll. "Can we go home now, Daddy?" I asked.

Father leaned forward, the pores of his tanned face more indented outside the shadows. "Soon," he whispered. I stretched my arm out a bit, but couldn't reach far enough. Like the next iron rung of the playground monkey bars, Daddy was something I longed for but couldn't reach.

"Rest," I heard. Father's eyes scoped the windowpane, the floor, the cabinets, until his eyes glazed over and he traveled in thought. I sniffled and rubbed my little nose, my tiny fingers soft and moist. The mattress made a crunching sound. The stiff sheets grated. Father remained undisturbed. My head throbbed. I felt around for blood and found none. I turned to the pillow to find a drop. I pressed on my tummy through my hospital gown. "I'm thirsty," I mumbled. I coughed into the ugly blanket. Daddy still didn't look. "I'm thirsty," I repeated, suddenly shivering.

Father blinked then, two times rapidly, and turned his head.

"Where is Mommy?" I asked.

With a look of reproach, he said, "I couldn't tell you."

One tear found me. My heart thumped in my ears.

Father got to his feet, strolled across the room, surveyed the hallway beyond the door, and returned.

"When's Mommy coming?" I queried. His eyes shifted to the empty chair and back to the open door.

"You know your mother," he sighed. I soaked in Father's view. He wavered at the outskirt of the bed, busying himself with the loose change in his short pockets. He shifted his body weight from one leg to the next. This became my life for the next hour—Father's every move.

Until the time came for Father to dress me in my bloodstained clothes.

Father carried me in his arms through the double-glass hospital doors. The threshold opened wide into the summer night air. "Your mother is finally home," he grumbled.

"I'm sorry, Daddy," I whispered.

"Why?" he asked, hoisting me further over his shoulder.

I didn't answer. I was too busy counting the bugs surrounding the street lamp. I wondered why they always went for the light, when it was clear that their friends were dying.

Father mumbled something in frustration, and then, having found his car, set me gently onto the back seat. Inside, I took in the scent of coconut suntan lotion and leather upholstery cleaner. "We'll see each other soon," Father offered, before making his way to the front of the sedan. I touched the back of my head, stroking the bandages with my fingers. I curled into myself and stared down at my stained yellow shirt. The crimson blood in the front was shaped like a butterfly. "Soon," I repeated. "Soon, little butterfly."

12. Proverbial Foot in Mouth

I wanted to write about *death terror*. You know that gripping existential fear that we all subconsciously suppress but still surfaces in subliminal ways in our waking hours. Or in my pathetic case, the all-encompassing dread of death that bypasses the subconscious and just haunts me pretty much twenty-four seven. But I figured the subject of death terror would be just a little bit too bleak for Valentine's Day. I tinkered with writing about this term that I've coined—*flash-sense*—an extreme sensory experience a person has when he or she gets a flash from the past that seemingly connects the past to the present in one blast. But that would have been a long, boring list of all these fragmented memories that have been coming back to me at locomotive speed since my diagnosis of Asperger's Syndrome. And although I *superdeduper* love lists and will gladly write you one anytime (and edit your diary while I'm at it), I didn't think a list of my current flashbacks would interest you much. And so I asked myself, *What would make me happy to read on Valentine's Day?* I scratched out the idea of love and gushiness—because seriously how many people want to read about a middle-aged married woman proclaiming her love for her husband? (Besides my mom.) And thusly, I was left with the old fallback, something I've always been super good at doing. It's one of those hidden talents that catches people by surprise. Sort of like a cute, cuddly kitten hacking up a fur ball. Yes, I thought for Valentine's Day I'd treat you to a couple foot-in-my-mouth moments. Like the first time I met my roommate's brother (who had just graduated from college with a teaching credential), and I exclaimed, with a full-mouth smile and high-pitched giddiness, "Congratulations! The chances of you getting hired are great, since you're an ethnic minority and a male!" Or the time a friend invited me over to her parents' home: "Oh, your house is so big and lavish and fantastic! (squeal and clap hands) Is this your dream house? Is this your dream come true? I wish I had a house like this. It's so perfect.

Did it cost a lot of money?" (Insert pause) "Oh, did I forget to introduce myself?" And that morning, not too long ago, that I asked my son's math teacher (in front of her students), "Do you actually like math?" And after she responded with an adamant but very odd-sounding *yes*, I still (perpetually clueless) responded, quite loudly, "Really? I don't."

Hmmm? And I hadn't yet figured out I was an Aspie? Go figure. And my all-time favorite to date has to be when my long-ago neighbor arrived home from his extended trip to Mexico to see family, and I responded, off the top of my head (never a good thing): "Wow, I bet you're glad to be home because it's so DIRTY there."

13. SHIRLEY TEMPLE

I had some quesadillas at a sports bar that probably wouldn't have qualified as food.

A bar? Are you crazy? (Perhaps.) A group of classmates at the university that studious me attends were headed out for a celebration. (I just deleted an entire paragraph about my theories of why people drink.) This was my first invite to a bar in eons. My little voice (inside my head) was excited, and she said, "Oh! This could be a fun experiment! We could blog about it!" She was all sweet and convincing and giving out all these facts, like how I needed to be brave and bond with my peer group. We had a little argument, Little Voice and I, as I stood in the elevator stuck and not going anywhere, with four of my classmates. After a good five minutes, I queried aloud, "Hey, did anyone press the button?"

We all had a good laugh then, and Little Voice used that as further nectar for her warped plan. When I arrived at the noisy, crowded sports bar, the only place left to perch was in the far corner. Which would have been tolerable, maybe even preferred, except I had to sit by two gentlemen from class. And my least favorite social thing to do in the whole entire universe, both discovered and undiscovered, is to engage in small chat with men, particularly men I hardly know.

In retrospect this situation easily merited ordering a glass of wine. But nooooo! Little Voice (in my head) was adamant that I had to be the real me and not compromise my normal behavior in order to attempt to fit in. (She's on some trip with that lately. It's rather annoying. Years of functioning without recourse through role-playing and pretending, and now she has to go and be all *real.*) Thusly, against my really-wanting-booze judgment, I ordered a Shirley Temple. And then to further torture Little Voice, I ate two very-bad-for-me cherries. While Little Voice was going on about the health hazards of red dye, I ignored her and pictured myself cuddled up at home watching the television series *Breaking Bad.*

But soon, I was interrupted with the same old tapes playing in my head: *What to say? How to say it? When to say it? How to sit? Where to look? When to smile?*

Blah, blah, blah. I did receive a tableful of laughs when I mistook the miniature trivia-game-playing contraption (one of seven the waitress plopped on our table) for an automated teller machine (ATM). I kept asking, while holding my little blue machine up high, "How does the machine know what I ordered for dinner? What buttons do I press? How does it know me?" Before looking for the slot in which to slide my bank debit card.

It's nice to know that the whole over-my-head quality I had in high school hasn't changed. (Sorry, I know I do this a lot. But what does *over my head* mean, literally? Is it facts flying over me? Am I ducking? If I stood up taller or jumped, would I reach the adequate information?) I ordered a Shirley Temple instead of my standard water. (Usually bottled or sparkling water, but bars usually don't have that. I think it's a conspiracy to make patrons order alcohol.) I ordered a Shirley Temple because in first grade I lived right around the block from Shirley Temple Black. I used to walk up to her wrought-iron gate daydreaming about getting her autograph for my spy notebook, while contemplating why she changed her last name. I ordered the soda for the sole purpose of saying, "Shirley Temple." But no one knew that. Just like no one knew I can't stand soda. The bar visit wasn't as terrible as it could have been. I managed the small talk okay. Overall, I'm pretty darn proud of me, and even thankful to Little Voice (just don't tell her), because I faced a huge fear without a friend by my side.

14. BEHIND THE CURTAIN

I remember years back looking up at the wide-open sky and wondering where the universe ended and, more so, where I began. I recognized I wasn't just my flesh and bone, and was so overly aware of the inner core of my being. I felt as if I were walking a narrow line between this realm and the next. There was turmoil at home that left me with a general uneasiness, but there was another, more defining, uneasiness building—an unsettling recognition that there was much more than the grown-ups could explain or even venture to understand themselves. Such knowing at a young age carries with it an insecurity and a reckoning of the uncertainties of the world, an acknowledging that reality isn't what one's peer group believes. There was a stepping out of sorts, a separating, at this point in my life—a kindling of new insight that propelled me onto the other side of the street. As if I were standing alone, isolated and curious, observing my playmates across the way. I could hear them. I could even speak, and they would acknowledge my presence, but I couldn't join them. My thoughts were a deep canvas: a three-dimensional painting I could step into and live. From my side of the road I would watch with wonder and interest, recognizing my own separation.

It was then—about the time most kids were discovering the wonderment of aboveground pools and slip-and-slides—that I was discovering the limits of my mind and the *unlimitedness* of the universe. I had wanted desperately to understand where I belonged and where I fit in. The others were all different. It was as if I had been given an alternate pair of lenses in the way I interpreted the happenings around me.

As time passed, I became increasingly more inquisitive and interested in adults; for I secretly hoped one of them would have an answer. I searched out a guide, even though I knew not what I was searching for, or even that I was searching. As I grew older the feelings inside of me also grew, filling up every inch of new space. In fact, I was so abundantly filled with emotions that at times I felt as if I were drowning inside my own self. I could hear things by then, too. And see things—things no one else I had encountered could. I grew lonelier. Though there were people nearby, I nonetheless remained isolated in thought. It seemed that no one understood me. For years I longed to be like my classmates. I came to see them as narrower and straighter, like the letter X, so that nothing could fill them and leave them gasping for air; wherein I perceived myself as wide and curved, like the letter O, so that everything and anything could use me as a vessel.

The later years were painfully difficult. When the teenage trials came, I felt bombarded and stampeded with emotions. If there was ever a time I believed I was from another universe, it was then. I played a game—that is how I saw it. I pretended to be someone. I was lost, lost on some stage, trying to find where I'd hidden my true self. I still feel as if a part of me is hiding somewhere, afraid to come out entirely for fear of misunderstanding and judgment. The tender part, the piece that doesn't understand in the smallest degree the cruelty and harshness of this world—she remains divided and alone, hidden behind the curtain.

15. EXPEDITION JOURNAL

Day One: Upon receiving my diagnosis of Asperger's Syndrome, I have subsequently clung onto the title. Beginning to understand the implications of diagnosis.

Day Two: My diagnosis now qualifies as a life preserver, as the term "Aspergers" appears to be keeping me afloat as I relive aspects of my past and evaluate my perception of reality. Mental connections observed. Huge relief in finding a semblance of answers, coupled with a preponderance of flashbacks. Mild degree of depression. Reality shifting.

Day Three: Uncertain if clinging is beneficial. *Is this need to grasp onto a title indeed part of my Aspergers brain or part of my soul's journey?* Many questions emerging.

Day Four: *If Aspergers is a man-made diagnosis, does it exist?* Still clinging to label.

Day Five: I've met others who recognize me and validate my experience. I have found my people. I am proud to have Aspergers! I no longer care if I am clinging. Most earthlings do not understand me.

Day Six: Preparing for trip to Planet Aspie. Confirmation received: I am of alien descent. Leaving behind all prior diagnoses, roles, and identities in hopes of forging ahead to new frontier. I have reclaimed my spaceship. Excited. Final good-byes to cruel Earth.

Day Seven: Takeoff! Less and less grounded, but filled with hope.

Day Eight: Landed. Assimilated successfully with my kin. Partying, connecting. Don't miss Earth one bit or anything I left behind.

Day Nine: Trouble breathing. Don't know how much longer I can survive away from blue planet. I fear if I depart from here I will lose clarity of self and multiple connections in new community. Gasping for air. Disappointed and discouraged by predicament.

Day Ten: Breathing remains labored. Beginning to reconsider options. I miss Earth. I miss who I was. Understanding my identity, views, and reasoning have become obstructed and marred by the mere act of defining myself as an alien from Planet Aspie. Forgotten who I was.

Day Eleven: I've been forced to make preparations to leave this planet after a radio signal I picked up from Earth on a social network frequency: "Isn't it strange how folks pigeonholed by their labels want to be recognized for their labels, yet don't want to be pigeonholed by labels?" Resulting consequence: Self-absorbed and in a feeble state of wounded ego.

Day Twelve: Ego attachment to Aspergers identity is still very strong as I buckle in and prepare for departure back to home planet.

Day Thirteen: Touched down on planet earth. Immediately reunited with vital parts of self. Collecting parts of personhood that I left behind. Mourning loss of identity. Breathing still labored.

Day Fourteen: Planting a new garden of identity that hosts a multitude of vegetation. Seeds in place. Breathing normal. Earthlings are loving indeed. Aliens no longer exist. All beings on same journey.

Day Fifteen: Successfully integrated all Aspergers traits back into the whole of my personhood. No longer in need of a self-definition to exist. Breathing is divine. Flowers are in full bloom in garden. Welcoming beauty. Anchored in awareness. Seeing others as a reflection of my perceptions. Continue to learn.

Day Sixteen: Working on accepting and loving all parts of self. Witnessed another earthling blast off to Planet Aspie. Will remain in garden waiting for her return. Sending her light and love.

16. BRAIN, LITTLE VOICE, AND ME

Have you ever been in one of those relationships where the person is highly intriguing, passionate, and overall seems like a very likeable guy, but for some reason you can't stand to be around him? That's the type of relationship I'm currently in. Only it's not exactly with a person—it's with my brain!

Brain and I, we go a long way back, yet I'm still trying to figure him out. Sometimes I try to understand Brain more by comparing him to other brains. For instance, just the other day I asked my husband, "What are you thinking about?"

He responded, "Nothing."

And I said, "What? You're joking. Really? Absolutely nothing?"

He thought (or did something) for a while, and then answered, adamantly, "Nope. Nothing."

Now by this time I'm laughing, in that annoying I-do-know-better way, wanting to knock my knuckle on his head and say, "Hello, in there!"

Later, I asked my eldest son the same question, and his answer mirrored his father's. "Well, what were you thinking about a few minutes ago, then?" I asked.

"I don't know, Mom. Leave me alone. Nothing important." (He's fourteen.)

Now, get this. When I asked my middle son, "What are you thinking about?" he gave me a thirty-minute dissertation.

Can you guess which one has Aspergers? I didn't bother to ask my baby boy; he was too busy securing plastic wrap over a clear plastic cup that he'd carefully filled with the blood he'd collected from his bloody nose. He was saving the blood for future science experiments. I easily guessed what he was thinking about.

Movies are *interestingly annoying* with Brain. There are times I have to press the pause button on the remote during a film because I'm so excited by the fact that I was actually enjoying the show for five minutes straight without Brain interrupting! This is a super big, explanation-mark deal in my proverbial book because usually when a movie is playing (some 99.99 percent of the time), the Little Voice in my head (LV) and I are carrying on an entire conversation. I noticed today that LV is starting to have a full on personality—which causes my stomach to rumble somewhat in fear because I fret I may end up with yet another neurological disorder. And there's only so many LV and I can keep track of.

I picture LV like Laverne from the long-running series *Laverne and Shirley*. Like Laverne, LV has letters monogrammed onto her tight sweater and she's totally clueless that her sweater is too snug. So she looks like a *loosey goosey* even though she doesn't mean to appear that way. She's like me, like the time when I wore those glossy yellow shorts during freshman physical education class that were way too short. Yet I hadn't a clue why the boys and girls were calling me those names. Not to *should* on LV, but she should have a question mark right alongside her LV monogram. It's all about inquiry with that chick.

Here's the typical repertoire of clauses she chooses from while I attempt to watch a romantic, carefree comedy: *Is that the director's first movie? I wonder how much that actress got paid? Is this a box office hit, for real? Wow, nice hair. Maybe I should get my hair cut. Look, did you see her pause for a whole frickin' five minutes to let the other person talk? How does she do that? Is that normal? Is that what I'm supposed to do? Oh my goodness, do you think she realizes what the plastic surgery did to her face? That can't be her? Is that her? Should I pause the movie and find out? I want that tableware. Is that materialistic of me? The blue is so pretty. What color is that? Cobalt. Cobalt is a strong-sounding word.* Which leads me back to the whole "why I wouldn't want to be my brain's friend" argument.

17. VIGNETTE, BLUE, AGE 4

Everything inside was blue—the seats, the ceiling, the floor, even the steering wheel. I tugged on a string from the backseat cover, wrapping layer upon layer of blue taut around my finger. This midafternoon it was my tiny index finger that turned a slight shade of indigo.

"Nothing to get hung about," Mother sang out smiling happily, as if the coming rain had already washed away her worries. She didn't have a singing voice, never had, but the effort and soul were there, the wanting and the need to sound good. Inside the rearview mirror, her eyes, the color of amaretto, glimmered reflecting the narrowing sunlight. From the back seat I hummed along to "Strawberry Fields Forever" and jingled my clear-red plastic piggy bank in the air, lifting him up and turning his gaze outside. High atop the rolling, grassy hills the enormous oaks stood like rows of fresh-cut broccoli, rich and green—the bold color before the broccoli is boiled to a dull olive. In the shadows of the day, tall eucalyptus trees were sprinkled between the weathered fruit stands, their silvery leaves rustling, fluttering up and back, yielding to the autumn wind. I winked one eye, then the next, and then winked several times to form patterns of gray, brown, and green. A gust of moist wind pushed in through the side window, tossing Mother's chestnut hair and bringing a sharp scent of diesel smoke and wet asphalt. In the box next to Mother, the framed photograph of my Labrador Sugar smiled up at the blue ceiling. Nearby knickknacks, either too delicate or too cumbersome to stuff into moving boxes, rattled. The tip of Mother's cigarette sizzled inside a circular lighter, and with a click of the knob the music faded away.

I scratched my leg at the point where my knobby knee stuck out of the navy-blue stockings, then flapped away a puffing train of cigarette smoke. The sound of spinning rubber against wet pavement reverberated. Up ahead on the highway a truck squealed to a stop. Mother plunged down on the brakes. A crystal bowl chimed. I leaned forward, bracing myself against the sudden jolt and then slunk down and huddled on the floorboard, listening to the soothing sound of the windshield wipers swishing back and forth.

Mother looked over her shoulder with a wide smile—her high-boned cheeks, pink, her dark eyes, easy. Both the top and bottom rows of her teeth were crisscrossed, but I did not notice her imperfections as much as the kindness in her eyes, the soft, approachable twinkle. From down below I grinned up, all of my little teeth showing. Mother sighed in relief, eased her grip from the steering wheel, and pressed on the gas pedal.

"It's raining again," she said, in a singsong voice. Plink, plink came the rain. I loved water in all its forms—the intricate crystals of ice, the cool running streams, the shooting and whistling steam of geysers, and especially heaven's tears, the rain. Mother snuffed out her cigarette. It was the last cigarette of her pack and almost completely gone, but there was still enough of it left for her to save. Mother was that way; she liked to hold onto things, even after they were mostly gone.

Gray-white flashes of road flickered beneath me. I leaned in close to the floorboard, sending my finger through the nickel-sized hole in our blue Dodge Dart. A fleck of rusted floorboard broke off and fell down the hole, and next was the foil from a stick of gum. Minutes later, I clapped in amazement from my seat as my wadded tissue shot up from the back end of the car and drifted away into the cloud-soaked sky. I crammed a stick of gum down next, then leapt onto the back seat and pointed as the gum wad shot out across the highway. I'd found a secret passageway.

A misty rain traveled to the back seat, tickling my cheeks. Above, the sky was painted thick like my nana's old front porch, the top colors peeling away to expose an undercoating of dense gray. Without warning, a drumroll of thunder accompanied a trumpeting of raindrops. I shivered and hid my plastic piggy beneath a small blanket. Mother rolled up the window, cranking her hand around several times, before returning the full of her attention to the road. I pressed the side of my cheek against the window, taking in the coolness. An octopus-shaped cloud opened its enormous mouth and swallowed the sun. I breathed out and steamed up the glass. From somewhere inside myself I recognized a wanting, a feeling which manifested itself as an announced emptiness in the pit of my stomach, like I had never had that grilled-cheese sandwich for lunch, like everything I ate had been poured right out of me. I imagined melting through the window, through the rain, and moving far ahead of the uncertainty of the day. But I remained where I sat, watching my own dark eyes stare back at me.

As the car slowed and my heart sped up, I held onto the familiarity of the ride: the twist of the fabric ring around my finger, the bumping of the knickknacks, the swishing of the windshield wipers. Mother watched herself with one eye in the rearview mirror, applied her cranberry-red lipstick, and brought our car to a final resting place on a sloped driveway. "Shit," she said, in a voice she had meant to be much quieter. "Where are my cigarettes?" She opened and closed the glove box before turning back with an apologetic smile. The windshield wipers stuck midway on the sprinkled glass, as if frozen in time.

Stepping outside of the car, Mother stuffed her brush into her purse and the shirttail of her blouse into her new pleated skirt. During the time it took her to open and close the car trunk, I wrestled with the snug opening of my knitted sweater, first trying to slant my head sideways, then slipping in the wrong arm, and lastly finding my way inside the thick beige wool, with the inside on the outside. That's the way it would have to be—inside out and lopsided. There was no time to start again.

Mother opened my door. "Come on, beautiful," she said, as she held my little orange suitcase and stared out across a grassy yard. I set one foot down on the driveway and then the other, working my way out the best I could, all twisted in my sweater. The air outside was nippy and unusually cold for October. I looked up at Mother before jumping out and running across the driveway with my piggy bank, moving forward with an energy made of mystery and newness and the finality of reaching the end of a long journey. I bounded across the walkway and landed full force on the wet grass, setting my thoughts on the freshly rinsed snails near the marigolds. The rain puddles drenched my socks. I giggled and pulled down on one pigtail. A clown squeak sounded in my shoes, an unexpected noise which caused me to smile the rest of the distance up the concrete path.

"Come," Mother said, from where she stood on the high front patio. I looked across the walkway and tracked her. She flattened her wavy hair and pulled back her narrow shoulders. "Let's go," she said, with a motion of her hand. I liked her fingernails, how they tapered evenly at the ends like miniature red candles. Giggling, I sprinted ahead.

After I reached Mother's side, she tapped on a screen door framed in avocado green. Within seconds, a lean stranger with sandy tresses stepped out to greet us. He embraced Mother's petite frame, taking her into him. I peered up at the tall man's pressed beige shorts, inching my eyes upward, noting his skin was crumpled sandpaper and the hair atop his head remarkably shiny and stiff. Freckles abounded so that I could not connect the dots that led from fingers, to arm, to neck, and continued up the entire canvas of his chiseled face. To a large extent he resembled an oversized wooden doll, for there existed a solid and inflexible aura about his entire character. The rigid man released Mother. His hazel eyes met mine. Deep creases formed along both sides of his nose. I swallowed, and it felt like I had outgrown my throat.

"Honey, this is Drake," Mother said. She ran her fingers through my freshly cut bangs and then continued. "Drake is your stepfather. Can you please shake his hand?" The man reached out his large hand to meet mine and I accepted the coarse clamminess.

I thought of my own father, my real father, the man who cut pictures of dolls out of magazines and then lacquered the faces to cardboard so I could have a doll poster; the man who sewed on the red yarn for my Raggedy Ann doll hair; the man who went down the curving yellow slide with me in his lap; the man who wore a fuzzy, rust-colored robe at night with a long belt which trailed behind him like the tail of a lemur. I thought of my father, until Drake cleared his throat.

I looked up and pulled my hand back. Drake flashed a brief smile of straight white teeth. Mother gave a crooked grin. I lowered my eyes to the patio floor, wiped my hands on my sweater, and tracked a zigzagging crack that led from the concrete steps to the side of the house.

A few minutes later, inside the unfamiliar house, I removed my wet shoes and socks and stood by the front door. More words followed then, but not words I found. Those words, the adults' chatter, drifted out of my reach. The only word I was able to grab a hold of was "stepfather," and that word alone confused me, as my eyes searched about the place for any sign of steps. Standing there, feeling the cold of the hardwood floor rise up, I nuzzled my piggy inside my twisted sweater. Then, leading my eyes past Mother, I looked about the unfamiliar room, taking in as much as my senses could carry. A burning log inside the fireplace hearth crackled. A large grandfather clock ticked. Everything else appeared brand new. The couch, the chairs, the coffee table, the drapes, the decor—all sterile, as if neatly unwrapped and kept in place. I looked up at Drake. His back was facing me. I looked at his starched shirt and starched hair. I looked at his starched house. And I reasoned the obvious. I decided somewhere in Drake's orderly home there had to be some drawer or shelf unkempt, some shoebox of secrets. And it would only be a matter of time until I accidentally opened it.

18. HELL OUT OF DODGE

I awoke heavyhearted; this led Sir Brain to take us on a detour from reality. He chose the path of words and focused on the origin of the word "humor." Why? Because I used the word "humor" in a sentence. (Sigh.) And that led frenzied Sir Brain away like a string of yarn does for a kitten. Brain's string began at the word "etymology," which means the origin or development of a word, affix, phrase, etc., and the string ended with the word "black bile." *Yucko-mania*! If Brain hadn't allowed for a detour into reasoning forest and instead left me in the moment, I fear I would be profusely apologizing for the spattering of snot and tears all over the computer screen. You see, Sir Brain and I are quite distraught. (LV hightailed it out of here and sent us a postcard from Maui.) Matter of fact, just last night Sir Brain was a daredevil speed racer for three hours straight, clad in his black leather jumpsuit and riding his cranked-up dirt bike through tunnels and across perilous ramps. He had a lot of processing to do. And when I woke up, *we* endured two more hours of it. The good news is the tears have cleared and hope has set in. There's a seedling sprouting at the belly of my soul and stretching to the open sky. "What happened?" you might ask. Well, I got the hell out of Dodge! ("Get the hell out of Dodge" was possibly inspired by Dodge City, Kansas— a rough cattle town depicted in Western films in the mid-twentieth century. The US Marshal in the television series *Gunsmoke* used the phrase; however, some claim the marshal never said the word "hell" because you weren't allowed to swear in shows back then.) In actuality, I got the hell out of the university that I was attending for my degree in mental health counseling. Kaput! We gone! And I am never going back. Never want to see my professors' faces again. I am too upset to even know how to begin to explain. Though there are a few distinct swear words I'd like to stick on the subject, but I won't. For now, I think I'll treat myself (and Sir Brain) to an overdue retreat.

19. Growth Points

Last night I was up late. I was typing a letter in therapeutic fashion, with no intention of giving the letter to the recipients. I was planning on sharing the letter with you, until I woke up this morning and decided the process of writing was healing enough. And then I thought to share another letter— which took about four hours to write. It outlines, in a professional and factual tone, the demeaning words one of my professors launched at me after class. I was very much an innocent in the situation. I offer this fact with sincerity and clarity. I would even swear on something or another. Typically, let's say 99 percent of the time, I can see the error of my ways, and how I most definitely contributed to an outcome. But in this ghastly situation, with the professor, I was a victim. I decided in the end not to present either letter publicly because I began to understand the motives behind my writing. I realized I wanted your attention. I wanted to elicit pity. And then I thought: *Is that the vibe I truly desire to put out there?* The good news is I'm about two hundred times stronger than I was forty-some years ago. Because I figure I've been challenged by significant events at least four to five times a year, ever since I can remember, and that I have gained one point for each challenge I have overcome; which puts me somewhere between the vicinity of one hundred sixty and two hundred growth points.

20. I AM ELEPHANT

Days like today, I want to find the highest mountain peak and shout in my loudest voice, "I am elephant!" I want to charge forward with my tusks at a massive pile of hay. Stab and stab with all my might, until no barrier is left, only scattered remnants that the animals can feed upon, digest, and carry away.

I hate—if I ever were to hate anything—the aspect of being misunderstood. I hate that my son is being misunderstood. I hate that I am misunderstood. I feel as if we, as an Aspergers *species*, have been set up for failure. As if we are supposed to make ourselves less genuine in order to not threaten others' norms. I understand we represent the unknown that exists outside the comfort zone of many individuals. And when we stand there face-to-face in conversation (the anomaly, if you will), others often perceive us as an entity that requires some degree of change or adaptation on our part. Yet I question: What is it about the way I think and function that requires alteration? What if the way I think and function is ideal? Why is it that the majority believe their way is the right way, when all about them the world is falling apart from war, famine, lies, manipulation, blackmail, disease, hatred, bigotry, and poison?

These named leaders play these games using their tricks. Wherein I, coming from a place of honesty, am perceived as a threat. Is the feeling of "threat" erupting from others' insecurities, or perhaps from the uncomfortable feelings that arise when one's foundation of what is believed to be *the right way* is confronted? Perhaps the way communication is currently played out is from a very limited and self-centered scope, wherein there is this unspoken dance in which I am expected to filter what I say, how I say it, when I say it, and how much I say in order to not risk causing discomfort to someone else.

Assuming I am reasonably self-aware (which I am), and I have no intention to cause ill will or harm (which holds true), and that I have generally mastered the basic social norms of avoiding rudeness (which I have), then what other rules must I add? It seems the other rules of communication include this basket of techniques, such as buffering and balancing, that enable the recipients to feel better about who they are, or at least not any worse. It seems a game where the first priority is to not make waves, to win the person over, to sound confident, and to sprinkle evidence of high intellect and likeability in order to allow the other person to feel comfortable enough to maybe begin to trust.

Why is it that if I accurately and purposely reflect what another individual wishes to hear and see that they then embrace me and wrap their tentacles of interest about; yet other times, when I am entirely authentic and I share without pretense, plan, or caution, I am questioned, perhaps even distrusted, judged, singled out, ridiculed, or admonished? Why is it some people want to converse with clones of themselves and make me into their egocentric mirror, instead of knowing me?

The way I see it, conversing is like driving down a dangerous road where there are warning signs at every turn: *Beware! Make sure your words are continually reinforcing the other person's identity, perception, and worthiness. Avoid offending, weakening, or threatening a person's idea of truth. Know that complete honesty triggers alarm in people. Understand that ultimately most people you approach already don't trust you, and you have to build and build trust before they will. Even then, know there will be people who will never trust you.*

If communication is based on a scale dependent on levels of trust, then the participants are continually establishing and refining how much they trust one other in order to determine what to share and withhold. If withholding information is the norm, then I question the integrity of the establishment who dictates such norms. If one were to say, "Impossible! If we all spoke our truth the world would fall apart," then I would ask, "Is the world not already falling apart?" The majority's opinion of what counts as the correct mode of communication appears backward and disproportionate. This dictated "right way" to communicate—the approach where people say what is expected in order to get at some unspoken goal and/or where people only speak after deciphering levels of trust though evaluation and judgment—appears manipulative, preplanned, and superficial.

And why is there a limit to what we are supposed to reveal? I understand donning clothing to conceal the taboo of the naked flesh. I can abide by this norm by cloaking my body. But to understand the taboo of sharing the naked truth—I can find no such cloak. I do not know what to cover my truth in.

21. ZOMBIE

My husband's snoring sound: ZZZ-Zzzz-ZZzzz-hn-oink-GGggoofffh-Ppwwbhww- zZZzzzZZ. Did I mention it's five in the morning? I'm thinking Brain (Sir Brain) is up because of the upcoming IEP meeting (Individual Education Plan) scheduled for my middle son at his school later today. That and the fact that the little voice in my head (LV) had this running dialogue about our life force's dependency on my body's internal organs, and how at any second our heart could decide to give up, or even explode. Sir Brain wasn't totally freaked out until LV added the whole aneurism (brain explosion) probability to the equation. That's when Sir Brain packed two rectangular, 1950s-style suitcases and stood up on his toothpick legs, and proclaimed, "I'm out of here!" Until LV explained that he was the brain and couldn't leave. Which bothered Sir Brain to no end, as he didn't understand how he wasn't a separate entity beyond a complex body organ. LV and Sir Brain are still debating on that one.

I wrestled with the thought of staying in bed, until LV brought me back on the hamster wheel and reviewed repeatedly (think copy machine spitting out one thousand copies) the fact that I didn't show up to my college course yesterday. Thusly, I rose with puffy, slit eyes, appearing as if I'd been born and raised on a planet without sunlight. I mounted the stairs like a zombie while listening to LV chat it up, in her California valley-girl dialect, about how I don't have to be from another planet because I live in a little town in Washington, a place primarily absent of sunlight. And now I'm here typing, while LV goes over with Sir Brain (who is frantic about exploding) about how yesterday was the first day in the totality of more than seven of my college years that I purposely missed a class without explanation. Indeed, I haven't missed a college course since my beloved Nano's funeral—the year *Rain Man* was released. So, understandably, LV and Sir Brain are a wee bit perplexed about me basically playing hooky from school. Although, they are quite aware that we have left the university but can't withdraw officially yet, because we're waiting (and waiting) to hear back from the authorities that be to see if I have to spill the beans about how I was woefully treated before I can get my tuition reimbursed. I'm thinking it's not too early for a glass of wine or a horse tranquilizer. What's your opinion?

22. THERE IS NO IT!

I do this thing where I personify objects. For example, this may get a little gross, but if two globs of minty-green toothpaste are clinging on for dear life in my bathroom sink and one glob is washed down and the other glob is still there, I feel sorry for the lonely glob. And sorry for the other glob that I washed down the grimy drain, too. Fearing what awaits him. Notice the *him*. Nothing is an *it*. There is no it! I even sometimes feel sorry for fruits and vegetables, like when I'm shoving cucumber peelings down the garbage disposal to their impending doom. When I used to fry (massacre) sliced potatoes in a cast-iron pan, when I was about the age of eight, the potatoes would make a squealing noise, like they were crying in agonizing "you're killing us" pain. It was actually just the horrible sound of oil sizzling, but I felt for those particular potatoes. Sometimes I removed the ones that cried the loudest, but then I didn't know what to do with them. Because who wants to be put in the garbage? All this personifying is a big part of the reason eating and cooking is sometimes challenging. It's probably why I don't ever care to empty a jar completely or don't finish the last pages of a book. Who wants to be brought to an end? Personification is likely why I don't eat meat—although, oddly enough, I have never felt sorry for chocolate. This marvelous discovery, this whole personification thing, explains why the other day I was actually wondering how the strings of celery must have felt as they were traveling through my digestive track. Sounds loony, right? I pictured the strings like they were on some water slide that ended in a tomb of bubbling stomach acid. Who does that? Well, supposedly sometimes other Aspies do that! So there! It's okay, I suppose, that I feel sorry for crumpled paper that didn't get tossed into the bin and is now stranded on the floor, because there are other earthlings that also feel sorry for the paper. What huge compassion I have. If you can understand the compassion I have for inanimate objects and food, then can you imagine the immense compassion I carry for animals and people? It's phenomenal.

23. WOUNDED SPIRIT

In totality I've likely cried one hundred times more in these last weeks than in the last few years. I'm upset and have a gnawing tummy pain. The feeling stems from the act of leaving another brief email message at the college I am (I was?) attending. I've yet to be withdrawn from the class with the meanie professor. This leaves me in an unsettling position, without closure and without finality. I'm an INFJ (Myers-Briggs personality type) and a harmony-seeking idealist (Keirsey temperament). What these personality traits boil down to is that I need frickin' closure! I'm so nervous inside. I've been waiting for the phone call for over ten days. I was very conscious about not calling the university too much after I received a slap to my self-esteem from one professor who told me that my two (count them: two) emails stretched over the time of one week—seven days apart—were too frequent and urgent. As loony as I think the professor's judgment was, no matter, I'm hypersensitive about contacting anyone at the university now. I'm thinking it's getting to the point that I ought to share with you what's going on; only there's a little part of me who wants to not burn any bridges, not point fingers, and not rouse attention to the situation. I struggle with what I can share, what action constitutes grounds for taking care of myself and sharing my story, and what is best kept in private. The dilemma in what to write all comes down to my tendency to overshare and then eventually regret what comes out.

24. Ten Myths about Females with Aspergers

ONE. Aspergers Is Easy to Spot: Females with Aspergers are often superb actresses. They've either trained themselves how to behave in hopes of fitting in with others and/or they avoid social situations. Many grown women with Aspergers are able to blend into a group without notice.

TWO. Professionals Understand Aspergers: No two people are alike. Professionals have limited experience, if any experience, with females with Aspergers. Professionals have limited resources, limited prior instruction and education, and little support regarding the subject of Aspergers. Coexisting conditions with Aspergers are complex. Females seeking professional help are often overlooked and sometimes belittled or misdiagnosed.

THREE. An Effective Diagnosis Tool Exists for Females with Aspergers: There is no blood or DNA test for Aspergers. No one knows what causes Aspergers or if Aspergers is actually a condition, and not just a way of looking at the world differently. The diagnostic tools, such as surveys, are based on male-dominant Aspergers traits that do not take into account how the female's brain and the female's role in society differ from the male experience. Diagnosis is largely based on relatives' observations and individual case history, and is determined by professionals who often do not understand the female traits of the syndrome.

FOUR. People with Aspergers Lack Empathy: Females with Aspergers usually have a great deal of empathy for animals, nature, and people. A female's (with Aspergers) specific facial features, body language, tone of voice, laughter, and word choice might result in an observer misjudging a female's (with Aspergers) thoughts, feelings, and intentions. Women and girls with Aspergers are often deep philosophical thinkers, poets, and writers—all attributes that require a sense of empathy. Females with Aspergers usually try very hard to relate another's experience to their own experience, in hopes of gaining understanding.

FIVE. People with Aspergers Are Like a Television Character: Many individuals have learned not to compare an ethnic minority group to a character on television, because such comparison is a form of stereotyping and racism. However, people are comparing male fictional characters on television to females with Aspergers. This happens usually without intention to harm, but out of a desire to understand. People with Aspergers aren't living in a sitcom. There is a need for a greater degree of understanding beyond observing an entertainer.

SIX. Aspergers Is No Big Deal: People with Aspergers often face daily challenges. There is no magic pill to make an Aspergers brain think differently. People with Aspergers see the world in another way than the majority. Females with Aspergers are not different in a way that needs to be improved. They are different in a way that requires support, empathy, and understanding from the mainstream. Aspergers is a big deal. The diagnosis can bring varying degrees of grief, acceptance, depression, confusion, closure, and epiphany. Here are just a few of the conditions a female with Aspergers might experience: sensory difficulties, OCD, phobias, anxiety, fixations, intense fear, rapid thinking, isolation, depression, low self-esteem, self-doubt, chronic fatigue, IBS, shame, confusion, trauma, abuse, bullying, and/or loss of relationships.

SEVEN. Aspergers Doesn't Exist: Aspergers does exist. There is a subgroup of females all exhibiting and experiencing almost the exact same traits. If there is no Aspergers then something dynamic is happening to hundreds upon hundreds of women; this something, whatever one chooses to label the collection of traits, requires immediate evaluation, understanding, support, educational resources, and coping mechanisms.

EIGHT. There Are More Males than Females with Aspergers: In regard to comparing females and males with Aspergers, just like our history textbooks, more males are in the spotlight than females. Males are typically the doctors, professionals, and researchers of Aspergers—males that do not have Asperger's Syndrome and who obviously aren't females. Thousands of females with Aspergers remain undiagnosed. Hundreds of women are searching social networks and the Internet daily for answers, connection, and understanding about themselves and/or their daughters.

NINE. Females with Aspergers Don't Make Good Friends: Females with Aspergers are all different. Just like everyone else, they have their quirks and idiosyncrasies. Many females with Aspergers are known for their loyalty, honesty, hard-work ethics, compassion, kindness, intelligence, empathy, creativity, and varied interests and knowledge base. Females with Aspergers, like anyone, have the capacity to make fantastic friends, coworkers, and spouses, if, and when, they are treated with respect, love, understanding, and compassion.

TEN. Aspergers Isn't Something that Affects My Life: More and more children are being diagnosed with Asperger's Syndrome. Adult males and females are realizing they have the traits of Asperger's Syndrome. The rise in Aspergers is a financial strain on the educational system and medical system. There are very limited resources and support systems available to assist people with Aspergers and their families. There is probably someone in your local community who has Asperger's Syndrome.

25. University Villains

Today I'm quite gleefully typing in my pajamas and socks. This is good, or rather beneficial, this rebel mood I'm in. Because today is the big day I've been both anticipating and dreading. I'm pretty darn proud of myself that I haven't blurted out in writing all that has transpired recently at the university. I like the mysteriousness surrounding what I have offered and the respect I'm giving the villains. I'm feeling okay about calling them *villains*, even though I know we are all God's (Universe's, String Theory's, what have you's) creatures. I know these people have taught me plenty, especially about how I don't want to lead and teach like them. And I know these lessons will carry me far and that the experience has already given me that extra sheet of armadillo layer across my soft-bellied spirit. Still, something feels so delightfully good about calling them *villains*! Some words for villain are "antihero" and "contemptible person." I picture a little ant with a small red cape that reads *HERO* going up against a grotesque giant in a huge white nappy (diaper) that reads *Anti-Hero*. And I envision the ant winning by some divine intervention from the Roman gods. I like the term *beyond the pale*, too. It's a term related to contemptible, and means an unpardonable action. I believe I am in the right to say the professor was *beyond the pale*. He was outside the acceptable and agreed upon standards of decency. And dang it, if I have to constantly adjust my actions and phrases to make others feel comfortable, then he ought to have at least had decency.

In symbolic summary, last night I dreamt that I parked my ten-speed bike in front of a quaint, suburban neighborhood house. When I returned to retrieve the bike, I found it broken into two (repairable) parts. I knocked on the door of the nearby house. An older man answered. The man explained that he took the bike apart because I left too much of my bike sticking out in his driveway. I hadn't. He then offered to fix the bike for a large sum of money. I knew he was applying trickery and trying to gain from my loss. I declined and instead had him carry the pieces into my van. I drove away. Hmmmm? I wonder how my subconscious is feeling about my dumbass professor?

26. A Shame

I can't see myself striving in an educational environment where teachers are compartmentalizing individuals based on their own narrow and biased theories, where they are desperately lacking in current theories and accounts regarding Asperger's Syndrome. And where they have no interest at all in learning how Aspergers affects individuals. A place where I was queried by a licensed mental health therapist: "Are you happy you have pronounced to the world your brain and your son's brain are broken?" A place where I was told that under the theory of *family systems* that I had "likely manifested my own Asperger's Syndrome in order to feel closer to my son." A place where I was accused of taking my child to a psychiatrist, "So you [I] can put him on medication and not have to deal with the real issues." (Not that it matters, but my son isn't on any medication.) There is more I could share, but I think this paints a clear picture. I am left perplexed and unsettled. I am concerned that this faculty will continue educating hundreds of counseling students. And I have been turning over in my mind why Aspergers is something I was cautioned to hide. Yes, I understand that by telling my professors I had Aspergers that I was treated differently than the average student, some would conjecture harshly. But is the solution for me to remain quiet and in hiding? Is that what minorities have done in the past to be heard, to be seen, to achieve equity and justice? Is Aspergers such a widely misunderstood condition that I should retreat in shame?

27. VIGNETTE, JUSTICE BLACK, AGE 5

Mother was always tenderhearted and carried an inherent soft spot for the underdog, lost, and forlorn. Where in some ways she failed me as a protective guardian, in other ways she opened my mind to the diversity and beauty of the world and the necessity of accepting others unconditionally, despite societal norms and expectations. As I've grown older, I've come to appreciate Mother's innate ways of gathering up the needy and gracing them with adoration and attention. My childhood dog was no exception.

It was a stormy evening when Mother spotted a sopping wet dog shivering in the dark corner of the alley outside of her workplace. Without second thought, she scooped the timid stray up into the safety of a warm blanket and brought him home. My new shaggy best friend first peeked out at me from beneath the towering statues of smiling Stepfather Drake and winking Mother. He was quickly named "Justice Black." A name Drake, a practicing attorney, took much pride in.

Justice had been abused, we would later assume. The evidence found in the way he retreated from strangers—ducking under our coffee table at first sign of threat. And in the way his demeanor was consistently accommodating.

From day one Justice was at my side. He was my constant companion and fiercely loyal—my own at-the-ready, kinky-haired mutt. Justice ran away only twice that I recall; the first time was only days after his arrival. But Mother was quick to bring him back. She fervently knocked on doors, took out a newspaper advertisement, and posted "lost dog" signs all over our affluent, suburban neighborhood. I can still picture the kind man with a fatherly smile who opened his front door and how Justice was seated at his side—bathed and appearing stately with a satin, blue ribbon wrapped neatly around his neck. I remember when we brought Justice back home, how I'd sat on the front porch and nestled my face in his freshly washed fur, breathing in his return. And how later we'd shared a vanilla ice cream cone, taking turns with the licks. The second time Justice left would be years later—and the last.

Most days of my youth with Justice beside me were filled with outdoor adventures, from tree climbing (with him on watch below) to inching our way under yellow school busses at the bus yard (to spy on strangers). I remember one particular bright day, with my face tattooed in tomato sauce and specks of scented marker, when Justice Black and I skipped across the neighborhood street to the wide-open field. The sky that afternoon was a crisp cornflower blue and the air a bouquet of fresh eucalyptus. There in the field, we galloped together through the high grasses toward the aged stone wall that lined the perimeter of my mother's vegetable garden. I carried with me a prized tie-string sac filled with pebbles, seagull feathers, and anything else that caught my fancy. And Justice, he housed a rolled-up treasure map inside his silver-studded red collar.

On this day we were fierce pirates. I did not care much for princesses. I much preferred my jelly-filled Stretch Armstrong doll with his rubbery skin and big muscles that I could yank and yank and still not pull apart. Barbie dolls, I had discovered, had heads I could pop right off.

In the field, we stood tall on the garden wall while keeping our eyes out for rival pirates. At the day's end, as was my daily tradition, I recited the American Pledge of Allegiance with my right hand over my heart, shouting the last line, "And *Justice* for all!" Justice moved closer then, nuzzling his pointy chin into my side and wagging his ticklish tongue. In return I embraced him, taking in the foulness of his breath along with the tenderness of his amber-colored eyes. I imagined our ship had taken sail and an opposing fleet of ruthless pirates was approaching just off of our port bow. Justice, with his long, jagged teeth protruding from his sideways grin, kept careful watch. When we'd outsailed the pirates, we played hide-and-seek beneath the shadows of the burly walnut trees. Only Justice, being a dog, still could not comprehend when he was supposed to cover his eyes and count.

After a long day of romping in the field, from the front door forward, I tugged at Justice's stiff collar with all of my might and nudged him toward the bathroom. From there, I led him to the edge of the tub and heaved his body up and over the side. Leaning over, I pressed my face into his fur.

Justice parked himself there for all of sixty seconds, just long enough to shake crazily and cover me in ticklish white foam, before he broke free and sprinted into the hallway, slipping and sliding at each and every turn across the hardwood floor. I found him all sopping wet under my bed. He looked ridiculous, his rump high in the air, his fur appearing to be parted a thousand times over, and his twiggy tail waving—a garden sprinkler on full speed.

Admittedly, I sometimes wished for a dog of grander stature, a fierce canine to protect me from danger. But I only let those feelings sit when I was frightened. More often than not, I was extremely grateful for Justice. He was my warm blanket on cold nights. He was a pliant creature, a survivor, and a constant in my days. And I loved him with all my heart—the only way a child can ever love her dog.

28. VIEW FROM ATOP THE TRIANGLE

Yesterday I overate. I grounded chocolate pudding brownies into mocha-almond-fudge ice cream. I had bread rolls and garlic bread, hash browns, and other carb-filled delights. When I wasn't eating I was stuck to my computer—hinged to it, as if we were one. I couldn't pull myself away from my interests as I sat there on the couch, essentially immobile. I felt entirely alone and useless. So much so that I Googled "Why it's okay to be lazy" and "Why it's okay to do nothing." I felt guilty. I analyzed why I had this guilt, but the analysis made things worse. I knew what I should have been doing, such as exercising, showering, taking my vitamin supplements, spending time with my family, going out into the fresh air. But I couldn't do anything. I was trapped. I couldn't even change my stained shirt or bend down to pick a crumb up off the floor.

These types of days, when I am overcome by fear and fatigue, are nothing new. I've had them since I was a teenager. The challenge is I'm not a teenager anymore—I am a mother and a wife. Roles that bring with them responsibilities beyond my own needs.

Yesterday wasn't the easiest of mornings for our family. There was some turmoil, and the spike of energy in our household left my brain sprawling, as does any type of unexpected event (particularly emotional upheaval). And no amount of cognitive tools or talk could dissipate my discomfort.

Yesterday the anxiety stayed with me. Yesterday I hated myself. I hated myself for my lack of willpower, my messed-up emotions, my inability to relax, my constant, constant challenges. I hated life. I was angry with how my analytical ability and extreme fluid intelligence put me into overdrive of self-analysis and remorse—my own thinking setting me up for failure.

Today, I am substantially more clearheaded, and in looking back I understand a bit more about how I relate to this world. I understand how Maslow's Hierarchy (a triangle of human needs) relates to this individual. I have concluded that, in many ways, I don't have a reliable sense of security and stability, and overall lack a sense of freedom from fear and anxiety— there are moments of serenity, but they are fleeting, always temporary. In addition, my sense of belonging is limited as a result of me believing that I am not upholding to the rules, expectations, and norms of others. I question my actions, my motives, my own belief systems. I upset my spouse; I neglect my family; and being a lover comes with challenges. It is true that I achieve mastery sometimes in my writing and in my ability to love others, yet there remains an underlying fear about people's judgment and rejection. I doubt my ability to be enough.

On the other hand, my self-actualization is intriguing—this is where my metaphorical (Maslow's) triangle is top-heavy. I do pursue my inner talents. I do pursue creative endeavors. I do feel fulfilled by my interests. Thusly, it appears my self-actualization is reached from a different avenue than the norm. I do not progress up Maslow's allegorical triangle. Instead I take a ladder, lean it against the triangle, climb up, and bypass the center to reach the top. I pursue my talents because that is where I find refuge. In this realm, atop the triangle, rests my freedom and power. Atop the triangle sits my obsessions, fixations, passions, joys, and extreme love. And that explains where I was yesterday: I was seated on the top level of the triangle, high out of reach.

29. THERE'S NO SUCH THING AS NORMAL

The idea of this concept called *normal* is one of the grandest illusions of our time. There is no *normal*. Normal doesn't exist. All definitions of normal are debatable—as are the definitions of typical, average, and ordinary. Normal apparently means behaving like most behave. But who are these most? And how do they behave? Show me the model. And please don't point to a television program.

The definition of normal is particularly alarming and highly debatable when considering the *Diagnostic and Statistical Manual of Mental Disorders* (DSM), a guidebook for mental health professionals. (Often referred to as "the mental health clinician's Bible.") Most mental health practitioners categorize and diagnose patients/clients by referring to the *Bible of Abnormal*—my word for the DSM. No surprise that the definition of normal changes with each publication of the DSM.

I'd like to see a *Bible of Normal*. I mean, if a whole thick book can list "abnormal" descriptors, then shouldn't the opposite book be available? Of course there is probably no profit to be made in a book on normal behavior. No big surprise, considering the times we live in, to discover the DSM is driven by the machinations of the pharmaceutical business. In fact, it's rumored more than half of the experts who compile the DSM have ties to the pharmaceutical industry. And other experts have other financial ties, such as research monies. Thusly, the current idea of *normalcy* is spawned from the introduction of psychoactive drugs. Beyond the tantrum I just had, I am also a wee bit confused about the current definition of Asperger's Syndrome. The limiting definition is based on only male subjects. I'm a girl last time I checked.

30. UN-FRIENDED

I was an only child, but I wasn't a lonely child. In my younger days I always had some type of friend; whether a cousin, a schoolmate, a daughter of Mother's friend, a neighborhood boy, or an imaginary spirit friend, I always found company. My favorite friends from my youth were freckle-faced, skinny Keith from kindergarten and Chris and Jimmy, the towheaded, cowboy-hat-bearing twins from first grade. I can still see Keith's Wonder Bread peanut butter, banana, and mayonnaise sandwiches, and the energetic twins leaping over their Kermit-green couch with toy guns in hand.

Making friends was never an issue—before I hit puberty. In my youth I had a natural cheeriness and good nature, and a downright quirky humor. I was clever, too—scrawny, hyper me creating multipage skits and stories, and directing recitals on a whim. I often liked to pretend I was a teacher, counselor, or a restaurant owner, and instructed my friends on the proper ways to behave and what to eat. (I guess in some ways, not much has changed.) I was a confident director and group leader. In retrospect, I recognize my rigidly enforced play structure and peer-management style enabled me to acquire a sense of order in an oftentimes-unpredictable world—mechanisms that served well to reduce my innate apprehension. But back then, I just did what came instinctually and tried to make the best of any given situation; for instance, there was the time I happily justified not only collecting dues from a neighborhood club I'd formed, but also using the spare change to buy myself poor-boy sandwiches at the corner market. Then again, I paid out my constituents from proceeds raised from yard sales that I both organized and ran.

For most of my younger years, as Mother would adamantly confirm, I was unusually cheerful—pending mayhem, major change, devastating loss, and what have you. (In that way, I haven't changed much either!) Puberty—well that was basically a dark, bleak splat in my lifespan. Think two-gallon inkbottle dropped down from the Seattle Space Needle. And as far as adulthood goes . . . well Sir Brain and LV (little voice in my head) jumped out and basically didn't know how to shut up.

As an adult I have lost a number of friends due to my behaviors and lack of a friendship manual. I lost one friend in grade school, as well, that I can remember: Elizabeth. But that's because her father didn't much approve of the happenings in my home. I missed her, and even named a stray cat after Liz. Today, there are two specific adult-friendship losses that stand out. One very close friend (the tea-sipping-on-the-porch kind, where you spill out your guts and cry in each other's arms), she suddenly stopped returning my emails and phone calls, and then *un-friended* me on a social network site. No explanation. No closure. No reason. Just erased me from her life. Kaput! Gone! She wouldn't even glance my way at social gatherings or outside the schoolhouse. At this time she only lived a block away from me. I mean I could see the tile rooftop of her two-story house from my front door, if I stood on my tippy-toes. And I'd even taught both of her children. Of course, in my defense, she brought closure to her last *best* friendship in a similar covert fashion. And in her defense, at that time in my life, I was a full-blown conglomeration of phobias and drama. The other person that ditched me without explanation was the only pal I made the first four years of college. We did everything together for a few months. She was the first to reassure me if I was thirsty, then it was okay to waste a buck at the mall on a drink. And the first to tell me my ankle-length jean skirt wasn't suggestive, as I'd assumed. But she disappeared. One day, without warning, she just stopped returning my calls. And when I phoned for the tenth time, her father informed me that his daughter was too upset to talk and no longer wanted anything to do with me. I'm still clueless about this one. Though I gather it was likely my obsession with a new love interest, coupled with this new bloke's unflattering character traits, and my tendency to put myself in danger when it came to dating. Interestingly enough, these two friends both have the same name. I'm not super fond of that name anymore.

31. NOTHING BUT A HEARTACHE

At any given time, from the age of thirteen to twenty-seven, I tried to have a best friend and a boyfriend. This pair of people anchored me—the best girl and the best boy. In some ways people would consider me lucky, as I seemed to attract the handsome boys. But some handsome boys, and boys in general, I later discovered, could be bad boys, too. Many people on the autism spectrum have reported that they didn't have a romantic relationship until later in their life, if ever. Me? I instinctively clung to boys starting at the age of five. Probably as a result of the raging hole I carried—a direct byproduct from the absence of my father and the busyness of my mother.

Living in a world of ghosts, haunted houses, and prescient dreams, while having extreme sensitivities to people, places, and things, left me longing to cling to something, if only for a sense of safety and retreat. As I reached my teenage years, I became akin to a high-quality plastic cling wrap. I'd seal a male over with my entire essence and remain stuck there in full-grip mode. I remember thinking I was experienced with relationships. Keen on how they worked, what to do, and how to keep a *man*. But I wasn't. I was weathered for certain, rusted around the outside like a metal pole set out in the rain one too many winters. But I definitely wasn't experienced. I hadn't the faintest idea of how to take care of my wants and needs, beyond lassoing a male to do things for me. I was quite pathetic, in an unintentional, hadn't-meant-to-be way.

By my early twenties, after graduating from college with honors and starting my first job as an elementary school teacher, I was deeply ashamed of the woman I'd become. More times than not, I didn't know the role that I played in life, didn't know my lines, or even where to find the script. From one moment to the next, I was changing; in one scene I played the part of the dedicated schoolteacher, in the next, a desperate fool holding onto whatever man she could get her hands on. A fisherman in the game of love,

I'd learned to bait my hook and cast my pole but hadn't known to catch and release. Each man I met who showed me the slightest attention soon became my new love interest. I was fortunate in high school to have had two boyfriends (at different times) that treated me tenderly and with respect. However, in later years, I dated men from all walks of life, most of whom were extremely damaged in some way or another. And all of whom were addicted to something or someone.

The worst part of being with a man was not what they ever did but what I let myself do. I made my bed and I slept in it. And I fooled myself repeatedly into thinking I was content. It didn't matter if the bed was too small, or too big, or if it had lumps. It didn't matter if the mattress was missing altogether and that I was made to sleep on the cold, hard floor. It only mattered I was in the bed, or at least what I'd thought to be a bed. My mind fooled me. My heart fooled me. My logic fooled me. While all along, my spirit wept. There has never been such a horrible part in my life as the years I walked half-blind to my own wanting. In essence I was a prisoner, unable to move without dragging and tricking myself in any given direction. Best to stand still in one spot—best not to move an inch—if that was possible. But it wasn't. I had to keep going. I had to keep stepping somewhere.

32. DEAR MONSTER

Self: Monster of the dark, why do you come to me at night and steal my joy so readily, and leave me shaking—a small child, lost, alone, and terrified?

Monster: I steal nothing, young heart of mine, which you do not wish already stolen, that you have not already offered on a table for me. Nothing you have not called me forward to retrieve and swallow whole. Nothing you do not already miss because you never allowed yourself to seize it. This fickle mind of yours is so solid in one truth and then the next. How bitter the taste to savor something that is already abandoned.

Self: Monster, I do not understand. How do I wish anything to be stolen?

Monster: You speak of love. Love, love, love. You cherish love. You want love. Yet when this love is given to you, you know not what to do with it. Instead, it is as if you spit on love. Spit and spit, unwilling to even grasp the idea of someone loving you. And yet you say you love? Ha! I laugh in your face. I spit in your face. If you loved, then you would gladly take this love they give.

Self: Monster, this is not true. You live in a false illusion. What you see is the fantasy world. You cannot see my world. Only muted shades of black and white. You see no colors. You do not know what I feel and what I bring into me.

Monster: Then why don't you take in what these people tell you?

Self: Monster, I do not know. I want to. I open my arms and hands and heart and mind, and I want to. But I cannot feel it, any of it. Everything of this world feels numb. This world of love. Everything seems a ribbon or prize, nothing that I am worthy of. I cannot take these prizes when I do not feel I have been a participant in the race or contest. Yet life feels so very much like a contest wherein everyone is struggling for prize. And I don't want to be like this, craving one prize after the next. Constantly striving. I just want to be.

Monster: But you don't take at all. You don't accept at all. You are this constant giver who will not receive. And that makes you a monster, too.

Do you not see? The greatest gift is to accept what others give, to with open hands reach out and accept their truth as your truth. This is not absolute. This does not make them right or you wrong. This does not make you prideful. This makes you real. And yet you partake in this dance where you cannot accept, cannot stand to feel. What is it you fear from these feelings? What do you fear?

Self: Dear Monster, I fear loss. I fear if I collect anything—friendship, objects, compliments, words, or thoughts—that they will eventually be lost. People leave. People perish. Objects come and go. Opinions change, and words; they are *shapeshifters* based on the speaker and witness.

Monster: Yes. Yes. But you miss the greatest point, the finite reason that your theory, your way, is flawed. For if you spend your whole life not accepting for fear of loss, then you spend your whole life losing from fear of accepting. You set yourself up from the start to suffer loss over loss, without remission, wherein if you were to open your hands and let some slip into your possession, then chances are you will hold onto some and lose some. But then again, even the lost was once had. With your way, nothing is ever had. Why are you so afraid to feel?

Self: Dear Monster, if I let myself feel, I risk everything. If I let myself love, I risk everything. If I let myself think for a fraction of a second that I am special, I risk self. I do not know the fine line. I do not know how to remain humble and how to accept love at the same time. I know how to give love. I know that well.

Monster: No, you do not! You do not know how to give love. You think you do. You think love is sacrifice. Love is not sacrifice. Love has no feelings, other than love. Nothing that pulls and tugs, digs or plunges, nothing that burns or confuses, nothing that makes someone hurt is of love. You are not giving love; you are giving fear. You are giving what you think love is. You are giving a safety net, a security blanket, a voice to calm the potential storm. Do not look at people as if they are about to explode or cry or reject. Look at people how you want to be seen. How do you want to be seen?

Self: Dear Monster, I want to be seen as a loving worthwhile being of light. I want to be seen as important and special. I want to be held over and over again, in kindness and affection. I want people to come to me for shelter and I want to receive shelter. I want to be weak and strong. I want to be happy and sad. I want to be me in totality and to be loved unconditionally.

Monster: Then you have your answers. Let people see your light. Let people see you are important and special. Let people hold you in kindness and affection. Let people be your shelter. Let people love you unconditionally, in all your states. They are trying, but you are not letting them, dear child. That is why I steal from you at night. For you leave everything out on the table like scraps for the dog. And I smell this waste. I smell this discarded love. And of course I come after you. I am hungry. I am starved. I am the monster that is you, who refuses to eat, and instead cries that there is no food. You feed off of ghosts and cry of starvation when there are plates full all around you. How can you point fingers at me, this monster, who only comes out crawling when he is called by your bitter woes? You ring anger's bell. You ring sadness's bell. You summon me time and again with this feast of forgotten love. And I take. Of course I take, because you will not.

Dear Monster: Friend indeed, a part of me. Here to show me what I cannot see. How I trick myself into thinking there is something in the shadows stealing and haunting my dreams, when in truth I am my own shadow, my own monster, my own robber of hope. How I do remember now, my familiar face—the hideous claws—the fang-like teeth—how I remember hiding them onto myself so I could face the world. So long ago, I hid you, Monster, my fierce protector and guide; so long ago, when you were once beautiful—a lovely song, a summer's sweetheart. How I hid you and disfigured you, and made you this hideous teacher to blame. And now you come out in truth and I take your hand. I see your beauty. Your eyes. Your hair. Your breath. The very essence of you. You are beauty from the dark. I am beauty from the light. And together we make days upon days, birthed out of wholeness and completion. Nothing is as it seems. Nothing at all. When even the darkness is me.

33. VIGNETTE, WINTER BITES, AGE 14

I used to sing, "Let me entertain you. Let me turn you on"—when I was ten. I didn't carry a barometer for appropriate behavior. I loved the song and I loved Natalie Wood. In my mind these were the perfect lyrics to bellow out in the center of the middle school cafeteria (while swaying my hips about and tossing my long auburn hair). I didn't outgrow my tendency to be perpetually clueless when it came to fitting in with the mainstream, which led to big trouble as I entered my high school years.

From the moment I stepped foot on the high school campus on the East Coast, I was targeted. Where my classmates were all dressed in their Sunday best, I, being from the West Coast, was dressed in an Ocean Pacific T-shirt and Levi blue jeans. In the hallways and during physical education class, the boys whistled and commented on my figure, some of them shouting out obscenities. The girls were no better—clicking across the hallways in their high heels and colored slacks, whispering secrets, intentionally ignoring me, and rolling their eyes in disgust. Being as embarrassed as I was to look people directly in the eyes made the situation worse; I came across as conceited and stuck-up. If the kids weren't calling me a *slut* to my face, they were claiming I was a *snob* behind my back.

I survived by hiding out in the back of the classrooms and penciling the entire lyrics to the song "Hotel California" across my desktop. Since relocating to the East Coast, every song that mentioned California, the West Coast, or even beaches became my favorite.

I suppose, in the long run, I acclimated to their ways within a few weeks' time, but I never assimilated. I learned how to style my hair in tight ringlets, spending an hour every morning to form the perfect curls. I babysat the neighbor children to earn money to buy colored pants. I purchased one pair of high-heeled shoes. I adapted to the local style of makeup—packing layers of foundation onto my face and edging the lower section of my eyes with a thin wisp of black liner. I cleaned up well. Just not well enough.

The boys still hooted. The girls still jeered. But I was able to make a friend in Rosie. She was a chubby brunette who was obsessed with the color pink—hair ribbons, clothes, sneakers, and feather-tipped writing pens—everything pink. She lived with both parents in a two-story, tastefully decorated home and had, what seemed to me, everything a girl could want. However, Rosie was very inexperienced when it came to the subject of boys.

Rosie was the friend who helped me initiate my first meeting with my freshman crush, Jeff—a popular Italian boy in my homeroom class whom I fell in love with as soon as I spotted him limping down the homeroom aisle with his crutches. He was lanky and thin, in that just-sprouted way, so that all the parts were there and developing daily into more manly features. I think what got me, what made me want him the most, were his dark brown eyes, the ones that matched mine, and of course his leg cast.

Rosie had graciously delivered my love letter to Jeff and later waited by the phone with me for his response. And she had been all caught up in a dancing flutter when Jeff called and asked me to *go steady*. After all, by peer standards, he was the most popular freshman boy on campus: a star athlete, drummer in a basement band, and strikingly handsome. There were a good couple of months where I was on cloud nine. Rosie and I did much together: slumber parties, MTV videos, garage parties. And I spent each afternoon at Jeff's house listening to him drum out music and then *making out* while pretending to watch the soap opera *General Hospital*.

But everything fell apart by the time I experienced my first snow flurries. I had dropped down a few clouds by then—actually, out of the clouds completely. I plummeted, breaking my head open, like I had when I was a small child and fell off my sitter's shoulders backward onto the hard concrete; only this time there was no hospital and no one soothing me with kind whispers.

It was a frigid day when Rosie wore her fuzzy, hot-pink sweater—the first day I understood how winter can bite. Dressed in her padded shoulders of fuchsia and matching leg warmers, looking like she was auditioning for a part in *Flash Dance*, Rosie greeted me at our usual table in the crowded school cafeteria. I arrived harboring a languid expression. The week had been horrendous, with one enormous and hostile junior girl barging into the science room during the teacher's lecture and shouting, "You're dead after school, slut!" And a couple mean-spirited freshman boys having had poked fun at my glossy, yellow gym shorts as I bent over to retrieve the volleyball. And let me not forget the French teacher who had informed me my grade average was a C−.

Rosie brushed the sleeves of her gaudy sweater and frowned deeply before tossing her big hair back. I assumed she was still disappointed over the news that the boy she liked didn't want to *go steady* with her. Before I had a chance to take a seat at the cafeteria table, Rosie barked, "Here!" A folded pink paper floated down. Giving a raised brow, I reached over and retrieved the note. By the time I read the first pink words, Rosie had grouped in the corner and was gawking alongside a gaggle of giggling girls. There was a raw burning in my throat. I opened the folded paper. The pink letters read: "You are a stupid slut. I don't know what any of the guys see in you. You are nothing but a cheap whore and nothing special. You think you're so hot, the way you shake your ass and the boys all watch. It's only because you are easy. I don't know why anyone would ever want to be your friend. Jeff is only with you because you are a slut. If you don't believe me, ask anyone. Your X-Friend, Rosie."

34. YESTERDAY'S FUNK

On the way to school today my youngest son exclaimed, "Wow, It's so dark outside! So much rain. Look at all the puddles. I wonder if more ducks will be here soon."

I'm convinced the city I occupy in the state of Washington is runner-up in cloud coverage to the town where the popular series Twilight takes place—a dark place where vampires want to live.

I like to walk. I am very thankful for these two functioning legs. But the majority of the time, in these here parts, a stroll in the neighborhood means sopping wet shoes, drenched clothes, and a rain-slapped face—and that's with an umbrella. Plus, this born-and-raised-in-California gal is still adjusting to the temperature change. Where I used to live, if the temperature was forty degrees in the morning, it typically rose up to sixty-five degrees by the afternoon. Here, when the temperature is forty degrees in the morning, sometimes it's only forty-one degrees by midday! What the heck? I actually sleep in my day clothes many nights because I'm too cold to undress. And I've developed quite the close relationship with my space heater. Even my socks and me are buddies.

Yesterday I was in a ginormous funk; lack of sunlight and the dark, drizzly weather came up first, for feasible funk-reasons. My iron and vitamin D deficiency came up second. Followed by my other physical ailments (hyper-mobility joint syndrome, endometriosis, fibromyalgia, etc.). But primarily what came to mind were all these grade school events I've had to attend as of late. There's been a bundle: violin concerts, choir, plays, student conferences, and so forth. Events with crowds are hard on me. I am strongly affected by others' energies—in person, online, or across the states. Who knows, I'm probably triggered by energy across the nations, planets, and multiverse. That would be just like me, to be affected by another dimension's being, like some obtuse, prematurely balding barber in Transylvania fretting over an infestation of cockroaches.

35. FASCINATE

This morning on the way to the gym a state trooper pulled me over. He gave me the star treatment: flashing, swirling lights, and sirens. I felt rather important. Especially when I pulled away because I thought the trooper was signaling me to park in a safer place. That's when the sirens got super loud and made a noise I don't think I've ever heard before. I felt like a fugitive. It was rather exhilarating and not nearly as scary as I'd imagined. I'm thinking I'd make a good villain or superhero, or someone who dodges the justice system. I take all the flashing lights as a sign from God that I shouldn't exercise anymore. I don't care if you disagree. I'm feeling very powerful after my run-in with the law.

Speaking of cars, I was a bit naïve a few years back when I was still single and bought a red Mustang on a whim, only because I thought the Mustang was pretty. I obsessed about the license plates for three days straight. I wanted the plates to be personalized and charming and creative. I came up with several ideas. I can still see the long list. (I solicited people for their top choices.)

It came down to two names—REDAPPLE (I was a teacher) or FASTEN8. I chose FASTEN8 because I thought the word was so clever. The FASTEN meant to fasten a seat belt and the number 8 is one of my favorite numbers. And I thought my car was fascinating, and actually that my whole creation of FASTEN8 was fascinating! My husband was the one who finally explained, some two years later, why men would slow down when I was driving my red Mustang, and nod their heads, and wink at me. I thought the looks were because of the nifty spoiler I put on the end of my car or the new automatic opening moonroof. Did I mention I was obsessed with my car?

My husband explained, "When people read FASTEN8, they aren't thinking about seat belts and how clever you are."

"They aren't? What are they thinking of then?"

Insert what you think my husband said here: _____

"Oh? Oh. OH!!!!"

I don't personalize my license plates anymore.

36. LOOMING DEMISE

There's a reason I didn't go into the medical field, besides the fact that I faint if I look at a needle. I don't do well with illness, disease, or sickness of any sorts (or thoughts of being attacked by a killer species). I do fine with driving my car, walking down dark alleys, crossing bridges, and climbing up to high places. I just can't deal with physical health conditions—well at least not rationally. The common cold sends me into a tailspin: worst-case scenario, *worser*-case scenario, *worstest*-case scenario. In the course of my four-decades-plus of living, I was certain of my imminent death at least five times per year. Looming demise total equals—two hundred times. Give or take a death or two. (Sir Brain is at his calculator now.) And I'm not talking a passing thought. I'm saying a good two- to three-week sickness-induced death terror cycle. And with the invention of Google God, I've also had hours of adrenaline-pumped investigative research.

Last year, about this time, I was certain, *dead* certain, that my heart was going to explode from a genetic disorder. When I was younger, rabies was my big fear. I never ever should have watched the depressing classic *Old Yeller* in third grade; after viewing the movie, my hamster-bit finger led me to check my mouth for foaming saliva hourly, for a month! Watching Hitchcock's *The Birds* was another faux pas. Remember the killer bees? Well, I do. I believed for years the bees were approaching in a swarm. Bloody noses are notorious fear buttons, ever since I saw that character on a television show, with a bloody nose, bleed out and die. My fear of the C-word started after my kindergarten teacher died, and I still have trouble writing the word. Which ironically sucks because it's my astrological zodiac sign. Four times during my life, twice as a teenager and twice as a young mother, doctors suspected I had C or pre-C. No cause for alarm in all four cases, but the panic that ensued during the waiting period was insurmountable. You know what really bites? Working at a homeless shelter and having a child infected with a lethal blood disease bite your leg through your denim jeans. The doctors assured me my chances of contracting the disease were almost zero;

still, they wanted to be certain. My most laughable approaching-doom fear happened when I was nursing my firstborn in the late hours of the night, and I'd stare down at the dirt in the corner of my toenail, and know with certainty I was going to die of toe fungus. If you bring in the big guns like MRSA, I so freak out. Any infection is MRSA. Hives? I'm certain I'll suffocate from severe allergic reaction. Menstrual cycle off a day—I have growths on my ovaries. To make matters worse, doctors have wanted to remove my uterus and my gallbladder and to do a biopsy on my kidney. None of which happened. But the fact that they recommended such procedures makes me think I have bad parts to begin with.

If you've got your wits about you, you've probably gathered I have a wee bit of a phobia to illness in any form—real, made-up, and imagined. What many do not understand about this illness phobia is that no amount of exposure makes a dang difference. With exposure therapy, if someone is afraid of bridges you can slowly and decisively assist her in overcoming the bridge fear. A common therapy strategy might be first showing pictures of bridges, next playing with toy bridges, later taking photos of bridges from afar, and then crossing a small bridge over a creek. If therapy is effective, then the person eventually will cross a bridge as a passenger, then drive assisted, and later cross alone. Sounds logical. Doesn't apply to illness: First look at pictures of people who are sick, next play in filthy area, later . . . not helping! And getting sick over and over again doesn't help either. Done that.

I'll bid you farewell with my latest encounter (a result of LV's and Sir Brain's conspiring, no doubt).

Me: "Well, now that you suspect I have hypothyroid, I guess I should mention that I've been having trouble swallowing. I read that's a symptom, too."

Dr.: "Oh." She pulls out a lab slip. "Well then, we better get an ultrasound for nodules."

Me: "Nodules? Can I die from nodules?"

"No."

"I can't?"

"No."

"What is the worst-case scenario?"

"If they find nodules, the protocol is to keep a watchful eye on them. If they grow, they'll likely drain them. But nodules are not deadly."

"Oh, good. But what about cancer? Could I have cancer? Or did my blood tests rule that out?"

"No, your blood tests didn't rule that out. But thyroid cancer is very, very rare."

My eyes grew super big and I swallowed hard.

Dr. added, "And the cure rate for thyroid cancer is almost one hundred percent."

"Oh!" Huge sigh. "Thank you so much for adding that. How long will I have to take the pills?"

"For the rest of your life."

Long pause.

Me: "But what if the end of the world comes? How will I get my pills?"

37. FAKE IT OR BREAK IT

Sometimes my writing is another player in the game—this game I've played since I was old enough to know that if I was nice enough, funny enough, and interesting enough then people would pay attention to me. And in turn, if I exhibited too much honesty, was too revealing, or too straightforward, people would reject me—or worse, simply disappear.

You see, a woman with Aspergers remains a constant actress. There is no escaping this. And to me this is the thorn of Aspergers. I continually scope and evaluate. I look at others' actions and responses more so than many can imagine. Some of the observations breed questions, a continual whirlwind in my mind. I wonder the simplest of thoughts, such as, "What was the motivation behind that person's comment?" Or I have more complex thoughts, such as, "What is the motivation behind my statement?" My mind forms a tumbleweed of sorts, spinning and rounding the field, pushing up dust and debris. The child in me watches in fascination. And the observer, the one avoiding the tumbling of thoughts, tries best to steer away. Still in the distance, regardless of my view, the tumbleweed loses its balance in the wind.

Some might advise, *Say what you want. Who cares what people think?* If only *I* were so simple. Yet this is one of the biggest burdens I have: thinking about what you are thinking about me. It stems from wanting to be seen, be valued, be loved, and be recognized for who I am. It stems from not wanting to be misjudged, misinterpreted, misunderstood, ostracized, dejected, alienated, stabbed in the back, and persecuted. It stems from a lifetime of recognizing I don't quite fit in with the mainstream, and that if I don't learn the norms—the unspoken rules—and then pretend to a degree and assimilate, I never will fit in. It comes down to the options of fake a little or break a little. And I've been broken. And the little bit of faking leads to a little bit of guilt and continued self-analysis and reasoning of how to be a better person.

38. REALITY AND EXISTENCE

Last night I had dreams flooded with majestic panoramic imagery, in which I floated weightlessly in delight—dreams in which some entity telepathically painted living pictures containing the secrets of the universe . . . Before you second-guess my experience, note that I did inhale half a bar of chocolate with espresso chunks yesterday, and I am on this new pig hormone for my hypothyroid; thusly, I can only conjecture what is occurring at a cellular level. Crazed by caffeine or hormone overdose, or not, the dreams were mighty spectacular. Beings of light revealed that the world as we know it is a grand illusion. We are creating our own reality. They explained that through my thoughts, I create my experience in this world. In my last dream of the night, I was a passenger on a large, windowless tour bus at a wildlife park. I was struggling to take photos of the upcoming buffalo and my camera battery was missing. A man sat across the aisle examining my actions. I quickly pulled out a notebook and began sketching the buffalo, until the man across the way said gently, "Just be. Enough. Just be."

Today I am pondering this notion of nonexistence—the nonexistence of time, and the nonexistence of months, and the nonexistence of anything and everything. I am examining the manifestation of reality, how words and symbols and sounds create. I'm thinking on my middle son's recent inquiry: "What if an animal exists that is a different color or form than we know and we don't yet have the capacity to see those specific colors or forms? Is the animal then invisible to us because we don't recognize those aspects? And in truth, does the animal even truly exist, if we cannot conceptualize it?"

Regarding reality and existence, a corner of Buddhist philosophy explains how we can never quite see the whole of ourselves and postulates that if we cannot see the whole of our being, then it follows that we cannot with validity claim we (as a singular being) actually exist in whole. The whole of me is impossible to capture on camera, in the mirror, or even from the viewpoint of an observer. There is always an aspect of me missing, perhaps the soles of my feet or my backside. I am never in completion. And nothing I set eyes upon is in its entirety either. As hard as I try, I cannot see the whole of you. I cannot see the whole of nature—the whole of a tree or a flower. However I search, there is always an element of the wholeness missing.

39. THE DAY I LOST MY BUTT

I was with a crowd of people the day I lost my butt. I searched everywhere for my butt. In desperate need of a butt, I clasped my hands over a stranger's butt and then I tried to fit her butt onto my butt. But her butt wouldn't stay on.

When the stranger asked, "How does my butt fit?" I responded, "Too small." And with a frown, I sighed, shrugged my shoulders, hung my head low, and gave her back her butt. As I walked in embarrassment, I covered the place my butt had been with my hands. Sometimes I slid across the floor to hide my missing butt or I squatted down and walked low to the ground. When I sat, I placed my hands beneath me on the chair to protect my flesh where my butt had once been. Other times I sat on my knees. Off and on for an hour, I searched for my butt. I asked, "Have you seen my butt?" I looked under my chair for my butt. I looked in corners and underneath people's legs for my butt. Later, in desperation, I found a microphone, and again asked, "Has anyone seen my butt?" No one had seen my butt.

After the butt incident, for weeks my three sons would peer from around the corner at random intervals and ask, "Where's your butt?" It didn't matter where I was in our home. I could be sitting on the toilet, climbing the stairs, or cooking dinner, and someone in our house would inevitably ask, "Where's your butt?" I will always remember the day I lost my butt.

My butt is back now. My butt actually never disappeared. I only thought my butt had vanished. In reality I'd been hypnotized on stage at the state fair to believe my butt was stolen. I believe at times we all think we've lost our butts, or at least we believe we've lost a portion of ourselves. Many of us think an essential part of us is missing or lacking. We believe we aren't worthy, aren't enough, aren't special, and aren't lovable. When in actuality we came into the world fully equipped with everything we need. Our butts are firmly attached. Nothing is missing and nothing has been taken away. We are worthy, we are enough, we are special, we are lovable, but we forget. When we think we are lacking that is like our mind tricking us into thinking we have no butt. When we think we are lacking, we walk the world like our butts are missing. We hang our heads low, we hide, we search, we ask, we fear and worry. We trick ourselves. We hypnotize ourselves into thinking we are lacking when everything is right there where it is supposed to be.

40. VIGNETTE, HOLDING ON, AGE 5

If I were to turn back the pages of my life, to the first calm years at my stepfather's house, my days would appear wonderfully simple and sweet, and in truth they were. It was a time when a gentle thread of calm and security weaved through my days. A brief moment I fondly remember and continually reflect back upon, perhaps in an attempt to regain some semblance of normalcy, or to remind myself there was some good. There weren't any worries about money. My stepfather Drake was an attorney and helped the city officials acquire land for approved projects, which sometimes meant property owners had to give up their homes. It was rumored much later, when I was an adult, that Drake's firm was actually responsible for my great-grandmother having to abandon her house for demolition to make way for a multilevel parking garage for tourists in Monterey.

Back then, in the early 1970s, Drake's two teenage sons lived with us, and his two teenage daughters visited us on the weekends. I can recall the friendly sisters setting me in front of them and braiding my long brown hair. And remember how I would sit for hours at the foot of the bed with kind David, who was deaf, drawing pictures of hearts and butterflies with my assorted pack of fruit-scented markers. It was the oldest brother Zachary, better known as "Zoomer," who taught me how to ride my first bike—the bike with the green banana seat and the wide yellow handlebars with white streamers. I can recall my first solo bike ride, vividly. It was a hot day in August, my second summer in Palo Alto, when Zoomer held the tail end of my bike and shouted, "Look straight ahead and keep your hands on the handlebars!" I had wobbled forward, screaming, "Promise you won't let go! Promise you'll hold on tight!"

"I won't let go! I promise!" Zoomer had hollered in response.

While pedaling fast, I glanced back several times. The first and second time, Zoomer's floppy brown hair and toothy grin were still there, but by the third turn every inch of Zoomer had vanished.

"You let go! You let go!" I screamed, and lost control, plummeting hands first into a prickly bush. After I gathered myself, brushing the leaves off of my shoulders and wiping my tears with dirt-covered hands, I cried, "You promised you wouldn't let go! You promised!"

Zoomer came running, then.

The second summer at Drake's would end with the start of the school year. I don't recall much about my initial years at school, not much beyond the terrifying fear I felt when Mother dropped me off each morning and the terrifying fear I felt when my kindergarten teacher died. What I do remember with clarity is the back room of Mrs. Stockman's house.

After kindergarten let out each day, I'd run out of the schoolyard, freeze at the fence, and wonder if perhaps my father would fly down from the sky and rescue me from the grimness of Mrs. Stockman's. To the average child, Mrs. Stockman's place—a two-car garage insulated and converted into a daycare— would not have seemed threatening. But to me, Mrs. Stockman's was painfully uncomfortable. The temperature was either too cold or too warm, the carpet stale, and the walls paneled in an unappealing burnished faux wood.

My chaperone, on the way to Mrs. Stockman's house, was a freckled-faced, pudgy-nosed boy named Keith, who I soon made into my best friend—a courting period that consisted of regular handholding, sharing of his gum (with the cherry flavor chewed right out of it), and a cola bottle filled with worms. Most afternoons at the sitter's I would lounge on the burgundy, vinyl-lined bench seat beside Mrs. Stockman's massive, wooden-paneled room divider, chew on my sweater sleeve, and analyze the animals camouflaged in the cottage-cheese-textured ceiling. Occasionally, I would listen to the older children's chatter and scribble down notes. Being the youngest in attendance, I was often excluded from the real secrets—the giggle-filled discussions that were carried on in the adjacent homework booth.

Daily, without fail, every fifteen minutes or so during the soap opera's commercial break, the garish, polyester-swishing Mrs. Stockman would appear at our side of the divider and attempt to bring things to order. In response to her authoritative presence, we would shut our mouths, smile, sit up straight, and make ourselves busy with our homework. Then, as the minutes passed, quick as a Polaroid flash, Mrs. Stockman would disappear. There was a definite ebb and flow to our world, where we the children were the ocean tide and Mrs. Stockman our moon.

Each weekday afternoon, I would hear our sitter wailing for some benign reason, like the soap opera baby being kidnapped from the hospital for the second time. Between her weeping hours, Mrs. Stockman led us through a large sliding glass door into her tree-lined backyard, much like she did with her little wiener dog, Peanuts. The slider was opened, she'd hand us our snack, and the slider was shut, with Mrs. Stockman still inside, and the huge hourglass on the television screen filling with sand.

One evening, after the parents had collected all the children, I remained behind at Mrs. Stockman's, wobbling from side to side on her high front porch. There, I paced, analyzing the word "sitter." At that point in my life, I assumed sitters sat a lot. Under the guttering light of the porch, Mrs. Stockman followed in suit, marching back and forth with a rhythmic swish of her polyester slacks. She would reach one end, circle, and return herself to the other side—much like a swimmer in a lap pool. After a few minutes of waiting, around the time I'd started wondering if babysitters actually sat on children, Mrs. Stockman began to screech, "Where is your mother?" In response, I kept my mouth shut and thought, if given the opportunity, I would bring my sitter back to the Woolworths discount store and trade her in for someone else.

"Where is she?" Mrs. Stockman asked in a demanding voice. I swallowed and tried not to cry. "You know, she should stop packing you apples for lunch. That's why your teeth are coming out all buck-like." Mrs. Stockman made another turn around the porch, taking me with her by the hand. "For heaven's sake. Here she comes. It's about time," she mumbled, adjusting her glasses and standing up straight with her customary I-don't-want-to-be-here-but-here's-my-smile-anyway greeting. I didn't smile. I didn't want to be there either.

Earlier in the day, Mrs. Stockman had spied me at the corner table erasing some pencil marks when I should have been in the backyard. She had stifled an evil growl and snapped, her jowls quivering—a bulldog dressed in blue. "So you are the one that has been making all these marks!"

"No," I had responded, meekly.

"Yes, you did, young lady."

I shook my head no and tried to explain.

But Mrs. Stockman interrupted and hugged her bulging hips. "Don't you fib to me! You can spend the next ten minutes wiping all those tables down. Do you hear me?"

"Yes, Mrs. Stockman," I said, in a whispered whimper.

"What did you say?"

"Yes, Mrs. Stockman!" I said much louder.

I went over this humiliating event as Mother somberly approached the porch. She was already apologizing before she reached the first step. "I'm sorry. I won't let it happen again. There was something I had to take care of at work." The cigarette in her hand toggled back and forth while she spoke. I tracked the smoke, wondering when the grown-ups would be quiet.

"This is ridiculous," Mrs. Stockman said, walking me forward and handing me off to Mother. "You can't just forget your child."

Mother's mouth opened wide, but no teeth showed. It was just one big black hole. "Forget my child? I would never forget my child. I told you this *will not* happen again."

I stared at Mrs. Stockman, and then at Mother, and then looked back at Mrs. Stockman. Her face eased a bit, so that the wrinkles along her jawline weren't as taut. "Just see to it that it doesn't! And for God's sake, take that child to the doctor. She spends hours bent over on the toilet constipated." Mrs. Stockman leaned into me and pinched my cheeks. A huge, false smile crossed her face. "Now, you have a goodnight, sweetie, and I'll see you tomorrow."

Right then I got the same chill down my spine as when I watched the flying monkeys on *The Wizard of Oz*.

"Say goodnight," Mother said.

"Goodnight, Mrs. Stockman," I obliged, and then sank into Mother's side, thankful for the smell of cigarettes and musk. A few steps away from the house, I whispered, "Mommy, I don't like it here." In response, Mother stood rigid, cleared her throat, and said, "We all have bad days. Mrs. Stockman has good intentions. And I promise I won't be late again." Then Mother leaned in and embraced me fully and kissed me multiple times on the top of my little head. I was picturing Zoomer letting go of my bike. "Don't let go," I said, as I wrapped my arms around my mother's waist. She rubbed my back in slow, even circles. "Just don't let go, Mommy," I repeated.

"I won't," she whispered.

And there we remained, in the darkening day, holding on.

41. Good-bye, Prude Dude!

Miracles are erupting. I'm engorged with passion! The prude dude in me is shrinking like a tornado has just smashed her into asphalt. Serpent power rise! I actually like the music my grandma used to play on the radio in her very slow-moving car—because it is stirring me in an erotic way. More proof? I used the words "erotic" and "engorged" and enjoyed it! Lately I can connect to every single song that has a semblance of a romantic edge. I've been delving into songs, living and breathing the lyrics, like some lovesick damsel in distress or a diving duck. Plunge, ruffle feathers, plunge, ruffle feathers. Every inch of me is longing for connection. Once a prude, not always a prude, I tell you! In high school, once returned back to the West Coast, I kid you not, on the bathroom walls more than one girl inked, "I want to be like *Sam* the virgin." Whether the restroom writing was fact or fiction remains a forever mystery.

The point is, I looked like a prude, acted like a prude, and was assumed to be a prude. I couldn't even say the names of private parts aloud—*hmmm*, writing them still causes difficulty. Don't worry, by next week I'll be able to write that particular word used to describe hot dogs—I'm certain. Passion was a no-no for a long, long time. But I'm done with the subdued prude dude.

"What's happened?" you might wonder. I know I was wondering. I've had crazy surging and purging emotional eruptions for the last few weeks. At first I thought it was the pig hormone I'm taking for my hypothyroid— karmic payback, in a beneficial way, since I stopped eating pork when I was eleven. But no, the pig-powers-that-be might love me, but this is something that even outdoes the power of Wilburs and oinkers everywhere.

My ongoing symptoms include: overwhelming and intense feelings surrounding everything; an extreme knowing that I have a right to feel what I want; pleasure seeking (safe and balanced); extreme feelings of passion and sensuality; reconnecting to and appreciating my body; longing to walk barefoot; improved energy, vitality, and health; a youthful glow; expanding personal relationships; achieving excellence in creative endeavors; enormous, indescribable hope; vibrating sensations; less sleep; thinking and acting remarkably different; self-transcendence; bliss; ecstasy; visions; clairaudience. If only I could bottle this! What's happening to me, as far as I can tell, is called a Kundalini Awakening (sexual energy). I'm no expert. I am a life student. But something booted the prude dude out and let the coiled serpent expand.

42. Aspie Friend

I have recently formed a friendship with an Aspie woman, and I have to say it is the easiest friendship I have ever had. Though it is long distance, we chat every day, sometimes for hours. What I notice about her are the same traits I notice about myself. Our lives and our thinking are so parallel that it is almost creepy. Essentially, we think and process the same way. We have the same worries. We see things in the same light. We both require the same security in conversation. We need validation and we give out the whole of ourselves. We are able to focus on one another entirely. Everything else can stop. We become priority. Talking to her is the easiest thing I've done in my life. She is genuine, open, and entirely honest. She analyzes everything she says before writing and then analyzes it again after writing—just like I do. She frets over her words. She wonders whether she is good enough for a friend, too intense, too different. She overcompensates with love and compassion to be certain I feel safe and understood. She offers help straight from the heart. She sits on every word, measuring the potentiality for miscommunication and the probable consequences of her message. She spins and loops about what she has said and how the words might affect our relationship. She thinks about me often throughout her day. She loves me wholeheartedly. She knows when I need her to sit and be with me, and puts aside everything else to show she cares. She takes the time to write to me. As soon as she knows I am available to chat, she comes my way with a smile, heart, or message. She is my soul sister, mirroring me in every way—and I so love what I see.

43. THE BEE'S KNEES

In the center of me is this awakening gratitude bursting anew like the perennial hyacinth after a long winter's snow. I feel like I'm twelve again, only much more mature, confident, wise, and damn sexy! I am dancing. I can't get enough of the outdoors. I am enjoying my friends as we guffaw a lot over girl talk. I am so excited for life and all life has to offer. I am very satisfied with who I am, where I have traveled, and what I have overcome. I feel like the cat's pajamas. And I'm moving toward my own style and own innovation. I'm chuckling over the silliest things, like this definition of "bee's knees"—coined circa the 1920s, "bee's knees" means something along the lines of very good, excellent, great, amazing. A bee's baskets for pollen are located near its knees, so when the bee's baskets are full of pollen they are filled with the *good stuff*. That just cracks me up! Filled with the *good stuff*! I feel filled with good stuff. I truly do. And of course this stuff turns into the sweetness of honey. I also laughed aloud at the less popular terms of endearment that never quite made it through the years—words like "the flea's eyebrows" and "the canary's tusks." I so want to call someone the flea's eyebrows, just once. "Hey, you sexy! Yeah, you! You, my man, are the flea's eyebrows!" I'd like to say that to a biker dude with a bunch of awesome tattoos just to freak him out. I am truly enjoying this rush, whatever it is. I don't really care anymore. I am happy. Balanced. Focused. And for the most part sane . . . just constantly aching. But hey, an ache in the loins makes for marvelous poetry.

44. LULLABY

I whisper thee a lullaby, to sing thy soul to sleep,
A gentle breeze of humming wings, to soothe and offer peace;
A place of solitude within, where angels touch the truth,
And carry forth to eyes of babes, the whereabouts of youth.
I whisper thee a lullaby, to sing thy hope to sleep,
With empty voice and quiet ears, to chance love never meets;
A place of gated reckonings, where nothing happens real,
And carry forth to mouth of one, the morning bells to heal.
I whisper thee a lullaby, to sing thy gape to sleep,
A blindfold made of atmosphere, to chase away thy sheep;
A place of dreams dried rapidly, where desire's last doth bleed,
And carry forth to heart of mine, the love that grows through seed.
I whisper thee a lullaby, to sing thy grace to sleep,
With pampered pains of yesteryears, to tender flames of weeps;
A place of casualty of want, where emptied withered cries,
And carry forth to joy of light, the rocking chair that glides.
I whisper thee a lullaby, to sing thy depths to sleep,
A phantom dance upon a land, to steer away the deep;
A place of missing merriment, where answered call was naught,
And carry forth to falling tears, the cloth that soothes what daunts.
I whisper thee a lullaby, to sing thy rain to sleep,
With hurricane of floodgates leaked, to erase what spirit keeps;
A place of choking roots of need, where thirst is met with blood,
And carry forth to angel's wings, a case to trap the mud.
I whisper thee a lullaby, to sing thy ache to sleep,
A hope that withered in the field, to scathe abandoned heaps;
A place of dreams collapsed in sun, where looker blindly turned,
And carry forth this crystal clasp, a salve to ease the burn.
I whisper thee a lullaby, to sing thy pangs to sleep,
With path of frosted glass, opaque, to find what's not to keep;

A place of past and future joined, where others spun and left,
And carry forth a winged dove, a chance for inner rest.
I whisper thee a lullaby, to sing thy angst to sleep,
A passion so engorged within, to move is giant leap;
A place of casualty of war, where battles never cease,
And carry forth the purest sheet, a bedding for thy grief.
I whisper thee a lullaby, to sing thy dreams to sleep,
With hope unraveled in the wind, to watch as chance does seep;
A place of deaf awakening, where prayers are left for naught,
And carry forth a candle white, a surrendering of thought.
I whisper thee a lullaby, to sing thy night to sleep,
A day extinguished by the dark, to fetch a ride and meet;
A place of lonely passenger, where single rides along,
And carry forth this arm's embrace, a haven for thy song.

45. SEARCHED

I searched a thousand love songs; I thumbed through printed prose;
I edged my mind round poems thick, all words that rhymed with rose.
In storybook or tale, the answer did not rest,
And so I tried with might, to search through nature vast;
From animal to tree, from sky to crumbled rock,
I walked from path to path; I tracked the soaring hawk.
In vain I hung head low, in sorrow and in shame;
I had not found the answer, and had to start again.
This time I looked at art—communicated form,
To marble, paint, and print, to oddities adorned;
To everything that came, to everything I saw,
I could not find the answer, not hanging on a wall.
My legs they soon grew tired; my heart, it gave a thump,
My mind, a spinning top; my throat, it felt a lump.
How could I describe you and show you how I cared?
Declare my adoration, when you weren't anywhere?
And so I found a tree, so very tall, and sat,
And took a deep breath in, and thought of this and that;
I reasoned and I volleyed; I cursed and threw a fit;
I hollered and I worried, and even gasped a bit,
Until the answer flew, smack straight into my heart,
And suddenly I knew how to piece together parts;
I found you weren't outside me, not anywhere I'd looked,
Not locked within the word, of any single book;
I see this clearly now, in everything you are,
The golden thread of hope, my brilliant shining star,
A source that danced within, my ever-waking dream,
Inspirer of wishes, interwoven in my seams.

46. SUCK EGGS

The tears keep coming—the troops from eons ago who gathered by the river, preparing to march onward, yet never heard the bugle's call. They come now, at my beckoning.

No one can figure me out, professionals and spouse included, so I rely on Google God for the answers. He is the king of Escapeville, his queen—a collaboration of nonfiction books in all forms. And I imagine the court and prince and princesses are documentaries, newspapers, blogs, websites, videos, and the like. I have been perusing the Internet looking for an appropriate word for how I feel about myself at the moment. I tried to find the root origin of "suck eggs" and concluded I am not a canine who has trouble with stopping myself from sucking chicken eggs. Nor am I in an uncomfortable situation that makes me appear odd. I searched for the word "suck" and ended up with synonyms like "drink from straw." I was about to ask Google God about "bitch" but decided I'd had enough of reading about dogs.

So here I am, debating about what I am feeling, who I am, and where I belong on this damn earth. The original title of this post was going to be "Why It Sucks Being Married to Me." But I thought that was just a wee bit too self-demeaning and seriously similar to aiming a firing squad at my ego. Not that ego doesn't deserve to be taken down every now and again; I'm just not ready to annihilate him altogether. I admit I'm not an easy person to live with. I sometimes wonder if life would be easier if I were single. Mostly so I could retreat in isolation and wallow in self-pity. I lived alone in my early twenties. I remember I was in a constant state of panic and fret. Anxiety lurched around every corner. I was even afraid to leave my apartment and walk across the parking lot to the laundry building. After teaching all week, I'd crawl into bed for most of the stretch of the weekend, too exhausted and nervous to leave the apartment, wondering how I managed to survive the week in the first place and fretting over how I'd survive the next. I've grown some in the last twenty years. I think I could manage a laundry facility okay. I wonder about all the other elements of life though. Too many to mention or even list. Don't get me wrong; I have plenty of wonderful qualities to offer a spouse. It's just that living with me is like living with a circus lioness let loose from her cage. I'm trained and all. I've learned how I'm expected to act. I try my best to obey the rules. I appreciate the food, shelter, and praise. It's just that I long to be free in the wild, without restriction, without having to follow a role, and without having to be someone I am not.

47. ME IN PARTS

Sensory overload can lead to meltdowns—which are akin to adult tantrums—a screaming out for help when one does not know how to help one's self. In considering sound, where many people can block out background noise and focus on the matter at hand, without distraction, people with sensory sensitivities, like myself, hear everything at once. There is no mute button. And there is no making the noise stop, beyond earplugs and escape. The other senses work the same. Textures irritate. Smells overwhelm and overtake. Sights hurt. And even the taste of air is unpleasant.

It appears there is something about my sensory and processing system that causes me to sense things in the environment in segmented, exaggerated parts. Instead of looking upon a crowd and seeing a crowd, I look upon a multitude of bombarding shapes and sizes, each movement as uncomfortable to view as the next. I am aware of everything happening, but everything seems to be occurring all at once. There isn't release. What would be a soft, unnoticeable hum to some becomes a piercing roar. It is as if someone has turned up the volume of every single one of my sensory organs. There is no relaxation, only the constant stream of shards—parts of chatter, parts of the ticking clock, parts of rattling. There are parts of smells, all sorted out and classified, not mingled, not forgotten. There are parts of tastes—the breath, the air, the fragrances, the chemicals. Sights are in parts; fragmented pieces that attempt to make a whole, but fail; a face not remembered, except as the shape of a wrinkled, wide nose and the color of dark, narrow eyes. Even the mind is in parts, continually breaking down wholes into subsections. Whole to parts is easy. Parts to whole is hard. Nothing is as it appears. Everything is in parts. It is the parts that bring agony, the endless parts that bring with them the impossibility of finding retreat in the whole.

48. FOR HEAVEN'S SAKE

As a child I'd make the sign of the cross when I spotted a dead animal. I didn't stop this ritual until midlife. To this day I have a strong impulse to bless listless animals on the side of the road. My Catholic grandparents taught me about the afterlife. They were kindly, hardworking folk—a deep-sea fisherman and a sardine factory canner. They were the constant givers of the coin-filled, piggy-shaped banks that I cherished in my youth. Theirs was a stable and reliable love, a safe haven I looked forward to every Christmas season. Nano was a funny, pot-bellied chap with a gruff voice that weaved tales about enormous and mysterious sea creatures through puffs of cigar smoke and a thick Italian accent. Nana, measuring a mere four feet ten inches and often smelling of a combination of bleach and Olay moisturizer, was the constant sweeper of carpets, the maker of all things sweet, and pincher of all things cheeky. Chances are I inherited a bit of my passion for creatures from my nano; he would curse and swear about the stray cats gathered on his back porch, and then later, when he thought no one was looking, go feed them by the handful. Their loving daughter, Aunt Fran, was another with a heart for animals and service—a heart for giving that far surpassed mine.

I still feel a sense of loss when I think back years ago to the time my childhood friend Jane collected starfish along the northern Pacific seashore. Halfway through her cruel plucking, I had sprinted up the steep sand dunes to her father's truck and hovered there in the camper shell, weeping. No one had listened when I had protested that the starfish were alive and suffering an early expiration. I remember the same grueling heartache, some months following, when I watched Jane's father and his companions take down birds from the sky.

I always had a love for animals—for anything living. Even for things most people thought to not be alive. One day it was an injured bird whose eyes were cold by morning. Another day a lost snail that had lost its shell, the next day a pill bug upside down, and some days the discarded garbage, needing a home. Yet with all things considered, the one I remember the most is the butterfly. She was a monarch. I found her in the gutter on a rainy trek home from third grade. Her wings were tattered and she was nearly drowned. I carried her home, cupped in the safety of my hands, and named her Jolie for her beauty.

At home in my bedroom I placed her in a cleaned-out pickle jar and watched her in awe as she stuck out her black tongue and lapped the sugar-water from a small lid. Her little wings were cast in masking tape. I observed her through the long night, ever so often turning on the light and checking on her. I loved her. She survived a full day in the warmth of my affection. When she passed, I buried her in the backyard under our fig tree and gave her a short sermon. This is the little girl I was: remarkably sweet and hopeful. I wish to go back to her, to kneel down at her side and say:

"I love you. I love you so very much. You are beautiful. So kind. So thoughtful. And I am sorry that you carry such a burden. I know how painful it is to love with all of your heart. I know how painful it is to want to help and to not know how. But you are helping. You are helping more than you know, my precious one. Look at me. Do you see what you have become? You are going to be a mommy someday, with your own family, and you are going to have what you need to take care of them. Precious child, your journey into adulthood will be very hard. There will be times you want to give up—so many times. And you will take many years to find your way. But you will. You will. I promise you that. And when you do, much will make sense. You will cry, very hard, like you are now with losing your beloved butterfly. But I will be waiting. I will be knowing that you will survive, that you will be strong, that you will love with all of your heart and get that love back tenfold. You, of all people, shall be loved. I will be here waiting on the other side of time with my arms open wide, and when we meet again in dream and in prose, I will embrace you. Thank you. Thank you for being you and going onward. Thank you for being brave and very strong. You are my living angel and I breathe for you."

49. VIGNETTE, LONELY HEART PILLOW, AGE 19

The sharp point of fear worked its way into me like the microscopic barbs of a seed-bearing foxtail. I believed with the coming of adulthood life would somehow get easier. I expected the load I'd carried from my childhood to shed into layers, to ultimately fly away effortlessly—to disperse across the sky like the seeds of a dandelion. Beyond the reach of my youth, I thought the answers would come, just as I'd expected my favorite show to appear when I turned the television knob. I wasn't silly enough to think I'd have all the answers, but I had hoped to have enough of them. I'd hoped to be less embarrassed in conversation and to effortlessly make friends. I assumed I'd finally feel comfortable speaking to others, be able to offer a gentle pat or welcoming greeting, without questioning my every action and wanting to run the other direction. Yet neither my age nor relocation altered my existence. My weaknesses had followed me as surely as my suitcase had hitched a ride in the trunk of my secondhand compact car and settled down for the long ride to Father's house.

The college-campus life accentuated my misgivings. At the sound of my own voice I noted how my inflection and intonation adjusted to a given circumstance, how around particular classmates I became increasingly goofy and outlandishly witty, and how around others I was a quiet hermit. I noticed, too, that I adjusted my persona, shifting my attire, my mannerisms, my opinions, and my likes and dislikes to match the climate of a given room. Once again, like before, I tried to become the girl I thought people wanted to see. In the years to come I would often think I missed the road to the joys of young adulthood, that after skipping over the innocence of childhood, I'd taken a detour and passed up the potential fun of college life. The chances were there, the opportunities, the choices; only they remained out of my reach. Where there might have been pleasure and friendships, there was only barren land.

I knew the cracks and lines on the college campus path like no other. There wasn't a time I looked up to smile or wave or interact outside of the classroom walls. Most of my passing time between classes was spent hidden in the bathroom stalls or staring at the mirror evaluating the flaws of my reflection. I had a set route leading from one bathroom to the next. I knew the hard sidewalk, the cold toilet, and the dirty mirrors. Those were my archetypal symbols for college. My only pleasure was found in the everyday eating of the egg-salad sandwich that I would purchase from the roundhouse campus deli—even though I feared I wouldn't be able to open the relish or mustard package without making a mess, feared standing in line to purchase the food, and feared the moment I'd have to make contact and pay for my meal. I remember wondering how all the students could look so happy, interact so freely, toss a Frisbee, and wave a casual hello—without fear, without effort. I wondered why I couldn't look up, couldn't smile, couldn't be comfortable in my own skin.

My only refuge came in pretending. Inside the classroom I played the role of the perfect student. There I could speak. There I would raise my hand. And there I would be admonished and criticized by others for acting like the teacher's pet or monopolizing the discussion. There was no place for me. Even the process of getting to the college campus was terribly complex. My worry list was far-reaching, stretching to the moon. The freeway, the off-ramps, the speed limit, the fellow drivers on the road, each and every thing terrified me. Finding a parking spot was formidable. I escaped through my imagination and creativity. I receded so far within the depths of my mind that I was able to bring out something of substance that represented the soul of me. Still, I was always hidden behind something. Always hiding.

I remember my college creative drama class. I had to write and perform a monologue about an inanimate object. The purpose was to bring the object to life. Which was easy for me because I already thought most inanimate objects were alive. I was never like the other students, not at all. I was the one voting to watch the movie *Gandhi*, while the rest wanted *Tootsie*. For the monologue in drama class one student stood up on stage dressed as a rock and finished his performance with: "I felt a chill go up my spine when she skipped me across the river." Another girl, who was garbed in the color pink to resemble an eraser, said, "I like the way it felt being rubbed all over the paper."

I was the last to perform. I was wearing all black with my head sticking through the center of a pillow. I still remember cutting the hole in my father's old pillow. When I stood on stage, snickers came. I breathed in, holding the edges of the pillow with my trembling hands. I began in a soft, wavering voice:

"I had a good life. David took me everywhere when he was a boy. In his room we heard bedtime stories and played fort. Each week his mother dressed me in a fresh casing. My favorite one had cowboys and horses. He was the best boy in the world—nice and smart and full of life. David used to say his prayers as he rested his head on me. Sometimes his friends came and stayed the night. Once David swung me in the air to hit his friend and another time he playfully threw me at his dad. Several times he hid his baby teeth beneath me. And later, as David grew older, I even got to see a little kissing."

The audience chuckled. I continued.

"Eventually, David and I went to college where we studied into the late-night hours. I was so proud when he became a teacher. It was then he would prop me up against his apartment wall and correct papers. We were so happy. But then something changed. Something the doctors couldn't figure out. Something that made David cry. David started coughing. He started being sick a lot. He started being home a lot. Then he began losing weight. I wanted to help, to fix him, but I am only a pillow. There were days my David could not pull himself out of bed. It was then that we spent much time together, but it wasn't the type of time either of us wanted. I sat by helplessly as David's energy slowly seeped out of him, leaving him emptied and a mere shadow of himself. I could feel his head and his arms on me—so much lighter, so much weaker. He became like a skeleton. I worried. I worried, terribly. I cried each night. I watched helplessly. Not even able to whisper, 'I love you.' After the sores came again, covering his face, David's family arrived and took us to their house on the high hill. I'd thought David would get better. But he didn't. And no one could help. At the hospital, loved ones came, each of them in their own way trying to make us feel comfortable. I absorbed the tears, grateful that I could at least offer this. Most of the tears were David's. Sometimes I caught others'. And I stared out with as much love as I could muster. In time, the sickness took over. My poor David could barely breathe. But I stayed right there beneath him. Always. Until there came a moment he could no longer fight. It was then he tightly clutched me, and I caught the last of his tears—heard his last breath. He whispered, 'I love you, Mommy.' Later they took my David away to a place they wouldn't let me go. And I didn't get to see him. They never brought him back. And now there is only me—a lonely, heartbroken pillow without his little boy."

On my last line I wiped my tears. The audience stood up and applauded, the whole room weeping. When class let out the professor explained how her close friend had just died from AIDS and how grateful she was for my performance. I can picture myself then—a twiggy little thing with my auburn hair swept in front of my wide, dark eyes. I remember the drama professor asking why I always hid myself with my hair when I had such a pretty face. And I remember feeling shamed by her question, feeling as if she could see past my façade.

After class I carried my hollowed-out pillow across campus, keeping a brisk pace with my eyes glued to the ground. During my undergraduate years I would never become what I had hoped to become. I wouldn't be a cheerleader or live in the dorms. I wouldn't attend one college event. Not one. I wouldn't be in a sorority. In the first four years at school I would make only one friend, a girl who would stop returning my calls after a few months. College would remain to me a dark hallway, a place I was forced to pass through to earn an education. A place I'd wear different masks and costumes while pretending to be whomever I needed in order to make my way through to the other side. A place where the real me was only seen once that I can recall—on that one day I stood as a lonely, heartbroken pillow.

50. SEEING ME

People often say I look familiar to them. Years ago someone thought I was that teacher that got convicted for shagging her student. Don't remember her name; it didn't help when the suspecting stranger asked if I was a teacher and I said, "Yes."

I've been told I look like certain celebrities—usually bad politicians or people who play dope dealers on television. That strikes me as odd, that people recognize me or relate me to others, because I haven't a frickin' clue as to what I look like. I do not recognize myself in any photo. My dear friend Steff, who is a photographer, says my facial bone structure affects my photos. She reassured me I don't need plastic surgery. I actually texted her from some hotel in Northern California in tears after a recent photograph, convinced I needed a nose job that very day. This week my dear masseuse Sue Happy (I call her "Sue Happy" because her name is Sue and she is perpetually happy) reassured me that in person I do indeed look like my photos. She said I don't look like me when I give *that look* though—a blank stare. Also known as my typical smile or what at least feels to me like a smile.

Every day my husband patiently answers questions about my looks. During a movie I might ask (during a crucial moment of the film): Do those look like my wrinkles? Do I look that old? Do I look like her when I smile? Is that my nose? Oh, is her hair like my hair?

Steff, that same photographer friend I texted, she has always said I am blessed with a gypsy-skin complexion and doe eyes. I like her. To make me feel better, she also has said, more than once, that *pretty* people never like photos of themselves because they appear different depending on the lighting. I really like her a lot. She also says I am a good catch. I love her.

To me, my appearance changes from moment to moment. Forget about the photos. Each time I look in the mirror I do not recognize myself. I particularly do not like my reflection in the car's rearview mirror or in the glass screen of my laptop computer. Some reflections accentuate all my lines and I appear to be a prune. I cry at prune faces. I do not recognize my eyes as the lids droop. And as I age, I wonder where I went. Not that I ever saw myself fully to begin with. But now it seems the person I never figured out is vanishing altogether into the folds and creases of flesh.

Not being able to judge how I look affects me in several ways. I can't apply makeup well. I don't know how. Lessons won't help. I can't tell if the shade is right or if I have put on too much or too little. Usually, I wear hardly any makeup. I do like watching my eyes change once I put mascara on my lashes, though. I'm like a little girl. I apply and then stare in amazement. It's like someone enlarged my eyes! When it comes to eyeliner, I can't tell if it makes me look older, wiser, sexier, or slutty. I do however notice that lately I have developed these distinct come-hither bedroom eyes. Don't know what's that about but I have some theories. Fixing my hair is difficult. I can't tell what it looks like. Hairpins at different angles, hair back, hair forward, hair wet, hair straight, hair curly—my looks alter depending.

I cannot grasp facial features of anyone. For instance, if an artist asked me to describe a person's face for a police sketch, I couldn't do it. I can't even describe my own children's faces. I was always fascinated in movies when the witness would tell the sketch artist about the nose shape, the eye distance, the lips, the hairline. It seems they have superpowers. I've been staring at my fourteen-year-old son's face for fourteen years, and I *still* couldn't tell you what he looked like, beyond the fact that he has big eyes like me, long lashes, thin dark hair, and a chin like his dad. The rest, all the in-between parts, below the hairline—the face shape, the nose, the lips, the brows—they all go blurry when I try to visualize my son.

I see things in pictures. I see things as a blurry whole or as a specific. For example, I see the wrinkles between the eyes, the bump on a nose, the ear that sticks out, the dot on a cheek. I am naturally drawn to the details like a camera on high focus. Then after a little bit of time, I focus out and see a semblance of the overall face. It seems I do not have a middle focus, only a very narrow or very vast view.

I've always studied faces, ever since I can remember. Last year my fixation was ears, particularly earlobes. I was trying to figure out what my ears looked like in comparison to other ears. I know my ears are unique—

elf-like—they stick out a bit and are chunkier on the upper part, and generally fleshy. Makes for good nibbling. It's been a whole year of ear studying and I'm still clueless. I couldn't draw you a picture of my ear unless I was staring at a photo and likely tracing it. I just started on my nose. I've been comparing my nose to other noses and trying to find a companion nose. My nose is a funny creature, constantly altering shapes based on the camera angle or the direction I look at myself in the mirror. When I take a photo of my face, my nose appears very European. Sometimes it's rather cute and pudgy. Other times, I know for a fact someone has put her nose on my face! I've been studying movies lately, pausing a film and looking at the actresses' faces, and noticing that their noses change too. It's not just mine. I've noticed how still frames of a movie star's face are so different from when an actress is in motion.

I'm still trying to get used to seeing me.

51. That Moment

I want to be that moment in a black-and-white film,
When man pulls woman into his arms;
I want to be that passion,
The lyrics in the love song,
That leave you gasping;
I want to be that instant when mother sees newborn,
And souls embrace;
I want to be that sigh,
As lost wanderer tracks the sun dripping below ocean;
I want to be that completion,
The final missing piece of the perfect puzzle;
I want to be that reason you sprint back home,
To find what was forgotten;
I want to be that breaking,
The mile marker when runner weeps,
And then pushes onward,
Strengthened;
I want to be that second,
When one first beholds his beloved,
And understands,
She is his answer;
I want to be that ache,
The final line,
In a love poem.

52. JODIE

During my first year of college in Northern California, I took an upper-division Psychology of Human Sexuality course on a whim, having had no clue that the subject matter would actually be about *real sex*! I chuckled this early morning, as I was reminded of the explicit adult films I was made to watch in the psych course and the intimate details I was forced to listen to during the class small group discussions. I recalled the term *penis envy*. A popular term back in the days of my early schooling that basically meant a woman's insecurity caused by her repressed subconscious desire to have the same package as a man. I giggled inside at the memory of going around in a circle during class and sharing our degrees of *penis envy*. Back then I was so malleable (still am) that any belief system that was set upon me I innocently absorbed as truth. Thusly, I went around for many years thinking I wanted to grow male stuff.

I often think back and laugh aloud over the times I was completely and entirely naïve. Like the many days I spent with my college friend Jodie. It was my fifth year at the university, during my teaching training, when I'd finally met an adult friend who wouldn't disappear on me. We befriended one another in the school gym, during a physical education (PE) class designed for soon-to-be elementary educators. Jodie was the friend who helped me paint a wooden beanbag toss—some odd-looking mouse- or catlike creature my father and I had sawed out of plywood.

When we first met, Jodie liked to tease me quite often. But I didn't mind. It provided ample opportunity to laugh at myself. Jodie's role was very much one of my protective big sister, even though I was a year older. I appreciated her frugalness and wit, and learned a thing or two from her about sticking up for myself. For my birthdays she'd come up with clever, economical, yet thoughtful, gifts. That first year of our friendship, she presented me with a miniature blue ice cooler and my own key to her apartment pool. Perfect for the hot summer days in the central valley. Although, I only made it over to the pool once on my own; I was much too shy to venture very far across my father's threshold. Jodie later became a vice principal—a role that suited her aptitude and spirit well.

It was amazing, back in the late '80s, when it turned out that my newfound friend lived in the apartments directly across from my father's house—only a skip and a hop away. Amazing again when I was the maid of honor in her wedding. However, the best memory remains the time she tricked me fully (and teased me about it for the following decade). When it happened, we were on our first walk together. It was a sizzling spring day with the hot sun bright on our faces. In my typical getting-to-know-you ("getting to know all about you") fashion, I was interviewing Jodie about her entire life. She was patient, or at least presented as such. During our stroll, Jodie informed me that she was from the state of Washington. On hearing her pronounce the word "Washington," with a tongue-rolling r sound (*Warshington*), I laughed.

In response, Jodie guffawed, raising her brow to imply I'd done something entirely incorrect and worth admonishing. "Why are you laughing?" she asked.

"Well," I stammered, "I just thought it was funny the way you said Washington. How you made it sound like it has the letter r—there's no r in Washington."

Jodie was unmoved in her expression; if anything, she appeared stern. "What do you mean?" she asked. She hit her thigh slightly and the crease of a grin edged upward on one side of her face. I watched with curiosity. Jodie continued, "Oh, you think I meant Washington DC. No. No. No. I'm talking about the state of Washington, the one up north. You know there is a difference, don't you?" Jodie faced me with a full smile.

I shrugged my slight shoulders and debated about what to say. Before I could speak, Jodie continued. "Don't you know the state of Washington is spelled with an r?" She spelled it out slowly and surely, "W-a-*r*-s-h-i-n-g-t-o-n." And then she said it again, but this time super slowly, "Warsh-ing-ton!"

I blinked, quickly. "What? No, it isn't," I answered, with my trademark nervous giggle.

Jodie continued, stating her case in a matter-of-fact way. She was so sure of herself. So confident. So . . . so . . . experienced! I reasoned I'd always been a bad speller, mixing up letters, omitting consonants and vowels, why not now? And here Jodie stood, from the state of Washington; she had to have known what she was talking about. Didn't she?

Jodie continued. "A lot of people get the two Washingtons mixed up." She winked.

"Oh, wow!" I said, feeling a bit relieved that I wasn't the only one who'd mistaken the spelling. "I never realized that." I breathed in and evaluated Jodie's expression. She seemed pleased with herself, but there was this awful silence. I quickly added, trying to save face, "Good thing to know, since I'm going to be a schoolteacher." With my last words, I settled back into the walk, glad to be corrected, and thinking more on my tanned legs than anything that had verbally transpired. It was nice having an intelligent friend.

Jodie nodded in agreement and picked up the pace of our walk. She held her silence for some time, at least a few blocks, until, after a brief moment of noise that sounded like a toad caught in her throat, she broke out in a husky, rip-roaring laugh. "Oh, honey," she said. "I can't make you go on thinking that." She laughed again, trying to catch her breath. "It was a joke. You were right before. There is no r. It's just the way I pronounce it." She laughed some more—her face as red as mine.

53. FAKE AND INAPPROPRIATE

"Do you think the title *Shag-o-rama* would pull in a lot of readers?" I asked my husband. I know just the thing to say to make him laugh. I'm gifted that way, in my off-the-wall goofiness and odd timing, whether on purpose or not. I'm starting to appreciate that about myself—my silliness and funny abruptness. I'm not ashamed in the least to proclaim that I often see the world through the innocent lens of a child and act childlike at times. I think the world could use a little bit more of whatever it is I have. If for no other reason than to crack people up!

When I was younger, people sometimes called me *fake*. To this day, every once in a while, adults question my intentions—sometimes that's a good thing and sometimes it's really not. (Insert emoticon with sad face.) I cannot pinpoint exactly what it is about who I am that makes me appear so out of the ordinary. Unfortunately, when I try to extract what people have said about me in the past, I can recall, at one point or another, a judgmental remark about pretty much everything about me, including my eyes, ears, teeth, hair, eyebrows, legs, and toes. So suffice to say, I am remarkable from head to toe!

Nowadays, at least a few times a month, someone gives out that familiar raised brow of suspicion upon meeting me. Just recently a new friend asked point-blank, "Why did you ask that? What do you want from me?" I'm not spending much time with her anymore. In my general everyday interactions, people typically pause to register what I am getting at. You should see their quizzical faces, all contorted and disfigured—like I'm indigo skinned or something! During some encounters, I long to tell the person who is reproaching with inquisition, whether indirectly or directly, that I seriously don't have this fictitious closet where I hide secret motives and trickery. That indeed I meant what I said, no matter how peculiar I might have sounded. In actuality, if I had the means, I would proudly flash open an imaginary beige raincoat and stand naked (for pretend only) and reveal that there is absolutely NOTHING I am hiding. But most people just don't get that. They conclude it's impossible for someone to be . . . like me.

It's actually funny (in the same ironic way it's funny that I was a dyslexic cheerleader with dysgraphia) that I cannot be myself without recourse, but that if I do fake who I am and act like everyone else around me (a.k.a. small talk and "normal" mannerisms, body language, tone, and subject matter) then I am trusted without question. Conclusively speaking, I am better apt to be trusted when I am not myself, which is very much a conundrum. To be or not to be? That is my life.

I giggle a lot, despite my circumstances. Laugh, too, when my peers point out the errors of my ways. Case in point, after my dear friend Lynny, a teaching pal from the good old days (waving at her wherever she be), came to spend the weekend with me, I learned quite a bit about myself. For instance: Don't take your vegan friend to dinner at a seafood and steakhouse restaurant, even if the place has a very nice water view. Don't forget to buy a box of Kleenex, so you don't have to hand your friend a roll of toilet paper when she is crying. Don't give your friend unsolicited advice about her relationship with her siblings, especially if you are an only child. Don't interrupt your friend in the middle of her serious talk by leaning across the dinner table, tugging gently on her long blond hair, and saying, "You have such pretty hair! You look like Rapunzel." Don't accept a wrapped present from your friend, examine the shape of the gift, and before unwrapping, proudly ask, "Is this a framed photo?" Don't interrupt your friend in the middle of a joke with the punch line, even if you are super excited that you figured out the end. Don't tell your friend that the previous owner of the house you live in filled the guest bedroom with wall-to-wall china dolls. Don't tell your friend you'll sleep in the same bedroom as her to make her feel safe, and then quietly tiptoe out when she falls asleep. Don't tell your friend your son sees the ghost of your dog in the guest bedroom and that you think it might be a portal to another universe because your friend will opt to sleep on the couch, despite the new pillow and new sheets you bought for the guest bed.

Back in my school days, I was often called a "dumb blond," even though I had dark auburn hair. Particularly when it came to understanding the punch line of a joke, the way in which I held certain things—like my pencil—and the manner in which I wrapped my entire mouth wide around the tip of a glass bottle when taking a swig. I understand now that I have an amazing knack for not catching onto the tiniest nuances of unwritten rules. I honestly don't know how a typical person absorbs thousands of hidden expectations without written direction. I can recall with a tinge of residual shame how, back in high school, a sisterly member of the cheer squad explained that it's not ladylike to sit on the ground at school (or anywhere else for that matter) with my legs sprawled wide open, especially in my cheer skirt. I'd never given a thought to how I sat. Never realized there were rules to sitting, too! I always just sat in a way that felt comfortable—that is, until people started telling me the *right* way to do things. In many ways I'd have been better off as a boy, I suppose.

54. TOTALLY RANDOM

Four teenage boys are awake at my house after celebrating my eldest boy's birthday last night. Their record bedtime is six in the morning. Of course letting my son purchase chocolate-icing desserts yesterday, that have enough sugar and preservatives in them to last until his hundredth birthday, was likely not a keen idea on my part. It is the first time I've actually bought that particular brand-name product, ever! I always feel weird filling my grocery cart up with junk food. I want to wear a sign that reads, *I normally do not poison my children but this is a special occasion.*

Yesterday's shopping excursion with my newly fifteen-year-old was painless—just a few swipes off the shelves. First stop soda, second stop large bag of make-your-fingers-orange chips, third stop Klondike ice cream bars, fourth stop donuts. Okay, I managed to convince him to buy some orange juice. Of course, I normally don't buy orange juice because of the lack of nutritional value and high sugar content. But considering what else was in my cart, the OJ came up on top as feasibly the only product that had real food inside of it.

This morning the boys are loud, very loud. My husband assures me that wrestling at this age is perfectly normal. They are testing out their manhood and showing who is top dog. I'm sure glad I'm a girl. I am not good at wrestling. I did warn them to stay clear of the fireplace hearth as they were throwing each other down on the ground. The first time I went into the daylight basement game room to see the boys, the first words out of my mouth were, "Wow! It sure stinks in here." I then opened the sliding door and turned toward the teens to smile. The boys looked at me like I was very odd. One boy shyly asked if I was indeed my son's mother. I'm not sure what to think of that comment. Who exactly does he think I might be? A friendly neighbor bringing junk food and candy to random children?

What an odd week. Everything felt like it just missed the mark, kind of like the whole universe was singing off-key and I was tone-deaf. So I didn't really notice but knew something was askew. My ankle went weak on me on my walk and I just about ate dust. Hip still healing. A friend visiting from California called me out of the blue and I totally freaked out because I had to change my plans for the day. But we had a grand time. Later my friend informs me she heard swear words coming out of my oldest son's mouth that she hadn't even heard before. That was a pleasant surprise. It was fun as well, watching her elderly father fall asleep with his finger still pointing to the line of text in his political book, after hearing from him that divorce is just a way to legalize prostitution, and finding out that he thought I was my sister. (I don't have a sister.)

The next day, after meeting my neighbor for tea, I get a text from my oldest son, five minutes into our much-needed conversation: "Please stop what you are doing and come home now! I cannot stop myself from punching my brothers." That was fun. And at that exact moment, what had to be the largest bug in the world flew into my face, and my friend and I both stood up and screamed and flapped our hands. Then the bug came back again. Turns out it was two black insects in the heat of romance. I still don't know what they were. But I do wonder what that would be like—flying and doing what they were doing. And today it was so very hot, some ninety-five-degrees hot. That's hot for here. We have no air conditioning. Our upstairs was eighty-eight degrees last night. Oh, and let me not forget this week when I took my two youngest chaps miniature golfing and my baby boy swung the club super hard and smacked a ball right into my ankle. Ouch! Afterwards, at the restaurant, a vegetarian trying to cut spare ribs for her son (that would be me) ended up sliding the ribs off the plate and smack onto the floor. During that dinner, a half-naked drunkard, carrying a toddler in his arms, rode by on a fluorescent green unicycle. (No joke.) And when we left the restaurant a fire truck was stopped in traffic with the fireman staring at me with wide fearful eyes, while I was staring at this scary man who had on sloppy white clown makeup, a red clown nose, and tattered clothes. He was attempting to do magic tricks by pulling out some type of raggedy colorful scarves from an old black wagon.

55. WHAT MY HUSBAND HEARS

What my husband heard today during our outing:

1. Do you think I look slutty? Are you sure? Do other women dress like this? Is this shirt too tight? I don't think I should wear this shirt in public. Does it make me look fat? How do you know I don't look slutty?

2. Look at my eye again. In the light. Can you see the pink in my eye? Does it look better? Are you sure? How do you know it is better? What if it gets worse? I think it feels better. Do you think my eye will be okay? Can you see the dry skin in the corner? What do you think it is? Look closer!

3. I am taking so many photos. Thank you for being patient. This is more of a leisure walk. We are stopping a lot. Later, I'll have to walk more around the lake. I haven't walked in two days. These shorts are too big. You are right. I should buy some new shorts today. These are too baggy. Yes, they are too baggy.

4. Take a photo here. Oh, stop here. Oh, look there. Oh, look at that tree. Oh my, look at that. Oh, look, look! Look up. Look at the spider web. Look at the water. Take one of me from uphill. I look better if you stand uphill. Not so much of my chest. You are showing too much of my chest. How do I look? Do I look okay? Can you tell my eye is pink?

5. I ingested far too much caffeine. I had that tea, and the chocolate bar, and the chocolate gluten-free cake. Feel my heartbeat. Is it beating too fast? Are you sure it's not? I think it's too fast. I'm okay, right? Feel here. I need to rest. I am tired. It's so fast. I have to stop here and catch my breath. This walk is not enough to burn off all the calories from the cake.

6. Oh, we should go this way, and when we get to the fork in the path then we'll need to go up and to the right. Otherwise we will end up on the wrong street. These maps are not designed well. We are educated and intelligent people, and we can't even figure these signs out! How are other people who aren't as smart supposed to figure them out? I don't mean that we are smarter than everyone. Well, you know what I mean. Maybe we should turn and go the other way. What do you think? . . . I told you this was the wrong way!

7. Are you staring at my butt and smiling? I can feel you smiling and staring at my butt. You are staring at my butt. And you are picturing grabbing it. I can see you. I am psychic, you know. This proves it. You are staring, aren't you?

8. Oh, it's a little Toto dog. How cute. Look at that Toto dog. Oh, he is so cute. Did you see that little dog?

9. I think I would like to have relations with a ninety-year-old man in order to give him his dying wish. Is that wrong to feel that way? To want to fulfill a man's dying wish like that? It doesn't feel wrong. But maybe it is.

10. You know if you cheated on me, I would forgive you. It would be okay. I know it would only be out of lust because I know I am sweet and you will not find anyone as sweet and as kind. So I know it would only be a physical thing. And by me saying this, it will probably make you less likely to cheat, because part of the reason men do cheat is because it is a no-no and forbidden, and you are not supposed to. So, really, since I'm giving you permission it takes the danger element out of it. But if me saying this to you makes you want to cheat more, then I take it back. You don't want to cheat on me now because I said that, do you? Should I take it back?

11. So there are different types of men I am noticing. There are married men who stare at other women and look to be thinking that they don't want to be married. But then there are men who look but love their wives and want to be with their wives, but they cannot help but look at other women. You're a man. All men look, right? And I understand if you have to look. All men look at other women, don't they? You look, and that's okay, but you do it in a sly, careful way. Some men aren't careful, and that would be hard. But if I was ever single, I would never meet the type of man I am attracted to because I'm not attracted to the men that stare in an obvious way. I'm attracted to the men who don't look or look really fast, and I would never know they were looking at me. So how would I ever know they liked me? You see, it would be hard for me because I like the shy guy who is a little insecure and doesn't know he is handsome, and those are the type that would never approach me.

12. What's your type of woman? Is that your type? How about her? You like women who are more like me, now, right? Before you liked tall and

blond. But not anymore. Do you know which of your friends I used to be most attracted to? Do you know why? No, not him. He is not my type at all.

13. If I die this is where I want you to spread my ashes. Right under this tree. Right here. Remember, okay? Here or at Mt. Rainier. However, this is much closer to home. Don't you think? This would be a good place. This is just as pretty as Mt. Rainier and that is a wonderful tree.

14. I used to date the most handsome men and it was so difficult. I would never do that again. They were handsome but not very smart. I'd walk in a room and all eyes would be on them and people would come up to me and say how handsome they were. And I knew those guys cheated. They had all these chances. It's no good dating a man like that. No good at all. Don't you agree? Oh, you are a good catch. As you get older, you outshine more and more of the men that are getting old like you. You are aging well, and they aren't.

15. I've loved you through thick and thin—mostly thick. Except for those two months you paid all that money to lose that weight, other than that, mostly thick.

56. EYE CONTACT (PICKING UP MEN)

I've been walking around the lake near our house once or twice a day. While I'm walking, I practice eye contact. Eye contact is not something I learn naturally and not something I ever feel comfortable with. Not something I enjoy, and not something that I like practicing. I taught myself how to make eye contact at the age of thirty-five. I first realized I had challenges looking at someone directly in the eyes the time I was attempting to glance up at a male sales clerk at a local take-and-bake pizza parlor. I got so nervous that I wrote a check for four hundred dollars instead of fourteen. He wasn't eye candy or even close to my age, but pretty much all males under the age of eighty and over the age of ten make me nervous. I didn't realize the error in my ways until the establishment cashed my check.

I get nervous looking at anyone I do not know well. Especially men. I have become much more comfortable with women my age and older, small children, and senior citizens. They feel safe. Every other age group, when I think about locking eyes, I squirm inside from nervousness. I now set my eyes just beyond a person or on a person's forehead in an attempt to appear friendly and approachable.

Lately, when I walk around the lake, I've been wearing sunglasses and a plastered-on smile. I listen to music and this helps me grin. And I remember all the smiles I've been practicing in the mirror. At first, my face fidgets all over the place while my smile tries to find a home. I am more comfortable with my mouth closed, though I think my toothy smile is prettier. So I probably look perplexed and intense when I smile. My hugest practice smiling comes when a man my age approaches while passing me on the trail at the lake. There are typically a couple dozen of men my age that pass on any given day. I have learned, through trial and error, to stare down the female if a couple approaches, before I glance very quickly at HER male. If I smile at the male first, I tend to get a very shifty, darty-eyed glare from the female. I find this interesting but logical. I have also found that men about ten years my senior tend to smile first, and even nod or say hello, while men my age look suspicious. This could be me jumping to conclusions. I wonder if I should start taking notes.

With every person that passes, I stand up straighter, glance slightly in that person's direction, and then look at the forehead. With sunglasses on I can hover there longer. Sometimes I get nervous and move my glance down from a stranger's chest to his upper leg region, which in retrospect maybe isn't such a good path for my eyes to follow. The whole time I'm looking I have a cheesy, closed-lip smile and I hold my breath.

I've been practicing smiling and was feeling fairly pleased with my progress, until tonight. Now I'm going back to the proverbial drawing board and trying to connect the eye-contact dots. At the lake on my last loop around, a man my age approached. He came up majorly close. I think he ran up to me from his car.

He said, "Hey," grabbed my wrist gently, and placed a small piece of folded-up paper in my hand. Between the "Hey" and hand grabbing, I figured this guy had special needs. He didn't, but that was my first thought—trusting soul that I am. And so I smiled big (with my teeth), wanting him to feel safe. As he stood there I unfolded the note and read it quickly. Kind of in shock, and not fully comprehending what I'd read, I fell back on habit and manners, smiled again, and said with a giddy voice, "Thank you!"

The note: Phillip. (His phone number.) I saw you checking me out! Text me your name.

Hmmmm. I think I might need some more practice smiling.

57. Vignette,
Good-bye Sunshine, Age 8

There were small, pressed dresses hovering above. Light spilled in through the bottom of the closet door in the shape of a crescent moon. From where I sat, the moonlight kissed the back of my hand.

An hour earlier, draped in my yellow, star-patterned nightgown, I had reached across the dining table and announced, "One plate for you, handsome Mr. Thumper, and one for you, dashing Blue Pony." My animal friends had stared back and smiled, Pony resting on his side in the chair (because he kept falling down with his bad balance) and Thumper with his paws on the table. "No arms on the table," I scolded, and placed Thumper on his rump. "That's better. Did you wash your hands?" They nodded. "Did you say grace?" They nodded again. "Good," I praised, picking up my plastic piggy bank from my chair and taking a seat.

"Good job," Mother had praised, as she walked in through the kitchen door. She plopped down a platter of cold meatloaf and a large bowl of buttered potatoes, and then lit up four tall candles. I held my plastic piggy up to my ear. "What's that? Let me see." I looked up. "He wants to know if he can come to the sitter's on Monday." Mother shook her head. "No, beautiful, you can't bring money there."

I shrugged my shoulders and tucked Piggy in my lap. Drake arrived home then with a parade of sounds: the jingling of car keys, the thump of a briefcase, the scuffling of dinner slippers, and the baritone of his voice. Five minutes later, with a pressed white T-shirt and a short glass of bourbon, smelling like minty soap and Old Spice aftershave, Drake sat down in his high-backed chair at the head of the table. He glared down with a cross of the arms and cleared his throat.

"Don't even start," Mother warned.

Drake swallowed his drink in five quick gulps.

Mother made a closed-lip smile and puffed up her cheeks. Her eyes were slits. She wasn't pleased. It was the same disapproving smirk she'd given when she went into the garage and discovered I'd taken the floppy salmon out of the fridge and placed him in a large bucket of water to swim. And the exact same look she had when my dog Justice snagged the barbequed steak from the table. And the same face she made when my stepbrother told her that he had found a baby rattlesnake in the garage and had let me watch from the doorway while he stabbed it with a pitchfork.

Drake gave Thumper an evil glare. "Is that thing clean?"

Thumper glared back.

I nodded. "I gave him a bath in the bathroom sink and combed his hair."

"Did you clean up your mess?"

"Yes," I said, hoping he wouldn't ask about Pony, who I accidentally had dropped in the toilet.

Mother put a slab of cold meat on each of our plates. I looked down at the meatloaf and examined the slivers of carrots and onions with disgust, thinking I'd rather not eat something multicolored and multidimensional. Drake chewed rapidly like he was late for something important. Mother chewed slowly like she didn't want to go anywhere. I didn't eat, just wiggled my food around my plate so it looked like I had.

Later, I brought Piggy up from my lap, a mistake Drake slapped away. Mother pounded the table, rattling ice and making the butter slide off the right lump of my mashed potatoes. She eyed Drake harshly, and then looking at me without a word tilted her head and moved her eyes to the far right. I swallowed, scooped up my cracked piggy from under my chair, and tried not to slide as I sprinted away in my yellow bunny slippers.

Soon after, in the darkness of my closet, Justice breathed in for the ninetieth time. I was losing count. I could hear them screaming. I scrunched my face up and squeezed my eyes shut. There were more mumbled shouts. Drake's voice echoed down the hallway. I imagined my stepfather's face like a swelled red balloon and Mother's screams a sharp pin. A burst was coming. Three seconds of silence. More mumbled stings. Three footsteps, and then thumps like a gorilla beating his chest—another boom. Mother yelled. Something flew, something breakable. I buried myself further into Justice's fur.

58. Why You Don't Want to Date Me

1) I used to sing a song about my grandmother's boobs when I was younger. I taught the song to my younger cousin. We would stuff our shirts with socks, cup our hands over our chests, and sing together, "Grandma's little boobies go boom, boom, boom, boom. Grandma's little boobies go boom, boom, boom!" It was a favorite party song. I choreographed the whole thing. On the first line our hands would shoot out in front of us. On the second stanza we'd drop our hands down with each boom, until they almost touched the floor. Grandma's boobs weren't little, and still aren't. Don't know why I called them "little" to begin with. But sometimes I still sing the song. Only now I'm crying in the mirror. (Don't ask me how this is related to dating. It just is. Boobs are always related to dating.)

2) I get super excited. Just ask anyone who has ever taken a walk with me. I like to process when I stroll. I like to process even more when I am first getting to know someone. I always apologize for rambling. And I always get the same half smile and bewildered eyes in response. People usually say, "It's okay." Only, I secretly want them to tell me they really enjoyed all my insights. That has yet to happen.

3) I am a very picky eater and will stress over where to go out to eat. Then when I finally do decide where I want to eat, I will take forever to decide between the three things on the menu that I might like. I discuss the pros and cons of each particular appetizer. I analyze the menu and point out to the waiting staff misprints and errors. I question the authenticity of the food description. I try to remember if it's *farm-raised* or *wild-caught salmon* that's better. I interrupt patrons to ask what they have ordered, and if it is indeed any good. I will taste your food from your plate without asking, especially mashed potatoes. I try to help people. Once I interrupted a couple's dinner and said, "Based on your conversation it sounds like your grandson might have Aspergers." No worries, I introduced myself first. The grandpa

wasn't too thrilled. I heard him say, "Boy, that lady has got some big ears on her!" I didn't take it personally because my ears weren't showing.

4) I will ask you many questions, such as: Is there anything in my teeth? Do I look bloated? How much do you think this would cost to make at home? Do you like the food? Are you full? Did you get enough to eat? Do you want dessert? Do you know soda is bad for you? Are you having a second soda? How are you going to work off all that soda? Are the refills free? Did you leave enough for the tip? How much? Are you sure? What do you think of the waiter's personality? Would you hire him? Can I have the rest of your potatoes? Want to guess what color I'm thinking of? Will you guess the number? Did you have a good time? Do you like me? Do you think I'm pretty? Why?

5) As a former teacher and mother of three energetic boys, I am programmed to play games for survival. While we are waiting for our food, I will likely engage you in a game of hangman, connect the dots, I Spy, and guess the animal. Electronics are not allowed at the table because I require your full attention. And it is important to follow *all* my rules. Don't even try watching television. Before we sit down in a sports bar, I will make certain there are no televisions in your direct line of vision, in an effort to not take away from our time together. Of course, I would question why you were taking me to a cheap sports bar in the first place.

6) I am not a meat eater and haven't been since 1984 (the year I was born). So, if you ask me to help you cut your meat, especially ribs, I will try to use a butter knife, and the ribs will fly across the table and plop on the floor. People will stare. I will then give you a look of disgust and tell you that I hate meat breath. Then I might, depending on my mood, remind you of one of the many documentaries I have viewed. I might even write the name down for you on a napkin. I will then eat your mashed potatoes when you are not looking.

7) I will compliment you. I will tell you that you have nice eyes or a nice smile, and mean it. I will likely compliment the restaurant staff, as well. Then I will stare at parts of your body that don't look perfectly to scale. I will point out the facial hair that needs to be shaved, the rogue eyebrow hair, the freckle that looks questionable, the blemish, the wrinkled shirt, the

old shoes, the nostril hair, and whatever else catches my attention. Unless you are a perfectly carved stone statue, I will find something to wonder about. I will obsess that perhaps you have a terrible disease or are allergic to something, and that is why there is a pimple on your neck. I will point out the bugbites on your arm. I will try to memorize your face. I will close my eyes and reopen them in an attempt to see if I can remember your hairline. Most of this I will do in my head and not say aloud. So I will be sitting there preoccupied, with a weird expression on my face and one eyebrow raised high, not listening to a word you are saying.

8) I will have to guess the amount on the bill. I will say, "Wait, wait, wait, let me guess!" Then I will calculate everything we consumed and add the totals up in my head, including tax. Then I will proclaim my guess. If I am within one dollar, I will smile so proudly. If I am wrong, I will go back and justify my answer, figuring out something I forgot—like the price of your soda. I will blame you for my error. Then I will lean over your shoulder to make sure you leave a 20 percent tip or higher; unless the service was terrible, then I will insist you leave 15 percent, exactly. If the waiter is exceptional, I will ask to speak to the manager about the wonderful service. I will tell the waiter first how great he is. And ask you to agree and nod. Then I will double-check the tip. I will still be worrying about the tip by the time we reach the car and ask you to verify we calculated correctly. I will then ask if you remembered the boxed leftovers on the table and ask you to go back and get them. If you have to use the bathroom, I will complain because I am tired and want to go home.

(I think this is best read to the tune of the children's book *If You Give a Pig a Pancake.*)

59. LET THE GRUMPY LADY PASS

"Guess what happens if you eat a raw snail? They have a parasite that goes into your brain and eats it. And our brain is not prepared for snail parasite. And you can't defend it. It's pretty much if you eat a raw snail, it's all up to the snail if you live or die. If the snail has the parasite, you die!"

I am looking at snails with new eyes now, ever since my middle son's enlightening comment. I have also reassured myself that the chances are null that I will accidentally eat a raw snail and die from parasites eating my brain away.

Words are powerful, how they can alter the way you once viewed a person, place, or thing—even snails. Words can change the course of a life. Proof positive, just yesterday I was strolling down the aisle in my favorite grocery store, pretty much minding my own business, when I spotted a blond mother with five small children. The oldest of her children, a young girl, was carrying her plump baby sister. The other three were little tots, all boys ranging in height by a couple of inches. I stared, because that's what I do when I'm processing. About a dozen thoughts came to mind. I examined the mom's facial expression and instantly wondered if she was happy or frustrated with the shopping excursion. I noticed two of the boys had little shopping carts and that as a collective clan the family had barely gathered any groceries—just a couple bags of snack food. I evaluated and reevaluated, concluding that the mother enjoyed the attention of onlookers watching her shop with her little crew of miniature hers. In fact, I am quite certain she liked the attention. There were several of us shoppers trying to maneuver around the little ones, a line of about five or six of us squeezing our way down the aisle. I was still watching and evaluating when I crept my cart forward. As I approached, the mom eyed me closely, and then turned to her troop and said, "Wait," putting her arms back in a stern gesture, "let the grumpy lady pass." Immediately my right eyebrow shot up. *Had she meant me?* I rolled my eyes up and gave a quizzical expression, and then moved onward. A few steps ahead, I stopped to retrieve a can off the shelf. I noticed another lady standing close behind. Feeling extremely self-conscious and flustered, I said, "Oh, I am sorry if I am in your way." She responded, "No problem at all. But maybe you can help me find the canned artichokes." We scanned together and I pointed them out with my overextended finger, while smiling big and glancing in the direction of the meanie mom, perchance to insinuate, "See how cheerfully helpful I am?"

Five aisles later, and I *still* couldn't get the meanie mom out of my mind. Was my expression seriously that sour? For a moment I wished to be an always-smiling golden retriever. By the time I reached the last aisle my thoughts were still wrapped around the incident. By then I had rationalized that the meanie mom wasn't a very patient woman and certainly wasn't showing an effective example of behavior to her children. But I also reckoned she likely was juggling a full plate and was having a tough day. I also decided, with a mischievous sneer, that her husband, if she still had one, probably didn't like her.

At the checkout area I found the safest checker I could—a round-faced, middle-aged woman with a friendly, natural grin. At the end of any shopping excursion, I don't look for the shortest checkout lines; I look for the least-threatening face. Typically, I chat it up with the grocery checkers while they are scanning my items. Conversation helps the time go faster and alleviates some of my anxiety. Not much makes me more self-conscious than a line of strangers watching me in silence. Especially when they are waiting with those daunting expressions, ostensibly cursing my high-piled grocery cart and wishing they'd chosen another route.

"I hope I don't look grumpy," I offered, approaching the checker. (Interesting conversation starter, don't you think?) I eyed the nametag "Marge" and then explained, rapid-fire, what had happened on the aisle with the meanie mother. Marge smiled and responded kindly, and we bagged the groceries together. I told her about Aspergers and the man at the park who gave me his number as a result of my practice smiling, and she told me about her grown son who just so happened to have Asperger's Syndrome. Turns out she homeschooled her son. He is now twenty and doing very well. We exchanged a lot of information in only a few minutes.

As Marge was bagging up the last of the food, she looked up at me sincerely, and said, "The main reason I homeschooled my son was because when he went to school he had to become someone he wasn't. He couldn't go to school and be himself and still be accepted. He had to let go of who he was. God made my son in perfection. I wanted my son to be able to be the person God intended." A bell went off in my head right then. My middle son was struggling in school even though he was attending part-time. His anxiety was very high and depression was setting in. I decided then and there to not send my son back to school and to instead homeschool him full-time (again).

Later that day, I calculated the probability of choosing the one checker out of a dozen or more that just so happened to have homeschooled a son with Aspergers. I then reasoned that typically I would have not mentioned the subject of Aspergers at all, especially to a random grocery-store checker, unless I'd been upset. I smiled naturally and wide with my teeth showing, repeating the silly phrase: *Let the grumpy lady pass.*

60. THE WHITE-MOCHA LADY

My youngest son made his way down the aisle lined with big, bulky, twenty-dollar televisions. "Those are ancient," he commented. We were at Goodwill, a national chain that sells used items. After twenty minutes of strolling together, looking at various treasures, and collecting a few home-school materials, I had explained to my youngest son, amongst other things, the complexity of college statistic textbooks and why he might not be interested in purchasing one today, the perplexity of eight-track tapes and how they don't sell new players anymore, the oddness of bowl-shaped old hair dryers that went atop the head, and the sad reality that this store didn't have used goldfish. As we wrapped up our mini-excursion and the mini-lessons, we stood in the checkout line to make our purchase. Seeing us there, a fellow lady customer motioned to our mostly empty cart and said, "Please, go first. You don't have much." I smiled and replied, "Thank you. I do that, too. Let people go in front of me. That was kind."

As she backed up her cart and we swapped places, I noted there was a Starbucks coffee cup in her cart. I don't regularly drink coffee. It turns me into a very dynamic thinker who believes she can solve all the world problems, if given an hour. In fact, during my walk today around the lake, I think I completed three blog articles in my head. (I had coffee today.)

At the store I turned to the young lady, motioned to her coffee cup, and said, "I left my Starbucks in the car. I can't wait to get back to it." As soon as the words left my mouth, I felt like a goof. I always feel like a goof when thoughts quickly brew and percolate in my mind, and spit themselves out before I have time to stop them. After I blushed, this kind customer, a woman about half my age (say twelve), began a full-blown monologue that sounded something to the tune of:

"I thought about leaving my coffee in the car. But I didn't. I brought it in. It's the same coffee I always get. I don't know why I always get the same flavor, *white mocha*, but I do. It's silly, but I always get the same. Maybe I should try more variety. I was going to leave the coffee in the car. I was. I wasn't sure I should bring it into the store. But then I thought, what if I die? I mean, what if I drop dead, and the last thing I think is *I should have brought my coffee*. I mean if you're going to die, you might as well have had coffee first. Who knows? This could be my last day, my last hour. And here I'd be dying without my coffee. And with the way my life's been going lately—lots of personal crisis and stuff that just makes me upset. Well, this coffee is a real treat, if you know what I mean. I need to treat myself, now more than ever. Plus, I'm anemic, and I get so cold. That's why I'm wearing this." She motions to two or three layers she's wearing and the high neckline of her cotton sweater. "I must look pretty silly wearing this in the summer. But my anemia, it makes me very cold. I shiver sometimes. I have to dress this way. That's why I'm shopping. This cart has my whole fall wardrobe. Can you believe it? The whole season, right here."

When she was finished, she grinned wider. At first I was speechless, as I watched my son's eyes grow super large and then shrink back to normal size. But I was certain to politely validate the lady before I set out to pay for my few items. Hours later, I was beaming; I visualized the woman with the multiple layers of clothing and her white-mocha coffee and kept hearing her words in my head. I couldn't help but to think that my big guy in the sky (multiple gods, or woman, or void, or flying spaghetti monster, depending on your belief system) was smiling down with a wink and saying, "See how grand it is to be quirky? See how grand to be you?" And I couldn't help but to like myself a little bit more.

61. BETWEEN THE POOPIES AND THE POPPIES

I have a difficult time understanding the middle ground. I am at one extreme or the other. I am a prude or I am sexy. I am trying wholeheartedly or I give up. I am excited or I am bored. I am starving or I have no appetite. I hyperextend my body backward or I hunch forward. I smile huge or I frown deep. I have extreme hope or I have extreme sorrow. I feel joy or I feel agony. I think I'm cute enough or I believe I'm too ugly to leave the house. I worry obsessively or I let everything go. I am overly fatigued or I have extreme energy. I cling or I walk away. I smother another or I want nothing to do with a person. I overshare or I clam up. I'm talkative or I want complete silence. I obsess or I walk away in disinterest. I am confident or I am insecure. I like myself or I hate myself. I'm trying to find that middle ground, somewhere between the poopies and poppies; between the crap and the sunshine; between the stench and the sweetness; between the ugly and the beauty—I just don't know how to get there.

62. VIGNETTE, MRS. CRAFT, AGE 23

A week before I met Catherine Craft and was greeted by her four little ones in a dream—their faces a blush and small mouths encircled with remnants of the faded pink of popsicles—I'd dreamt of a dark-haired lady guiding me from one room to the next of a colonial-style home. There we had walked together, with the glee-filled echoes of children's laughter fluting down the staircase. In real life I would meet Catherine a week after my dream, during my last years of college, and find her house to be much the same as my vision, with the element of joy spread out evenly throughout her dwelling like mortar across brick.

I lived my time under Catherine's roof as a summertime nanny, arriving in the morning and returning home to my father's house after suppertime. It was strong, where Catherine lived, unbreakable in most ways. But nonetheless a house embellished with slight hints of life's imperfections—just enough of the ordinary everyday hassles, such as minor quibbles and forgotten appointments, for the common visitor to feel at home. The house was always abuzz, with children and parents busying themselves with hobbies and responsibilities. As it was, there didn't appear to be a single space in the house that wasn't occupied with life. Even a colony of honeybees had once attempted to live out their days between the master bedroom's walls. I'd been there, with Catherine, to hear the echoing of a thousand buzzes through the aged plaster. That was one of the many days we'd laugh in astonishment together over the oddities of life.

We shared a certain connection, Catherine and I. While I'd had my dream about her and her home before we'd formally met, Catherine had been told, in an answer to prayer, that a kind and good young woman was coming to take care of her children. Because of our shared faith, and various other commonalities, through the years Catherine and I became fond friends, a relationship akin to a favorite aunt and a beloved niece. It was our unshakable close bond and shared confidences that made her death all the more painful.

When I initially heard of Catherine's illness I was a public school teacher of my own right and had bid good-bye to the nanny position some three years prior. I was renting a little apartment about twenty minutes up the hill from Father's house and drove down on Sundays to attend church at the downtown cathedral. On a midmorning summer day, during the last minutes of church, I discovered Catherine was ill. After hearing the news, I immediately drove over to Catherine's house to find an answer; expecting, for the most part that Catherine had been laid up with the flu or a head cold. What I would discover instead would be the biggest shock of my young life, not so much in the news, but in the way the finding played out.

There had been no warning, but then, with the coming of the news of death, no amount of preparatory time would seem enough. Still, the way I first heard of Catherine's fate had been a reincarnation of the days with my mother's boyfriend Ben, in the way I was to be knocked off my feet with the wallop of words. On my arrival, I found Catherine's husband seated outside the house atop a flight of concrete stairs. There alone, he was leaning forward with one hand on his forehead and his tousled white hair shadowing his face. I approached innocently enough, stepping up the stairs, while calling out and waving a cheerful "Hello." After my words reached him and he lifted his head, I stood still waiting for his response. But nothing came from his end—only a cavernous scowl. In return I stammered for words, not managing to say a single thing.

He remained silent and moved his head from side to side, leaving me to feel as if I'd spoken when I hadn't.

Needing to speak, I continued, superseding the growing lump in my throat. "I heard Catherine was sick," I offered. But my words did little except to cause him to sit up tersely and change his gray eyes from once vacant, to firmly disturbed.

My body took over then, letting the shuffling of nervous feet and trembling of hands preside. Seconds later he barked, and where he had once seemed frail and distraught, he now seemed born again. "Yeah, she's sick all right!" he shouted, setting his eyes down to the barren street below. "She has an inoperable brain tumor and will be dead in a month!"

I tried to maintain my balance with legs I could no longer feel. He continued, cursing God and His wrongdoings. Then placing the palms of his hands on his face, he said, in a muffled plea, "And she won't take the treatment, won't do anything to buy a little more time with us. They can prolong her life by a year, if she took the medicines, but she won't. She said she doesn't want her last days to be like that. Why does she want to leave us?"

He glared up at the sky, pushing himself up. And then, with heavy steps, he ambled down, turning once to wave me away.

My eyes reached out ahead to the high front porch, then back to his hunched back, and lastly up to the clear blue of the sky. A minute later, when my feet had found their way to the doorstep, Catherine answered, appearing as lovely as ever—perhaps paler and a bit tinier, but still beautiful. I couldn't yet catch my breath enough to fashion words. Catherine, only five feet tall and dressed in a slim, plain, black sleeveless dress, seemed more my little sister than my elder. Finding her warm brown eyes, I smiled weakly, searching for what to say. In greeting, Catherine's mouth folded into a light smile. I pushed myself forward past the threshold.

Inside, Catherine wrapped the weight of her arms around me. Behind us, her youngest closed the door. The words came then, soft and wavering, as we both told of our sadness—Catherine's utterance shaved with tears and mine in trembles.

"I am so afraid of dying," she said, whispering in my ear. Three of her children watched us from behind a shadowed corner. "I don't want to die. I don't want to die."

I could barely hold back my tears. I was made brave only by the sight of tiny, wide blue eyes below.

"Sit with me," Catherine voiced softly, leading me into the living room with the familiar touch of her smooth palm. "Stay," she whispered.

She would live a year, even without the medicines, but the disease would take its toll, invading her faculties and leaving her a hollowed being with much of her golden spirit long departed before her physical vessel left. I'd see her twice more, and in doing so wish I hadn't, for she preached irrationally about God's grace and the angels waiting for her everywhere from a platform of a much-withered and depleted mind. An older, less vulnerable me would have visited dear Catherine frequently and held her hand through the immuring days. Instead I—the damaged girl I was—chose to escape her emotions by forging a new relationship with a man she didn't even like. Indeed, by becoming emotionally entangled in a newfound person, I was able to cloak the encroaching loss.

A week after Catherine's passing, I had a dream. I found Catherine fully healed and at peace, standing outside a yellow school bus. She stood in line with many people. I was there as well, dressed in my nightclothes. Without hesitation, I politely squeezed into line and stood directly behind Catherine. As I stood there waiting, Catherine turned around and greeted me with an understanding smile.

"I think I'm dreaming," I whispered.

Catherine nodded. "Yes. You are, darling." She then placed her tender hands on my shoulders. "Child," she said, facing me. Her smile enlarged—her eyes bright, more beautiful than ever. "This is not your time. Not yet. Not now." I shook my head. I did not want to hear those words. "Please," I asked. "Please!" I begged.

Catherine smiled. Embraced me in her warmth. And then slowly let go, still holding me with her brown eyes. Then she smiled once more, a knowing smile, before turning around and taking her place back in line. Moments later she stepped forward, walked up the stairs, and entered the bus.

And slowly the door closed.

63. VERBALLY PROCESSING

I told myself I didn't need to verbally process anymore, that after so many days of writing I was good to go, that everything had been cleared and cleaned out of my head. I actually believed I was no longer troubled with multiple-leveled intrusive thoughts and intense logical reasoning, and cluttered ideas, and unyielding inspiration, and nonstop jibber jabber of the brain. I was a housewife, a mother, a cleaner of all things grime, and cooker of all things organic. I wasn't this complex person requiring repetitive processing. (Ha, ha, ha!)

I actually thought to myself, *I am a typical mainstream person and I've made up all this Aspergers mumbo jumbo in my head.* I actually thought and thought and thought. Until I realized I was thinking an awful lot. So much so, that I likely had Aspergers! I then reasoned that I might unknowingly be trying on the persona of an Aspergers person for size—actually inhaling and creating Aspergers traits because I needed an identity to function in life. That in truth, I was perfecting said *Aspergers*, as *Aspergers* was my new inspirational role. Yes, I'd garbed the facade to the state of complete lifelike amazement! And if this were true, if in fact I was convincing myself I had Aspergers in order to figure out my role in society, was that insanity? And what is insane? And who isn't insane? Or more so, who is sane?

Then after looping, I concluded, like I have done more than a trillion dozen times before, throughout this writing endeavor, that if indeed I was once again taking on the persona of an Aspie to feel safe in this world, as I need a role in order to feel secure, then indeed I must have Aspergers. Brain Pain! Hmmmmmm.

So last night I'm thinking, at the late hour of eleven o'clock, as I'm watching reruns of the show *Glee* and getting all tingly, like I get when I hear good music, that I ought not to have had coffee after the noon hour because then I can't sleep and my thoughts speed up like Sheldon on *The Big Bang Theory*. Then I'm thinking I relate way too much to characters on television, and how much more superb and *brainiac-ish* it would be if I related to characters in books. But I don't. So I'm stuck as a character on television.

So, as I'm processing, basically alone, while the rest of the household is sound asleep (including Spastic Colon, a.k.a. my miniature Labradoodle dog), I'm starting to get stomach pangs of growing anxiety, dread, and fear. I'm telling myself it's the dang coffee, in addition to my binge into the wheat zone. (I try to avoid gluten because it increases thoughts of impending doom, like dying of toe fungus or a nose pimple). I keep reassuring myself all is okay. That much of what I'm experiencing is biochemical, while cursing to the star-fairies, "Why do I have to be so frickin' sensitive to everything on this planet?" But the reassuring (and cursing) isn't working because the episode of *Glee* happens to be about the adorable school counselor having OCD and taking medication to ease her symptoms. And I get so tangled up on tiny amounts of anger when I hear the overdone, generic fallback overused by psychiatrists (when speaking of medication) that hums to the tune of, "If you had diabetes, you'd need insulin. This is no different." And in my mind I'm screaming, *Dang straight it's different. Diabetes is proven and shown on blood tests. It's in black and white. Plain as day. Mental challenges are not that black and white. It's not that simple!*

And that got me thinking, do I need medication? My husband would shout an adamant, "NO!" Because the one and only time I was on a low-dose antidepressant for muscle pain, I ended up in the psych ward with suicidal thoughts and a man who called himself "Jack Off."

At this point I'm exhausted but too awake to sleep. Next came the wave of panic that ensued after I opened an envelope—an envelope from the university I attended for one semester when I was focused on working toward a second master's degree; until I hightailed it out of the university on my own therapist's advice (and my inability to stop my crying and my trembling fear of returning). The panic I felt upon opening the envelope was akin to the fear spawned from my overall university experience. Inside was another bill. Which means once again I'll have to play phone tag to try to clear up the financial issue. And this sets me into a coffee-plus-wheat-induced terror state with doomsday impending thoughts. Deep breaths. Pause. Maybe I still do need to process through writing. Just maybe.

64. TRIPLE-CHINNED MONSTER

During the past few days, LV (little voice inside my head) has been analyzing actors on television shows and how their hair affects the way they look. In the meanwhile, I realized that at some point in my life I got the notion stuck in my brain that I truly look like the ugliest photos out of all the photos ever taken of me! In other words, taking the lot of all the photographs I've ever made an appearance in, the ones that depict me at my worst (gaunt and ghastly) are the *true* representation of me. And the rest? Obviously lies! (Thanks Sir Brain—you rock.) I mean, wouldn't it be nice for me to one day believe I always look like the best photo? But no! My little brain (Sir Brain) thinks I *must* look like the absolute worst photo ever! Of course, this is the same brain that somewhere along the road gathered the baggage that if I do not look beautiful with my hair unkempt, makeup off, and dressed in frumpy stained clothes, then I am not naturally beautiful. The same mind that played tricks and told me that if I wear makeup and fix my hair and take a nice photo then that is a lie, and fake, and not the *real* me to begin with. And thusly, if someone gives me a compliment while I'm *fake,* then the compliment is not real either! The same brain that told me all these years that when someone says I'm *beautiful* or *pretty* that the person is just saying that because truthfully I'm hideous and they are trying to lift my spirits. That, in truth, the entire world is in a conspiracy to make me think I'm lovely because when they look my way they feel sorry for me. Oh! My! Gosh! Growth, growth, growth. Just today, my son took a photo of me with his new camera, and for the first time ever, when I glanced at my image, I thought logical thoughts. I heard this in my head: "Oh, I have a triple chin because he is little and taking the photo from way down low. I look different in all angles and lighting. This is not a true reflection of me." Much better than my standard: "Oh, no! I can never leave the house again. I am a triple-chinned monster that everyone is pretending not to see!"

65. Processing

Processing: Take One

I can't simply think without establishing layers of miniature clans of dictatorships, hall monitors, and the rogue rebel here and there. I don't get to do that—the all-or-nothing factor out trumps the simplicity, and shovels heap after heap of soil into my already-marked spectacles. I don't get to see a straight-shot view. With all the leveled parts of my thought process, and all the interior battles at play for center seat, I am left askew, searching for the optimal view whilst my heart is still set on wishing to see straight and level. If this thought process sounds overboard and complicated and too fluffy, and perhaps profound, well indeed it is.

Daily, my crowded brain (Sir Brain) spills out impetuous and multiplex tangents of thoughts that are tangled, bundled, and laborious to decipher; because of these complexities, there are days when my own thoughts put me into a state of inertia. During this state, I do not feel comfortable in any part of my body, and it's all I can do to function and perform daily tasks. I might be in bed for the full of the day or might continually write in an attempt to pour out some of the vexation. Distractions do not work. Neither does the company of another, movies, books, or any type of distraction that might typically pull a typical person out of her thoughts.

When I visualize my processing, I see a heavy lump of muck. This lump is a representation of what I have seen, heard, or read. Whatever emotive response was triggered, it stirs and stirs my mind. All I can do at this point is to sit back and become audience to my brain—as it sifts, filters, dissects, chops, and dismembers this body of information. Then the body of data becomes whole again, and the process is repeated.

Most forms of processing occur in such rapid fashion that I don't initially recognize what is taking place. Other forms of processing take a few minutes or the better part of an hour. Some processing can take a day. Extreme processing can take the better part of a week! In example, sometimes I need to press repeat in my mind and cannot help but to rewind and review, and rewind and review, a past event. If a conversation is written in text, I might go back and reread the words in detail a half-dozen times or more. I will analyze certain words and theorize what was said—the plausible intentions and what might have been said differently. If the conversation was spoken out loud, I might recreate the scene and relive the experience multiple times. I will picture where I was sitting, what I was doing, and visualize the room and distinguishing elements about the environment.

At times, I use logic to talk myself through the upset or overwhelming angst produced from overthinking; I write my thoughts out or talk aloud. Sometimes the only way to relieve the discomfort is to phone a friend. Life doesn't feel real until I have expressed my thoughts. Or perhaps I don't feel real until I get things out of my head.

66. Processing Processing: Take Two

I am endowed with the capacity to triple think (or quadruple think). That is to say I can process several thoughts along separate lines at the same instant. So while one process is happening, so is another. In addition, there is a finite goal to this reasoning, in which the lines of thought are straight and contain their own predetermined want of outcome and motivation for completion. I am along for the ride like a passenger traveling on three trains simultaneously. The linear thinking on multiple parallel levels happens frequently.

A way to visualize how my processing "machine" works is to imagine a huge, lit-up, electronic computer grid, with me as a miniature person standing in the middle, or to envision a large framework of reality—a dynamic blueprint— such as those demonstrated in quantum physics. There, millions of avenues and routes of thoughts travel different pathways, reverse, recreate, and travel new paths again. Images and ideas bounce back and forth, inside out, up and down, and all about. Like a hokey-pokey dance of the mind—only it's not my right foot doing the dance, it's the whole of me. I cannot concentrate on anything else at depth until the processing is complete. Until then, I will wear a faraway stare and appear depressed, withdrawn, and deeply preoccupied, to the extent where an observer might ask, "What's wrong?"

What's wrong is that something has been seen or heard that has triggered an array of uncontrollable thoughts and emotions; that discomfort will remain until I go through the undertaking of analyzing, dissecting, and piecing back together what has occurred. This usually means I sleep less and wake up with an urgency to repair or fix the unsettled state. This usually means researching whatever triggered the current processing episode—whether through conversing with others, reviewing my prior writings, looking up facts and statistics, or rereading and rereading a written correspondence. OCD-like repetitive behaviors often set in, such as continually checking a social network site or asking the same question persistently, e.g., "Do you love me?"

I cannot say any of this is an easy process; however, labyrinth thinking is a highly remarkable experience, especially once the intricate processing itself is over and the relief follows. Sometimes there is no answer to be found and I grow exhausted of the thinking and rethinking and just let it go. Oftentimes I find solutions and new ways of viewing the situation, or I collect valuable information. Other moments, I am able to offer assistance to those with similar challenges because I've lived through my own distress so acutely. Overall, processing is an experience that still baffles and entirely exhausts me, as it runs away with my time, energy, and thoughts. Yet in the end, I feel filtered through. In many ways I am part of an elaborate filter system that locates the muck and junk, scoops it out, and leaves me cleansed and purified. It's an arduous affair to go through, but it's part of who I am and how I function.

67. THE PANTY DILEMMA

When the sales lady informed me, "You can't wear panties with this dress because of panty lines," I ought to have recognized I never would be able to go to my husband's work party without wearing underwear! Still, I bought the gorgeous dress that fit me like a glove and also showed off all my lady parts, hoping I'd get gutsy. (I was going to write "grow a pair" or "grow balls" but that just seemed plain ridiculous to mention when talking about a panty-free dress.)

My husband was with me at the quaint downtown boutique when I tried on the dress. He loved the dress. When I asked him about the shopping experience later, he chuckled and said, "Do you really think I could comprehend anything AT ALL after I found out you would have to wear no underwear!" As you can see, he was little to no help.

When I talked to my friend who lives in England, she said, "I don't think that's such a good idea, wearing no knickers to your husband's work party."

You think?

When I thought about creating an underwear-free zone under my dress, I was taken back in time to the months I had to share a small bed with my wrinkly, snoring grandmother. She never wore underwear to bed. Regardless of my panty issues, I brought the body-hugging dress home with high hopes.

The night before last, I spent an hour searching in the intimate undergarment department section of the store for stockings. I figured stockings would at least provide a layer. I found some nylons that made me gasp out loud: "EWWWW!" I didn't know they made stockings that stretched all the way up to the bottom of the bra line. The photo of the woman was outrageously odd, like some bipod mermaid in a stretchy, black, see-through suit. First no panty lines? Now no stocking lines?

I was beginning to wonder whom I was hiding all these lines from and for what purpose. Looking around the department store, I found all types of signs that tried to remind me of my inadequacy. I couldn't believe all the weird contraptions: bodysuits that sucked in fat, bras that pushed up stuff, and other thingamajigs I wasn't sure what I'd do with, other than take photos to send to my friend in England so we could bust up laughing.

My favorite was the attire that read, "Gets rid of muffin top." I didn't even know clothes manufacturers used that term. Oh, and one item promised, "Gives you instant confidence." I thought, *Wow, I didn't have to write. I could have just spent $19.95, slipped on this nude-colored leotard thingy, and presto—had instant self-esteem.*

After all the line-hiding regulations, I was surprised I was *allowed* to wear a bra. Until I saw these things called breast petals—tiny flower-shaped bandages made to stick to boobs, or at least the tips of boobs. I just about lost my composure then. Why would I want Band-Aids for my boobs? And, man, the peel-off factor when all was said and done. Ouch!

I ended up buying three different pairs of stockings to try on with the deemed "panty-free" dress. At home I tried to wear stockings with the pretty dress. I tried really hard. And then I cried inside because I couldn't pull it off. I felt like I lost a part of me, the panty-free pinup girl who never was. Sigh. Luckily, I had the black little nun-like dress I fell in love with a week prior to finding the pinup dress! And as soon as I slipped the black dress on, I twirled in glee. For this dress I could wear panties with!

When we first arrived at the party, only the owner of the company, my husband, and I were touring a section of the building (The Tacoma glass museum); the rest of the guests, some hundred people, had moved on into other rooms. The whole time (some fifteen minutes with the owner) I kept thinking to myself, "I'm so glad I wore underwear!" Thank goodness I didn't say my thoughts aloud.

Imagine the scene: "My smile? Well, to tell you the truth, I'm just so thrilled to have panties on!" As it was, I kept saying to my husband all night, "I'm soooo glad I didn't wear that other dress!" He just nodded. But I could see in his eyes what he was really thinking: "You have Aspergers. You are processing, thus the repetition of the same statement. However, I kind of wish you didn't have panties on."

68. FANTASY CYCLES

I have a very active fantasy life. I live more inside my head than outside. I am in control inside my fantasies; in there no one can get to me, see me, or judge me, unless I say so. And I always look fabulous! Outside of my fantasy world I am vulnerable.

Sometimes my fantasies nurture and fuel me. I am motivated and calmed by repeating the same scenario—perhaps a conversation in which I picture two people and their exact dialogue. There are days I can live inside of my head for hours, basically rerunning the same images and dialogue. I start from the beginning and then rewind and review the whole thing again. The fantasy itself could be only a few minutes long, but it is replayed frequently, and in that way it lasts much longer.

Sometimes the fantasy (or better yet imaginings) involves organizing, such as visualizing where my belongings will go in a future home. This type of active visualization and sorting is similar to mental *stimming*. Some people calm themselves (stim) by repeating the same phrase aloud multiple times or by the use of repetitive actions, such as clearing the throat or snapping finger to thumb. For me, in order to calm my mind, I sometimes visualize the same sequence of steps again and again.

When a fantasy cycle ends, typically because a future event I've imagined comes to fruition, or because reality sets in and what I imagined no longer seems feasible, I am sometimes left unnerved. If my fantasy is about a person, as was common in my teens and twenties, I might feel disappointed in some way. If I lose a person in real life (e.g., end of a relationship, relocation), who was also an active part of my fantasy life, then I feel a substantial loss at multiple levels—I feel a loss of the real-life relationship and I also feel a loss of the fantasy relationship. Always, without fail (unless concerning death), the loss of the imagined relationship hits me harder than the loss of the real relationship; primarily because I have more than likely idealized the imaginary relationship. I mourn the vivid images and quixotic scenarios I created and who I made the person out to be. I then might confuse the fantasy person with the actual real person, inflating another's character and exaggerating my own loss. A part of me believes the fantasy was attainable and very real. A part of me knows it was not realistically ever going to happen. But the fantasy-seeking part typically wins out, creating havoc and heartache.

69. MYSTICAL MUSIC PROSE

You are like music upon music upon music, a figure seemingly out of tune.

At times I think if I could only find your one song, the part that is truly you, then I could play you again and again, and dance, whether alone or together, in endless ecstasy.

Even as I tell myself you are complexity and spiraled wonder, I long to unravel you to the core—perhaps as some vegetable with heart or some flower with first petal.

I like to pretend you are easy to find, to see, to portray. For with easiness would come the grace of painting you into the shadowed corner of my existence, a mural to keep me safe, a walking space that requires no effort but touch. One finger slipped onto the wall of me and slid across your slivered silhouette.

For it is in my shadowed times I cry out for you, for oneness, for connection, for acknowledgment that I am as beauty, only because you are as beauty. Though in my days of sunshine, I too call out, reaching in silent gratitude and shimmering in your brilliance. It is then you are an effervescent glory to behold. A gift set amongst a fleet of angels with the finest and most demure of sails.

I have carved you within my soul light. Sat up constant nights awake in my dreary state, counting you like youth beholds her sheep. You leap across my chamber ceiling—a ghost set free in crimson carriage, bouncing through the valley of my imagination; your face bare except your kaleidoscope eyes; a barren tunnel of absence entering a rainbow of stars.

I see there, into myself, and breathe, my last glance of this world, the beckoning of your substance. Awoken, the days come with the joys and woes of worldly possessions explored and dried, withered and left for the illusion of promise they be. Awoken, the days come, with the sorrow and gratitude, the biting into what was once ripe, to find the taste of expiration and abandonment.

Still the bell chimes, in memory of laughter and in preparation for the surprises beneath my pillow. I harbor such secret dreams and cherished gifts. And to share them, I set you upon my shelf of butterflies and sing only to you.

You are to me the mystery of fantasy, the puppeteer with magical strings of grandeur, capable of contorting a stage of delight or drama of doom. I hone in on what could be called your goodness and try to trap your substance within my tiny womb—to bathe you in the babe's cocoon with my essence. Yet my attempts are futile, for you are not but one form, not but one song, but an orchestra drawn out into a long and distant parade.

I cannot keep you as beekeeper keeps bees. And so it is, that even in the ward of captive thought, your honey I cannot taste. For you are food to the masses, a delicacy set before the king of kings; royalty, in your very blood and bones, built up and made into something I cannot decipher nor replicate. You are magnificent splendor set upon the eyes of the mind. And I ride you, this child of the merry-go-round world, upon a horse ever-changing. Until spinning top stops, and I am flung out of your land into the stillness— made to watch alone, your partner for eternity—wavering outside and beyond, the mystical music of you.

70. THE UNION

She entered gently, the kissing sunshine on her shoulders sweet, a baroness of beckoning light within my dimly lit threshold. I greeted her, the doorman shy, and took my place at fair lady's feet, the honey-milk of her scent upon me.

My awakening came slowly, as the crimson rose blooms beyond time, opening bud after bud to her glory. She whispered; her words a chisel of feather soft, her eyes the ebony of compassion, her hand upon my surrendered shoulder. Touched, I wept, the tears inside cleansing wounds of sword, fractures of youth's mourned merriment.

My every cell moved, beholding this adorned child dressed in blue, the ocean maiden of the distant ages. Streams of aqua reborn merged forward, pushing the heart of past into the baptismal of present—a forest of water at my door.

Quaked, my very existence stood tall; quaked, the foundation of all truth and valor collapsed without fall, the boundaries, dripping as honey, disappearing into the depths of hope. I faltered in thought, recalling my place, my duty, and traced the outline of her shadow, a maiden with endless treasure, the illusion of end marking entrance to eternity.

"I am home. I am home," the whispers came, a tapping upon the window of heart, an opening to the view of victorious, to have found the mirror of me, the echo of my existence, to have found the palm of palm, and coming of my own dawn. To watch as her sunrise awakens the world beneath my flesh, calling upon the beast to rise and devour with gaunt hunger what is served. Dish upon dish.

Beyond the cage I sat, wanting and waiting, my crying her own breath, my need fulfilled at the calling of her name. The spoken word, a spell upon my lips, a taste upon my soul, to behold the beauty unwrapped before me. To behold the mistress of my ache, the mistress of my time and making, the sun captured within the capsule of opened spirit. To kneel before the queen of my own mystery and bounty, and melt into the vision as one, my every wish to rest within her endlessly.

Beyond captured, I retreated into gentleman's cave; even there the darkness dissipated, healing blood pulsating across the caverns. Everywhere—her redness, her sacrifice, her singing love—and I could not but help to taste her, the sugarcoated finger to mouth.

For she was in me, about me, and beyond, her essence the chalice of my life; and I drank and drank, until the ocean floor sat alone.

71. LITTLE SUPERWOMAN

Shortly after mother and I had moved out of Drake's house and into a tall duplex overlooking the school bus yard, I received a record player from Father. It was a gigantic silver contraption encased in clear plastic with a magical black arm that automatically moved back to its resting place at the end of every record. I remember replaying the only two records I owned at the time, over and over. I memorized the song lyrics to "Fifty Ways to Leave Your Lover" and "Blue Bayou," belting out the songs at the top of my lungs. And I remember pondering why it was that Paul Simon didn't truly list fifty ways to leave and why Linda Ronstadt kept singing, "blue by you." I figured Paul couldn't count and Linda was perpetually lonely.

During this time period, about the age of nine, it was my ritual to pull pointy thumbtacks out of the soles of my tiny feet. Not on purpose, but because I'd had a mind to go about rearranging my dog and cat posters—moving them from one spot on my white walls to the next. A habitual practice brought on by the tugging need to bring order to my room and to my life. Without fail, relocating my animal posters resulted in tacks slipping out of my grip and tumbling into the hidden dark of the shaggy green carpet. I can still remember the familiar sting brought on by stepping or dancing into a tack's secret hiding place.

I also recall with fondness the short stint of time where we had thirteen cats—three adults and two litters of kittens—before all but one cat "miraculously" found "new homes" in one day (thanks to Mother). Some afternoons I would shove all ten meowing kitties under my bedcovers and dive in for a fit of ticklish delight. Other times, against Mother's ardent advice, I'd steal my little hamster Whiskers out of his jailhouse and cuddle with him under the covers—that was before one of the cats found him. I still harbor some guilt in regard to the horrific demise of that little guy.

When I wasn't relocating my posters, dancing and singing, or attending to my pets, I was usually organizing something or another. My room was a palace of order and tidiness. It never was messy. My cherished stuffed animals (all of which I kept until my first teaching job) were gathered together in a straight row on my large queen-sized bed. There were over a dozen set out and displayed in birth order based on the day we first met. I can still visualize my favorites—a brown bear dressed in orange Hawaiian garb and a straw sunhat and two intertwined monkeys hugging. The girl monkey was pink. My trolls that were paraded across my mirrored yellow dresser were neatly organized by height of hair—with the potbellied, orange-haired fellow in the front. On the days I felt like Superwoman, I'd push my dresser across my room, leaning in with the full of my body weight and using my arms and legs as leverage. Little me, I'd stand in my doorway evaluating my room, all serious and business eyed, like an art investor measuring the symmetry and value of his prize collection. Until, exhausted from heaving things back and forth and never finding the right spot, I'd escape into my yellow submarine—a bright walk-in closet with a high, southern-facing, circular window. Inside were neatly organized new hardback books with colorful, glossy book jackets. I can still smell the ink. Each cherished book on my blue shelf was paired with another book of similar height and color. Mother had received the books free of cost from an editor friend—a large cardboard box piled high. As it was, I couldn't read the books because the three dozen or so treasures were all adult novels with words too rich for my eye's taste. Though regardless of their original purpose or practicality, basked in the sunlight and security of my closet, my books found me, and we'd smile together.

72. Communication Work

Partaking in conversation is often overwhelming. Not only do I have the nonstop chatter in my head dictating my actions, but I also question if I've done the communicating job right. I've done away with the sharp critical voice, thank goodness, though the expert coaches and evaluators are still up in the bleachers shouting out their observations. Take that along with the environment, e.g., chair texture and firmness, room temperature, ticking clock, talking children, music, air fresheners, and the feel of my own body (physical pain, taste in mouth, feel of teeth, tightness in body, muscle cramps, etc.), and I am struggling stupendously just to remain present. Add to that the act of following the contents of the conversation, in hopes of replying in the appropriate manner, and I'm ready to collapse. Plus, I always have this little voice inside my head (LV) that chimes in, "Can I talk now?"

During interactions, besides monitoring my communication, I am monitoring the other person I am speaking with and noticing miniscule "flaws," both in her communication style and in her physical attributes. Even the tiny hair on that freckle can be a distraction. Sometimes I have to come back and figure out what the person was saying before I was pulled into a freckle. Then I worry about her expectations, and if I am a good enough friend or listener. And then I wonder again, "Are you this distracted and bored when I talk to you?"

In addition, each word a person says triggers an avenue of feelings and avenues of thought. For example, at mention of the word "dog" I might think, *Did you say dog? Oh Scooby. I miss my dog Scooby. Have I told you Scooby died? Why did he die? Maybe it was . . . Oh, no! She is still talking and I missed most of what she just said. Should I tell her or just nod? If I nod is that lying? I should remind her I have Aspergers. Or maybe I should just pretend.*

That's just one word. Typically, a conversation has much more than one word. Online communication and texting is better than face-to-face communication. I can forgo a huge section of people pleasing and distractions. I can pause, skip sentences, reread for clarity, and take an extended period of time to process information. Heck, I can ignore the person altogether, go grab something to eat, and come back later. I can even scratch, fidget, doodle, or work on something else, and the person isn't offended at all!

73. THURSDAY'S PEE

I always have to pee at the least desirable times. Like right now, as I sit here in this coffee shop, dressed rather cute with my new white jacket that was initially supposed to accompany a dress I never wore—a panty-free dress. I'm all dolled up. And why? Why is my hair curled, my lashes too, and my lips a sweet watermelon color? Because it's Thursday, of course! As I sit here typing, I have a full panoramic view of the room. I can see the fireplace and, unfortunately, the man who set up camp right in front of my leather couch, across the coffee table. I've been battling his come-hither stares since his prompt arrival and wondering, *What's a girl to do?*

I have to pee because I had a huge cup of coffee mixed with organic hot chocolate mix. Can you say double yum? I had that to-die-for beverage earlier when at home.

Arriving at the coffeehouse, with all my perky self, I said to the lady behind the counter, a sweet young thing, "I'd like a decaffeinated soy chai latte, please!" I flashed a big grin. I liked the sound of my order. And plus, my jacket said it all: I am sexy, I am cute, and I am fabulous. See the bow in the back of my coat?

My face said the rest: See my big grin. I am so extremely comfortable here. Let me lift my brows to decrease my wrinkles and set my head so delicately to the right. Am I approachable, yet? Am I fitting in, blending in with the other humans?

The tall bearded man, near the young lady behind the counter, strikingly thin, likely a vegan extremist, eyed me fine and good. He spoke without words for a millisecond. Processing. Then he breathed out his thoughts, quick and easy, with a *smirkish* clear of his throat. "We don't have *decaf* chai," he said, with a roll of his eyes, before he scooted his frailness out of my line of vision. Though he kept watching me with his I-know-more-about-beverages-than-you stare. Deflated, I panicked and slid my thoughts to the right, examined, and tried to grasp my next step. Catching an idea, I said, as smoothly as possible, in spite of my nervous giggle, "Oh, yes, of course.

Chai is caffeinated." Then I felt doubly incorrect, remembering there is decaf chai tea in the stores; and for a moment, I was in the grocery market, away from this frightful man.

I was quite beside myself with embarrassment, realizing that I'd once again overreacted to the slight poopiness of a stranger. After the boob of a man (rather Zen of me, don't you think?) slapped down the tea menu in front of me, I had the keen impression he was fed up with my query-filled eyes. Sucking in my breath, I said, "Ginger tea," delicately, and tried to fluff up my sweetness. *Can't you see that I'm nice?*

With tea in hand, I retreated with imaginary tail between legs to my spot, and then struggled to figure out proper etiquette for placing down my items. Where to put my scarf, keep jacket on (looks cute, keeps me warm, hides my boobs) or take jacket off (keeps jacket clean, might be more comfortable), put laptop on lap, put laptop on table? Cross legs? And so on. Endless it is. Problem is, right when I got settled, that's when the stranger arrived. With some fifty other feasible places to sit, he chose to sit directly in front of me, in a position where his line of vision crashes and smacks mine. I can't even hide behind my laptop. The stare down begins.

So far, in the last hour, I've noted his outdated sneakers (I mean 1980s black checkered Vans) and his need to pull his hat over his head and nap. I've taken random glances when he wasn't looking, but really wished I had a note on the back of my laptop that read, "This is an experiment—I have Aspergers. Don't expect me to look you in the eyes or respond to your existence, unless you are a woman my age or very old and safe looking. Or a child. Or a dog. Or even a bird. But if you are a man, beware. You're invisible. Kind of . . ."

I really have to pee now. But in order to vacate my spot I will have the task of stuffing the laptop into my computer case. That, in and of itself, is difficult. I am not very coordinated. Stuffing things inside other things is not my forte. In fact, trying to fit anything inside anything is hard. (I'm embarrassed now, as this someone how once again seems sexual. Like I said, I'm twelve inside.) Think outdoor folding chair into folding chair's bag. Panic attack! I don't know which side goes in first. And then I get all bothered with everything that sticks and snags and acts stubborn. I often carry my portable lawn chair in one hand and the designated bag for said chair in the other hand. It's just how my life is.

I have to figure out if I am going to ask the very, very kind-looking woman at the table, diagonal to where I am seated, if she might watch my laptop. However, she is deep in conversation, and though her friendly eyes beckon me, I cannot help but visualize her running away with my laptop, all the while smiling in delight and screaming, "Ha, ha! You're overtrusting!" I am now starting to run through in my brain the very feasible scenario of what will happen if I do in fact piddle in my pants. I really want to keep my place, my cozy spot on the couch, so I am setting my book on the coffee table alongside my scarf and letting the thoughts of "new book" and "pretty, purple, ruffled scarf being stolen" saturate and then spill out of my brain. I take a deep breath, wondering if the bow in the back of my coat is in actuality cute or just plain silly for my age. Deep sigh, stepping forward while balancing laptop. Glancing back to reassure myself that my spot is still marked and claimed. Thoughts of a dog peeing on a bush to claim territory enter briefly. Wondering if anyone is in the bathroom and hoping I can reach the sanctuary of the porcelain pot in time.

Passing people, standing upright, trying to look confident. Knowing when I stand too upright that my body is bendy-like and I look like a stretchy doll. Smiling, knowing I don't feel natural when I smile and that likely my eyes are super wide, eyebrows raised, and I look freakishly overly caffeinated. "Squirrel. Squirrel!" The dog barked in full elation. That sums up my expression, surely.

Searching for bathroom key. The first threshold is reached. A sign reads, "The keys are near the dishes window." Back stepping. *Where is the dishes window? What is a dishes window?* Holding legs closer together. Calculating if I feasibly have enough time left. Found. *Which one do I take?* "Excuse me, Miss. Is this the right key?" Holding any random key up. Wondering how many bathroom doors there will be.

Next threshold. Go through door to find long hallways and more doors and more signs! Staring at a door with numbers that look like an old push-button phone. *Do I need a code, too? What if someone is already inside?* I hear water running. *Do I wait? How do I scan this frickin' plastic key card?*

A lovely young man arrives, and smiles. "Do you need help? Are you having trouble figuring out what to do?"

"Ummmm," I say meekly, with goofy teenage grin. "What if someone is inside? Do I enter?"

He is smiling, I think, but I can't tell because I am staring at my boots. He offers, "You can just . . ."

And POOF, the door magically opens as the other female patron exits, and I slip inside, red-faced and flustered and scolding my cute little kidneys. Mission accomplished.

Quick phone photo (a.k.a. *selfie*) of me, a relieved woman looking (not surprisingly) drunk and haggard.

As I'm summing up the last details of my excursion in typed print, the friendly-looking gentlemen to my left (lots of men in this coffee shop) pauses, then glances my way and asks, "Would you mind keeping an eye on my laptop for a minute?" Overly zealous, I accept. I must look trustworthy, I think. Or remind him of his mother. The irony of the handsome lad's question settles in. I spend the next five nervous minutes wondering what I would actually do if someone snatched up his laptop. *Would I chase them? Would I scream?* I panic. So much for designating Thursdays as my public outing days.

74. I Think He Likes Me

"I think he might like me," I told my husband, in reference to a man at a coffee shop.

"What do you mean?" my husband asked.

"Well, he was smiling and taking interest in me," I answered.

"Honey, he doesn't like you. He doesn't even know you. He might be attracted to your body or something about you physically. That is different from *liking* you."

"Oh," I answered.

The next day as I was heading out the door to go to the grocery store, my husband warned, "Remember, if a man looks at you because he is attracted to you, that doesn't indicate that the man necessarily likes you. You are a pretty woman who some men find attractive. But their attention doesn't mean they like you." I found his words to be a mixture of both comfort and confusion.

I am slowly, very slowly, learning the social innuendos regarding communication with men. I never knew there were this many unspoken rules. It's fair to say I've got the woman-to-woman social interactions down. Though now there seems to be this whole other guidebook regarding the male species. I think as a child, because I did not have the example of a stable father-and-mother relationship, nor brothers, or even uncles that I knew well, meant that I never had the chance to really learn how to interact with a man, except television characters and single men in my life I sought to make my husband (starting at age six). And I guess, too, the actions of predators, in combo with the uncouth behavior of some other males, added to my confusion of my place in the world as a female.

Today I feel so very alien and unprepared for Earth as I approach the male zone. To date, almost any adult male seems to put a magical spell of nervousness, meekness, neediness, and insecurity upon me. I naturally become a shy giggle machine, complete with batting eyes and flushing cheeks. And I still don't understand the nuances of male/female communication. I don't understand how much I should look into a man's eyes, how close I should stand, how I should smile, what my tone should sound like, what topics are socially appropriate. I don't understand what most people learn through experience or just know innately. I am starting to understand how I surely give out mixed signals, matching and mirroring a male, thinking that reacting like a mirror image is the safe and appropriate technique. In dealing with male encounters I don't want to come across as a prude, or rude, or stuck-up, or extremely shy, or as a flirt. I just want to come across as me. The problem is I don't know what that looks like.

When I returned home from the grocery store, I explained to my husband about my encounter with a handsome store employee that took place while I was trying to determine what dessert wine to purchase. In my retelling of the events, my husband took in the observations of my encounter and reported that likely this man was somewhat interested in me. He explained that if a man, instead of a woman, had approached and asked this employee about wine, the worker likely would have been shorter in his explanation, not have locked eyes the entire time, and not smiled and offered out his favorite wines for five minutes straight. He wouldn't have been standing as close either.

I still don't know. I told my husband, in all seriousness (and while slightly tipsy from the port wine in hand), that I'd like him to come to the store the next time, stand back an aisle or two away, watch how men approach and interact with me, and then report if they are flirting. He said, "Honey, I really don't take pleasure in watching other men pick up my wife."

Hmmmmmmmmm. Hadn't thought of that.

75. Light Returned

My husband and I both agree that a light has returned, a light I think I lost about the age of thirteen, when the fear of what life entailed set in. At times, I truly feel like I went away for a couple decades, just slipped out because life was too much. I don't know who took my place, but it wasn't me. I look back at this woman I was and I don't recognize her. I truly don't. I know she was in essence a part of me. But she wasn't me. I know the light returned because despite the trials of my life, I never gave up hope. I never let the world destroy my heart. I never stopped loving. I never stopped believing I could make a difference. Even when I wanted to die, I kept moving forward. I've known since I was a young child I would be called to be a healer, probably at the age of four, when I stopped eating lamb because I didn't have the heart for it. Probably again when I was nine years of age, when I hid in the bushes weeping because I couldn't comprehend the vastness of the universe and the depths of human suffering. Probably again when I was a teenager, and I would sit with people in convalescent homes just so I could be near the lonely at heart. I knew I was a healer when I became a teacher, and later when I served as an advocate for children with special needs. I knew I was a healer when I was called to write. What I didn't know was the profound effect the healing would have on my own life. I didn't know how deeply I would be blessed.

76. Dear Soul of Mine

I love you. I see you. I hear you. I believe you. I believe in your experience and perception. I believe in your efforts and hopes. I know you. And I adore you. There is nothing you can do or say that will change this. I have the potential to love you in all seasons, through storms, and through merriment. I will not leave your side, nor your heart. I am you. You are beautiful. And because you are so beautiful, a spring of fresh light and goodness, I shall always love you. There is only pureness in you. I choose this. I choose to see the glorious child you are. I see through that which is not you. I see into your true form, and this makes me weep with joy. How lovely you are, in all your seasons, in all your ways. How perfectly lovely, my adored one.

77. FIXATIONS, SPECIAL INTEREST, AND REGURGITATION

As I was driving home today I had this entire post (and the next one) play out in my head in six minutes. Sometimes I wish I had a recording device for my thoughts to enhance my recall and make the regurgitating that much easier. As I know, in recollecting what said brain was processing, I can never do the initial thoughts justice. The aftermath, or later resulting spillage, I reckon is more akin to a person who appeared a beauty at the start of the day, only to be haggard and worn by night's calling.

So here I sit—haggard in thoughts.

What was happening in my brain earlier was a symphony of processing and understanding. A further easement into the essence of this person I currently seem to be. I made it clear to myself, or some other source did (e.g., Jungian collective unconscious, alien brain lock, hot chocolate mixed with coffee—you decide), a greater understanding of my vast and complex mind. Here is how it looked, or sort of looked, untamed in form at best.

The thoughts that crossed my mind, or more so did wheelies in my brain, included the classification of *fixations* and *special interests*. Special interests are something that I always have that don't go away—ever. I find pleasure in special interests; and, to a degree, they are a means of release, escape, and comfort. My special interests have always centered on writing, poetry, music, reading, healing work/counseling, teaching, health/sickness, the meaning of life, and, to an extent, verbally processing with other people (a.k.a. I like to talk to someone beyond myself). I have had all of these special interests since I was a small child.

While special interests remain a stagnant part of my life, fixations come and go. I move through fixations like one might move through fad diets: one month this—three months later that. And with each new fixation I think: This is the one! This is what I've been waiting for. (Kind of like I did with men in my youth.)

In the last year alone, I have fixated on editing my writing, photography of nature, photographs of myself, (obsessive) mirror staring, poems specifically related to spiritual awakening, walking many miles, organizing my house, feng shui, cooking from scratch, and watercolor painting. Fixations on things always involve my active participation. There is a gray area in distinguishing whether or not I am actually fixated on the thing itself, the action, or the hopeful results. It's likely a combination. When I am fixated on something it preoccupies my mind. Everywhere I go I am thinking of this fixation to some degree, and in everything I do I am making a connection to how my fixation can feasibly be molded and blended into my current day. For instance, when I was a middle school teacher I wanted to make picturesque bulletin boards about the Inca and the Mayan cultures. In this case everywhere I went I was thinking about resources, primarily expired National Geographic magazines to collect, cut out, and use to create bulletin boards and slideshows. Other examples of resources for this particular fixation included used bookstores, secondhand stores, garage sales, libraries, etc. I couldn't tell you if my fixation was the creation of the displays, the need to teach, the collection of magazines, or the collection of knowledge about Incas and Mayans. I just know it was a fixation that lasted a few months. And then *whamo*, the fixation was gone.

78. Fixations, Special Interest, and Regurgitation Part Two

Two things about my fixations are the following:

1. They last a few months.

2. When I'm in the middle of a fixation, I have this constant dialogue within myself that goes something like this: "This is a fixation. It will pass. You are trapped in the cycle again. How can you get yourself out?" . . . Pause . . . "No, you are not. This is something you will do forever! This is your passion. You have found the *thing* you long for. This is it!"

I get lost in my fixations and use them as a means of escaping my overwhelming emotions, nonstop thoughts, and my anxiety. Of course my fixation has never been the *one*, the answer, or the new long-lasting special interest. The fixation always fades. Each of my fixations is like a light bulb of sorts. I do and do and do. I learn and learn and learn. I collect and collect and collect (or research, learn, play, partake, etc.), and then the light bulb filament burns out, breaks, and I am left with no interest whatsoever at all in a subject that once consumed my entire day—and mind.

During this time of *light-snuffed*, I might seep into a slight depression or sadness. It's akin to suffering a loss, only more abstract and unattainable in the manner of pinpointing the pain. I might have feelings of guilt about how I had been distracted and not present for my loved ones. And with the return to real life and release of the fixation, I will question, *Where was I? What just happened?*

There are two separate types of fixations I have: fixation on a thing, action, goal, research, hobby, etc., and fixation on a person. For some reason my person-based fixation lasts a long time. The thing I recognize now about fixating on a living, breathing person versus an inanimate object (activity, project, etc.) is that there is a definite, definable give-and-take—a dance, so to say—between two people, wherein the fixation gives back in a notable and concrete way, transforming continually. While I could drown myself in facts about an inanimate thing—say a freebie website (where I could learn all I could and order free stuff for months)—and eventually hit a point where enough is enough (because there is only so much I can learn and gather about a freebie site before I grow bored and disinterested), with a person, the situation is different. With a person, there isn't a stopping point until I am emotionally drained or suddenly seem to wake up.

79. ATTACK OF THE KILLER SHEETS

On arrival, my middle son said straightaway, "I don't like the smell of this place."

Upon entering the spacious motel, I tried to get into my place of Zen. In considering the room, I contemplated my good fortune. We had fresh water, shelter, blankets, warmth, electricity, and more. I snapped myself out of the disappointment zone without calling myself names like *spoiled* and *unappreciative*. I began to list in my head everything the motel had to offer, right about the time my husband came out of the oddly angled bathroom (toilet juts out and causes one to bruise knee when passing) and announced, "Don't forget to add that the floor slopes down at an odd angle to your list of 'why this place is cheap.'"

He knows me so very well.

So, I'm listing the positives off to myself: Internet connection. Oldest son has own bed. Even though I can't use my bath salts, as there is no bathtub, there is a quaint stand-up shower. Mold is only on the outside of the shower door. The smell of cigarette smoke, and what seems to be wet dog, is not too strong. There are other cars in the parking lot, which means other people stay here, too. No hair that I can see, dog or human. The sparkles glow that are set in the cottage-cheese-like ceiling. I don't think I can get asbestos poisoning unless someone jams a fork or something up there. The glass lamps painted poop-brown from the inside out that are all cracked and broken make for an interesting type of abstract art. I wasn't electrocuted when I turned on the lamp. The boys won't be fighting over television channels. The main door lock sticks and we can't use it, but that chain should hold up for the night. The light from the parking lot will serve as a giant night-light. We don't have rooms below us or above us, and on either side of our room are storage garages. The boys can be loud and no one will hear. We don't need to use the noisy heater that heats up the room too fast, especially since the curtains hang right over the heater, because if it gets cold, we can pretend we are camping. This would be a cool setting for a *Fargo*-type movie or for the series *Breaking Bad*. If anyone died in here, it was likely a long time ago. I haven't slept in a full-size lumpy bed for years. The lacquered wall art of trees reminds me of my youth in the 1970s. I have both thick socks and slippers on, so I'll be good to walk on the carpet.

I'm working on my list of gratitude when my husband chimes in, "And these walls remind me of my mother's family room." He's pointing to the fake wood paneling and laughing. I fake a smile and then whisper to him, "I probably shouldn't tell the boys to stop rolling in the bedspread because the bedding is likely not laundered, and adults could have done any a number of things on those covers, right?"

"Yes, hon. Not a good idea," he answers, with his trademark I-married-a-loon-that-I-adore shake of the head.

Right about then, my son who has Aspergers pipes in: "Have you seen what they can find with those special blue lights in hotels?"

My husband and I politely ignore him.

In the bathroom, after bumping my knee, I notice that there is no shampoo, no hair dryer, and no supplies beyond toilet paper, Kleenex, four wrapped plastic cups, and a stack of some ten miniature soaps. *Ten tiny soaps wrapped in brown paper?* I come out of the narrow bathroom and soon my Zen attitude is promptly invaded by a case of the sillies, and everything spills out of my head out loud in the form of a verbal tag game of why this would be considered a dive hotel. Of course, I won when I pointed out that there was no coffee or coffee maker. Still the little voice in my head circulated and percolated, reminding me to be grateful. After all, there was a Starbucks nearby.

This brings us to tonight, and me explaining to my husband why I couldn't sleep while in the motel. This is how the conversation went:

"Well, it wasn't really your snoring that kept me up. That was just a small part of it." I paused, not so much for effect, but because I knew I was going to bust up laughing, even though I was entirely serious.

I continued. "I couldn't sleep because . . . (searching for words) . . . I couldn't sleep because I was afraid I might . . . touch the sheets."

My hubby held back his chuckles. "But you had your sleeping bag, pillow, and blanket from home."

"I know," I said. "But I was still afraid I would accidentally touch the sheets."

Full laughter. "So you were lying there asleep and then you'd wake up with a jolt, look to your side, and think the sheets were monsters?" He stiffened his body straight out on the bed and pretended to be too terrified to move an inch. "But you were in a sleeping bag," he added.

"I know," I said, "but I was afraid if I fell asleep my arm might flop out and . . ."

My husband interjected: "And accidentally graze the sheet!"

"Yes," I answered, laughing hysterically.

80. Vignette, Collapsed Star, Age 9

It was an ordinary night for a child who had grown accustomed to the unordinary. My dog Justice trembled under the bed while the music of Led Zeppelin vibrated through the wall. Inside the sheets, all wrapped up in Mother's essence of Jean Nate bath oil and sandalwood, I tossed and turned. Then I laid listless and awake—a lump of boredom. I could smell the funny smoke again and hear bottles clinking. I pleaded with God, "Please make the people go away." All at once, a melodic voice called out, "Hello, little girl." But I knew the voice wasn't God, for I was certain my God didn't have a Jamaican accent.

"We didn't know you were in here, pretty lady. I'm sorry if we woke you," the voice apologized, as a figure approached Mother's bed. I leaned over casually on my arm, wanting to seem mature and interesting. "You didn't wake me," I responded, with a fake yawn, tapping my little chin with my tiny fingers. Justice let out a slight yelp. I was accustomed to seeing strangers in the house. I wasn't nervous in the slightest. I liked meeting Mother's friends. They were all interesting in that odd way.

The man with skin like chocolate syrup winked at me. I shot up—all big eyed and bouncy—and just about jumped out of Mother's bed altogether, thinking this broad-shouldered man would work quite well for a piggyback ride. Another man, with skin like milk, was grinning at the foot of the bed. "Sweet girl," he said. "We're not here to bother you. You just sleep." His voice was boring. But I smiled anyway, my rogue eyebrow standing at alert. The stranger with the milky skin stroked his hand across his dimpled chin and shifted his weight from side to side. His prickly face grew tight and then relaxed. "Ben asked us to get something out of the room for him," he offered.

"What does Ben need?" I asked.

The men didn't answer. Neither one. Instead they seemed to be playing a game, a pretend game of not hearing me. The chocolate man stayed at my side and spoke so low that I could barely make out his words. "It's nothing for you to worry about," he said, and then dabbed his forehead with a red kerchief. He continued, "I'm worried because Ben specifically told us not to wake you. And now, pretty one, you are very much awake."

My heart fluttered. I pushed my lips out in a perfected pout. The stranger at the bedside shuffled his feet as I drew my eyes to his tall forehead. He motioned to his friend to leave the room. "I know you won't tell," he said, with a quick survey of Mother's dresser. Then suddenly, his whole body lit up. And I could see an idea had found him. "Do you know how you can tell a star from an ordinary girl?" he asked, his melodic voice rising on the word "star."

I shook my head back and forth, curious.

"A movie star can close her eyes without fluttering her lids," he said.

I gave him a sideways stare and my best shifty eyes.

"I bet you could be a movie star," he said.

I thought of Shirley Temple Black and nodded in agreement.

"Try it. Try to close your eyes now, pretty girl."

I leaned back on my pillow and squeezed my eyes closed. Dreams of starring on the show *Love Boat* danced in my mind. Something rattled on the dresser. But I didn't open my eyes. The stranger sighed. Still I didn't open my eyes. I was that good!

The stranger's voice echoed. "You are perfect. You are a star. Don't stop now."

Self-elation oozed out of every pore of my body. I was on top of the world. I was extraordinary. I remained still, and then stiller, until there was only me, only my dreams, and I drifted to sleep.

I awoke refreshed and alive, and back in my own bed. I got up and looked in the bathroom mirror. I was pretty. I was good. I was talented. I was to be a star! I swept my arms back and forth and glided into the kitchen—the best of the best entering the stage in evening gown and princess smile. I waved as if on a parade float. I practiced my shy giggle. I batted my big eyes.

And then suddenly, my world stopped. Ben, he huffed. He hunched. He heaved.

I froze. And the stardom dropped out of me. Right then and there. Plop. I looked at Mother. I looked at Ben, her lover. And then I looked at my big toe. It was shorter than its neighbor toe.

"Shit," Ben said, scratching his stubbly round face. "Those assholes took the entire stash! All the cash, even your shitty jewelry!"

I peeked up toward Mother's unkempt hair. Mother shook her head and sighed. The scenes from the night before played out in my mind—the men—the room—my eyes—my eyes closed . . . I couldn't form words. The whole of me was frigid and stuck. The sting of one thousand wasps found way to my inner parts. I wasn't extraordinary after all, I thought.

I was nothing good at all.

81. Pointy Boobs

Yesterday I wore this fabulous red sweater. I was feeling very confident because I was having a good hair day. Plus my husband had been saturating me with compliments, at least twenty since daybreak. And after a hot sauna meditation and hot soak in Dead Sea salts, I was literally glowing. With my cheeks rosy, I set out to do errands. Time to redeem a gift certificate, a rebate check, and buy some food staples. At my third stop at a grocery store, while pushing my half-full cart down the snack aisle, I felt an itchy sensation at the nape of my neck. I reached down and found my sweater tag. My cheeks blossomed into a full crimson then, and all at once a rush of fear came over me as I realized my sweater was on backward!

I quickly, without calling too much attention to myself, turned my cart around and made my way to the back of the store. Retreating into the bathroom, I had a good look at my sweater in the mirror. I gasped while trying to laugh. But no laughter came. The way the sweater was set, with the backstitching in the front of me, made it look like I had two torpedoes jetting out. Before, while dressing at home, I'd merely thought the way the sweater set against my chest was just the way the sweater was made and that I ought not to have fretted about the design. I needed to get over my fears and wear clothes without insecurity. Who cares if the cut of the sweater accented what was naturally a part of me? But now that I could tell for certain the sweater was on backward, I thought for sure people would have noticed and would have been laughing, not only at my *backwardness* but also at my pointy boobs.

Inside the store bathroom, still contemplating my silliness, I twisted the sweater around only to find that my undershirt, a little sleeveless black thing, was on inside out! At this point I looked down at my boots, convinced I'd probably placed them on the wrong feet. I know it doesn't matter in the end. People at the crowded big-box store probably didn't truly notice, and if they did, they got a good laugh. And I'm all right with giving others a good laugh; nonetheless, I can't help but think about those two older men who stopped me in my tracks in the grocery store prior to my discovery, how they played dodge with my shopping cart, like we were two familiars partaking in a friendly game: "Try to get past me with your cart!" I can't help but think how ridiculous I must have looked with my front side all pointy and pronounced and all, as they tried to engage me in conversation and keep me from moving. It's just plain crazy, the way I cannot dress my own body, likely an aftershock of having never liked or played with Barbie dolls; I should have taken notes, or at least practiced.

82. I Wish It Were Tuesday

Phone call to husband: "I had a rush of fear that you are cheating on me. You aren't cheating, right? It's just my brain, right? You love me?"

Text message (paraphrased) to both husband and good friend Steff: "I have a scratchy throat and feel achy. I am worried that the cold I had is trying to come back. Other people have colds that come back, right? It doesn't mean my immune system is bad and I'm dying, does it?"

Phone call to husband: "Honey, I'm not losing my mind, am I? How has my memory been? Have I been forgetful? Do I seem like my brain is degenerating?"

Seems I've had coffee today. Racing thoughts and borderline paranoia about health and relationships. I tried to not have coffee for two days and quickly slipped into a state of increased pain, fatigue, and melancholy. With coffee (spiked with organic hot chocolate) my energy is tripled, my esteem increased, and my mood is mostly happy. I got a lot done this morning, with the help of the aforementioned caffeine and sugar combo. I feel satisfied when I get things done. I feel guilty when I'm a couch spud—which I am when my pain and fatigue is at its peak. I've been working to find balance, a careful ratio of just enough caffeine and not too much. I've been trying combinations of green tea and coffee and chocolate.

Everything in my life seems to be dependent upon balance and ratio. I'm often at one extreme or another of something, some experience or some thought. Everything and everyone affects me at some level. A new day is never easy. The act of waking and moving takes enormous energy. Not the opening my eyes part, but the actual being alive part. I'm not depressed, not normally, and I'm not lacking esteem or joy for the day. In truth, I like my life. I love my family. And I find great happiness in the world I've created for myself. Waking up isn't hard because of what is ahead of me or what's on my proverbial plate of opportunity. What is difficult about rising to a new day is the fact that I have to move, I have to think, and I have to make decisions. Some days I am immobilized for hours on the couch because the thought of having to make one more decision is too overwhelming.

Upon awaking, thoughts bombard me. For example: What is the best way to approach my day? What is the meaning of "the best?" Who established "the best?" Why are the establishers right? When will the best approach change? What are truisms and what are lies? What is the base of reality? Who am I? Where is the balance between giving and taking? When am I taking too much? Am I present enough, available enough, loving enough? I need to let go. I need to relax. I need to just be. But how do I turn off my mind? What should I do first? Should I shower? Should I move across the bed, around the bed? Straight to the bathroom? Should I rest more? Did I get enough sleep? And on and on and on. I awake to my thoughts, and my thoughts exhaust me.

I have managed to weed out most of the self-doubt and negative thoughts about myself. This is a great accomplishment. I have managed to interweave positive self-talk and positive affirmations into my day. This is helpful indeed. I have managed to find release through the creation of painting and writing. This is a comfort. I have managed to understand myself in great depth. This is useful. Yet I have not managed to decrease my intelligence, my ideas, the bombardment of what is, what isn't, and what mysteries have yet to be uncovered. And with so much going on inside my head, somehow my brain has forgotten to dissect and digest the basics.

Perhaps this is the executive functioning part of the frontal lobe of the brain misfiring or being disconnected at some level. As the basics—the seemingly easy aspects of thoughts—become lost to me. The fact that the day of the week is Tuesday slips away. The capacity to memorize times, dates, faces, places, names, and the like simply isn't there.

I have complex thoughts. I have the slipping out of common facts and knowledge, and then I have this need to classify and organize. Numbers are constantly on my mind: how they add up, where they show up, what they signify, how they can be shuffled and ordered. Apace with the numbers is previous data I've collected of the supposed rights and wrongs of *how to be*. The rights and wrongs of how to be a community member, a friend, a mother, a neighbor, a daughter, a lover, a wife, a cook, a writer, a shopper, a driver, and so on. I have this ongoing list of how I am supposed to be alongside an ongoing voice of how no one really knows how anything or anyone is supposed to be.

Simple things aren't simple. The task of buying shoes can be excruciating. I have the guilt of being able to buy boots when others cannot afford them. I have the questioning of whether or not the boots are saying too much or too little. (Does it appear I am trying to look young or am I looking foolish? Am I represented by these boots? Or is this a false projection of who I am? And who am I?) And then I am sad, standing there alone looking in the mirror, wondering why I can't just see boots.

Today, bombarded with thoughts, I forgot the day of the week. I went to my acupuncturist and he wasn't there. I called him and said, "I have written on the calendar that my appointment time is Tuesday at eleven. I think I might have made a mistake. I'm here and you are not. Please call me." He was quick to call me back. He politely said, "Yes, I have written down that your appointment is at eleven on Tuesday." Then he inserted a long pause, ample time for me to process. In response I digested his words. Soon a light bulb of recognition went off. Yes, indeed it was not Tuesday. It was Monday.

I was quick to respond, "Oh [giggle], I thought it was Tuesday. That's what's wrong. My apologies. I'll see you tomorrow." I hung up, convinced I was going senile or out of my mind. How could I know so much and think so much but not know what day of the week it was? And then the guilt, the embarrassment, followed by the positive self-talk and forgiveness of self, followed by the analysis of self-talk and praise. Followed by the wondering if I did the self-talk right. Followed by the thinking about thinking about thinking. My husband told me today that I am amazing. He praised my intelligence, my genius. I am happy he sees me this way. All the same, there are times, like today, I just wish it were really Tuesday.

83. MAY MY BOIL REST IN PEACE

I have a titanic boil right on the tip of my chinny-chin-chin. I don't usually get boils, at least not since I was a teenager. However, I had this streak of fixation of daily saunas followed by sea salt baths. The overheating, followed by drippy sweat, followed by the mineral oils in my last soak left my chin all hived up and splattered with a gigantic, painful boil. I forced myself to leave the house, certain the bulging cyst was a red-flashing siren. I was so concerned that during my three stops to different stores, I had to go to the bathroom to look in the mirror to make sure the ripening zit had not suddenly exploded.

The first bathroom visit was uneventful. The second time I had to wait and wait and wait. A kindly couple finally came out, an elderly man pushing a woman in a wheelchair. I immediately felt guilty for having thought there was a fart-filled man in the bathroom taking his sweet time and stinking up the place. I don't mind waiting when I'm alone. But the whole time I was outside the bathroom door, I was standing next to a young man. While lingering in this narrow hallway, I kept staring at my cellular phone pretending I was reading. Thinking all along that this guy likely thought I was addicted to my phone. I did all I could do to keep from making conversation. My only wish at that moment, beyond wanting the patron in the potty to flush and be done with his task, was to not have to look at this man at all.

It was finally my turn. Of course, I didn't really even have to pee. Nonetheless, I flushed the toilet just in case someone was in earshot. I noted there were no seat covers (empty) and no paper towels (empty). I was processing the missing paper products, in all my fluster, when I absent-mindedly left my phone atop the paper-towel holder (while I shook my hands). I had had to wash my hands just in case the person listening out for my flush was also checking in to see if I had washed my hands after doing my (imaginary) business.

When I returned to my cart and entered the produce aisle, I panicked fast. After checking my jacket pockets and emptying my purse, I realized I'd left my phone in the bathroom. *Crap.* I returned to the cramped waiting area. Someone was in the bathroom, again. I thought about my abandoned phone sitting helplessly alone and how I definitely needed to remember to log out of Facebook. Fifty thoughts later and the door opened. Naturally, it was the same man I'd been avoiding out of fear of human contact. He had my phone and a big smile. He handed over the phone and I mumbled some nonsense indicating thanks. Thanks to my boil, I'd spent a good twenty minutes in the store doing absolutely nothing beyond bathroom stalking.

Outside of the hallway I strongly thought about letting an employee know the bathroom was missing paper products, but I didn't want to talk to anyone. I decided to just keep my mouth shut. Of course, as I'm processing this need to not socialize, I grab onto an organic pear, and my thumb presses right through it.

"Yuck," I announced, loudly enough for the older lady next to me to overhear.

"Oh," she responded. "You really ought to take that to an employee. That's what I do when something like that happens."

I smiled, thinking of how unsolicited advice sometimes sucks. I slid the pear to the corner of the fruit stand and said, "I'm sure they will see it here. This way no one else will get their hands all sticky." I could see immediately that this stranger was not too pleased.

"I think there is a garbage nearby," she insisted. And then she glanced over again at the employee.

In retrospect, a braver me would have chucked the pear at the lady's face. Begrudgingly, I looked down at the isolated thumb-crushed pear. I made a face. I didn't want to touch it. I then felt positively foolish and offered an excuse—albeit a sort of lie (but not a full lie). I said, in an attempt to justify my pear-retrieval hesitancy, "Well, I really would rather they put it in the compost."

"They have a compost here?" she asked.

Therefore, yes, in the end I had to go up to the worker stacking groceries and explain about the broken pear. Though I was sure not to mention the toilet seat covers. Indubitably, I was overcome with anxiety and had to thusly spill out said events to the young girl ringing up my groceries. I explained to her all that had happened and she just kind of looked up quizzically, saying something like, "At least you found your phone."

I wanted to tattoo *socially inept* across my forehead.

My final shopping excursion event found me in the parking lot chatting it up with a lady my age. I was telling her all about my van door that would not close because the sliding-door latch was frozen over, and how all the way to the store my light was blinking on and off, and the van was singing a *ding-ding-ding* noise. She was excited to report that for the first time ever she couldn't roll up her van window because of the cold weather. "What a coincidence!" she exclaimed. I liked her immediately and noted this brief encounter as the highlight of my day.

84. THE STAR OF MY POST

I panicked this morning. I pulled my husband out of the bathroom. He was stripped down to his boxers. And I was mean. I don't like when I am mean. I hate it. At the core I am nice. But this mean, panicky part surfaces at times. She especially appears when I am feeling bombarded with change and sensory overload. When my normal routine is drastically altered, I get a bit crazed, and then my scale of unpredictable outcries is undeniably both potent and dramatic.

This morning the birthday sleepover for my youngest boy was almost over. There had been much noise and upheaval as the boys celebrated together and tore the daylight basement apart with their slathering of snacks and soda. I'd not fallen asleep until nearly two in the morning, and I'd cleaned and organized and shopped and prepared the entire day before. My husband had been a great support, as much as any human could be who didn't possess superpowers; notwithstanding, by morning, he, like me, was exhausted. And unlike me, he was ready to get out of the house and start a course of errands.

He headed downstairs to shower, while I was wrapping up the party and awaiting the arrival of the two last guardians to pick up the party guests. After twenty minutes of feeling a kneading, unidentifiable discomfort inside, suddenly a shock of revelation hit me—*two strangers were about to appear at my door!*

As I thought about this fact, I was bombarded with what-ifs, and what to say, and how to stand, and how to smile, and how to be, and how to stop my own very self-consuming fear of being seen by another human being. My anxiety grew. I wanted to duck under a blanket to escape and to not face anyone. Suddenly an all-encompassing fear bit at me like a disobedient hound. I logically processed. I figured this biting and uncontrollable fear was part of my Aspergers, part of how my brain worked, part of who I was and had always been. The feelings weren't unfamiliar, not even more intense. Nevertheless I was more aware. Still, even with the understanding,

I could do little or nothing to calm myself down. At any moment there would be a knock at the door and a stranger would appear. I talked to myself in silence. I reasoned. I tried to logically stop the worries and concern. I knew there was nothing to fear. Still I feared. I knew there was no threat. But I felt threatened. I wanted to run.

The doorbell rang. It was the first stranger. She was kind and courteous. We didn't have opportunity for small talk because her nephew had gathered his things quickly. I shut the door after wishing them well and sighed in relief. I felt half of the anxiety leave. Only one to go.

I attempted to self-soothe, to talk myself into the fact that I was safe. But I couldn't. Though half the anxiety had left, the remaining panic was fresh and alarming, clawing from the inside out. I just couldn't do it. Not alone. Not by myself. Not with all the uncertainties. Fear rushed in. I darted down the stairs in a state of meltdown. I was imploding and exploding all at the same time. The outside me, the observer who sometimes watches (and takes note of my behavior and who is often able to laugh or offer sound advice) had been swallowed up in the confusion of my emotions. I had to find my husband, make sure he was dressed, and get him upstairs right away. There was no time to wait. My soul was on fire! I found him in his boxers doing something in front of the mirror. I don't remember what. Everything was a jolted blur of chaos. "Please hurry. He will be here any moment, and you know how I am," I whined.

I looked my husband over and realized he hadn't showered. It had been twenty minutes and he still hadn't showered! "What have you been doing?" I queried, rudely. "This whole time you could have showered and you didn't. Why didn't you? Why did you leave me up there alone? Why? You don't get me. You don't know me. What do you not understand about Aspergers? What do I fear the most? What do I fear the most?"

My husband stammered with his eyes and braced himself against the bathroom door. I could see he was processing my emotional state. I could sense the familiarity of his experience, how he knew I was on the verge of freaking out and that his next move would either create a domino effect of me collapsing into hysteria or serve to bring me out somewhat from my spinning panic. He stepped closer and waited, waited in a way and with a skill I have not yet learned and doubt I ever will. I felt a reckoning of sadness, a knowing I was different, odd, and displaced on a planet where my skill set had never been completed, where my toolbox of communication skills was vastly depleted.

I wept inside, until the fear rose again. I went on fast with an unrelenting urgency. I knew what I was doing and what I was feeling, and it all felt ridiculous and unnecessary and unfounded and just plain stupid. Nevertheless, I couldn't help myself. I was trapped in a prison of jumbled thought and worry.

I said more, my words not chosen carefully, my panic taking the wheel. "You abandoned me. You abandoned me. You say, 'You take it from here. I'm going to shower,' and you leave me to face the strangers. You know how I am! How could you do this?" My eyes welled with a mixture of tears and rage. I was on the verge of flipping my husband off. About to mount the stairs and, with a quick turn of my back, turn and give him the finger. I was so confused. My emotions all jumbled and twisted into a crisis.

Regardless, I stood my ground, even as I saw another path of what I might have done, how I might have taken off as I told him off. I stared past him, fighting back the urge to yell, "I hate you!"

He didn't move or even flinch, but looked at me with such profound patience. I knew I was being childish. I knew at that moment he was the only adult in the house.

"Your worst fears are talking to strangers, especially at the door and to men," he replied. He then said, with a sigh, "I'll wait to shower. I'm coming upstairs. Be right there."

Within two minutes I was back on the couch, hiding behind my laptop, and my husband was in the leather chair twiddling his fingers and playing with his cellular phone. I said, "Stop picking at your lip. That bugs me." I said, "I don't understand. Don't you care? Why did you do this to me?"

He looked at me blankly and replied. "I didn't shower. I came up here for you because I love you." I waited for him to be triggered or upset or to show emotion. I needed him to be emotional. I needed him to take me out of my emotional state by means of his emotional state, to be able to focus on his wavering feelings and to blame him, in order that I might escape self-blame. I punched at him with my words. He didn't care. He didn't. He didn't know how to show love, is all I could think.

He got off of the couch and came to my side and held me. I didn't feel release. I'd wanted to blame him and make him act a certain way, thinking his behavior would bring relief. It didn't. He stayed at my side while I maneuvered through the stream on my Facebook wall. He was watching the posts, watching me, and in my space. I looked at him and said, "Thanks for the hug. Can you go away now? I don't want you near me. Please leave." I recognized the cruelness and impatience in my voice. I sensed my selfishness and sporadic ways. I couldn't help myself. I was in the middle of a meltdown, and nothing my husband did or said could help. My husband rolled his eyes and shook his head. I offered out some half apology for my behavior, knowing I'd been terrible. I tried to make him laugh. "Well at least you might be the star of my post," I offered. I don't think he smiled.

85. MANAGING SIR BRAIN: THINGS THAT "AIN'T" WORKED YET

Here is my experience, to date, searching for ways to manage Sir Brain:

1. **Exposure Therapy**: For years I thought if I just socialized more, if I just connected more and tried harder to be like everyone else, then my endurance level for social gatherings would improve and my anxiety levels would decrease. I believed that through repeated exposure things would get better. That has yet to happen.

I don't have a fear or phobia to any *one* thing or event; therefore, there is nothing I can focus on overcoming or having less fear about. My anxiety isn't caused by anything I can pinpoint. My anxiety is caused by the way I process the stimuli in my environment and the way I respond to my surroundings. I am hyperaware and my senses are turned up to the utmost degree. I am also, despite self-training and studies, unsure of how to act in a social gathering (e.g., how much to share, when to share, when to stop, when to respond, how to stand, how to look, when to be less honest, etc.); and as a result of my uncertainty, I have a constant inner voice (LV: little voice in my head) reminding me of how to be. I need and long for structure and routine. My fear can be reduced if the same events happen in a similar way. However, inevitably changes occur. To say I will get better with practice or exposure is not an accurate statement. First of all, I am not wrong or in need of improvement. I am uniquely wired. One would not tell a person with a visual impairment that if she kept staring at a picture on the wall the image would become clearer, just as one would not tell a person with a hearing impairment to repeatedly listen to a song on high-volume to improve his or her hearing. In the same line of thinking, one should probably not tell me to continue to go outside of my comfort zone in order to eventually gain a sense of security. I do not have the physical capacity. This is not biologically possible for me (or for Sir Brain).

2. **Cognitive Behavior Therapy (CBT)**: While Asperger's Syndrome often has coexisting conditions of generalized anxiety disorder (GAD), obsessive-compulsive disorder (OCD), and mood disorders, such as depression, Aspergers is not the sum of its parts. A person cannot be treated for the coexisting conditions and then grow out of Aspergers. If anyone says they outgrew Aspergers or "cured" themselves, then I don't believe they were Aspie to begin with—unless they've feasibly learned how to reprogram their brain. I do not think there is a way to change my brain; and as hard as my life can be, I don't like the idea of my brain changing. (Sir Brain concurs, nodding adamantly in fear and searching for his suitcases.)

Aspergers is not a mental illness. Why and how the condition develops is still largely unknown, though there seems to be an obvious genetic factor. While positive self-talk has many benefits and can decrease episodes or the degree of anxiety and depression, and perhaps even diminish some OCD tendencies, it does little to help with Aspergers itself. No matter how much self-talk I employ, there are times I still respond in a fight-or-flight manner. I do not want to feel anxious and do not choose to feel nervous; nonetheless, this is the way I feel. Self-talk and cognitive behavior therapy techniques can sometimes do me (and LV and Sir Brain) more harm than good. When I am panicking, no matter how many times I incorporate positive self-talk or implement cognitive behavioral techniques (e.g., replace negative belief that is a falsehood with a true reality-based belief), my body continues to respond as if I am in danger. When I do implement the self-talk, in an attempt to do the "right" thing or to "fix" myself, I then feel guilty when the technique I employed does not work. I then question why I was not capable of applying such a simple concept to my own way of thinking. No amount of practice, hard work, or scouring through books has increased the effectiveness of cognitive-based therapy techniques for me. And the more I use them and fail, the more I feel as if I am wired in a way that is wrong. What does help is letting go and realizing that the panic is something I have to go through, and realizing that when I am on the other side I will be okay. And recognizing there is nothing wrong with what I am doing or going through. It is just the way I am. So in a way I am using positive self-talk, but not in the traditional sense. I am not finding a false statement or belief and fixing it. Instead I am self-soothing and reminding myself I will be okay regardless of how I feel at a particular moment. I use my thoughts like a type of security blanket. The best thing for me to do in times of anxiety is not to retrain my brain to talk better to me (LV), but to retrain me to treat my brain better (Sir Brain).

3. **Controlling Shutdowns**: I can't control myself sometimes. I thought if I read enough and studied enough that I could reprogram who I am at a core level. Nevertheless I cannot change this elemental core of Aspergers; and if I feasibly can, the answer stealthily eludes me. I have tried every way imaginable to knock some sense into me when I go into a mode of shut down, and still there is nothing I can do, beyond pushing through the uncomfortable emotions. When my anxiety is at its peak, I become immobile. I become trapped in a cycle or loop of thought. And the odd part is, I know what tools to implement that should supposedly pull me out. I also know they won't work on me. I have tried. Nothing works to stop the anxiety when it is in full swing. (Think Sir Brain and LV diving off a high diving board over and over.) It seems I have to go through the crashing of waves to come out cleansed and regenerated.

Days filled with too much sensory overload lead to days of shutdown. During this time, life seems bleak and not worth living; however, it does not feel *hopeless*. I feel *fed up* more than anything else and exhausted by thoughts and life. My good hours are usually from when I wake up until midday. By midafternoon, I often become overwhelmed. (LV has been talking all day!) This is when I can do little more than sit on the couch. I cannot listen to someone talk for very long. I become like a computer with the memory capacity maxed out. There is no more room left for input. I have thought to scribe a list to remind myself during the high-anxiety, shutdown times of what I need to do to feel better. However, when I am in shutdown, I know that no list of any sort will help. It doesn't matter that I know why I am distressed and exhausted. Sir Brain is in lockdown. (Drowning and gasping for air!) I am protecting myself from short-circuiting. The last thing I need is logic or steps to follow. Cognitive reasoning only leads to further shutdown and retreat, and further bombardment. The only method that works is releasing control and letting myself go through the emotional process. If I do not let myself retreat, I will likely have a meltdown in which I shout and cry. I need time to decompress and be alone—time to process and discard of my abundance of emotions and thoughts.

4. **Displacing My Anxiety**. With self-recognition of Aspergers my behaviors have shifted. Despite this fact, Sir Brain's behaviors haven't changed. Before I didn't understand my emotions. Before a major event, like a party at my house, when I didn't know I had Aspergers, I would get extremely controlling and high-strung. I would order my husband around and start arguments. I would (subconsciously) create chaos in order to release the tremendous fear building up inside of me. My husband would often ask why I was angry and touchy before a party. I didn't know. I thought I was a controlling person and needed everything to go my way in order to be happy. The problem was I knew innately I didn't want to be controlling and I was never happy, regardless. It wasn't until I was diagnosed with Asperger's Syndrome that my behavior changed. Now, before an event, I no longer subconsciously create drama in an attempt to release emotion. I didn't consciously decide to change this; the change happened naturally. Now, I am hyperaware of why I am upset. I recognize my emotions in detail and the triggers that lead to anxiety. It might seem that knowing myself more would make the anxiety level decrease, but actually the anxiety is more intensified because I am no longer subconsciously utilizing displacement. I am not displacing my own dread about an event onto another event. I am not using or finding a scapegoat. I am not creating drama in order to diffuse my own tension. Instead, tension keeps building and I have no way to release it. Now that I am more aware of my own behavior and emotions, and the triggers, I do much more stimming, e.g., flick my nails, flap my hands, clear my throat, click my teeth, repeatedly saying "okay," and so forth. I also have anxiety dreams related to upcoming events. In addition, on the day of a happening I have extreme fluctuations of emotions and physical symptoms, such as hives and/or stomachaches. I am now taking in the full experience and my body is responding. I don't know if this is better or worse than the displacement. What is also happening is instead of "freaking out" before an event, I am often "freaking out" after the event. (Sir Brain and LV running around in circles in full panic after climbing out of the swimming hole, exhausted, to discover they are naked!) I feel very much like a child who holds herself together at school for the better part of the day, only to return home and have a meltdown. I have found, to

date, the best way to handle my anxiety is to not turn it into the enemy, or something to be eradicated and ejected, but instead something to be accepted. The more I fight the anxiety, the worse I feel, for there isn't any feasible avenue of solution that leads to rescue. I have to go through the discomfort in order to feel relief. The process is similar to a minor panic attack or adrenaline rush, but it passes. And the more accepting I am of the process, the quicker it passes.

5. **Making Plans**: Sometimes lists help, especially if there are no deadlines on the list. I like to make lists of chores or errands, and to cross out items as they are accomplished. I also like to rewrite new lists and to see how much the to-do items have diminished. Lists are my friends (and highlighters). Appointments on the calendar are not my friends. I remember my father was similar in his dislike of scheduled events. I would ask him if we could get together on such-and-such day, and he would typically respond that he couldn't tell me because making a commitment didn't feel comfortable to him. He did better with last-minute plans. I didn't understand at the time why my father acted this way. Today I understand my father better. He didn't want to make plans because he didn't want the stress of worrying about an upcoming event. I am the same way. I have been my whole life. The best days are days nothing is scheduled on the calendar. Even one appointment or obligation can cause anxiety for hours beforehand, sometimes even weeks. Without fail, the thought of having to pick up my sons from school each afternoon causes me acute stress. I leave at a set time daily, and the trip is short, easy, and uneventful; regardless, the stress does not dissipate. Usually two hours before a scheduled event, I start to become very preoccupied with the time and the steps involved in departing. I might glance up at the clock on the wall a dozen times during the span of thirty minutes. Simple tasks, like showering or getting dressed, feel overwhelming. It's not uncommon for me to spend the better part of an hour processing and reprocessing the pros and cons of showering. I often create a half-dozen scenarios of what sequence I should follow in preparation for my departure. Even before I've started the process of getting ready, I am typically mentally exhausted. When I view an upcoming event on the calendar, I experience a surging panicky feeling because I know in the near future I will go through cyclic bouts of fatigue, doubt, generalized anxiety, and feelings of inadequacy.

This seems contradictory in nature—the fact that I do well knowing what to expect and with routine, yet at the same time dread set plans.

I look forward to well-structured days indoors at home. However, the repeated isolation and lack of adult company can lead to depression and feelings of loneliness and "not enough." There is a continual pendulum of want inside of me. On one side there is the longing for company and stimulation found outside the home; on the other side, there is the longing to hibernate and to not have to experience the exhaustion and anxiety involved in going out. This pendulum moves back and forth. If I am not careful, I can self-punish by wishing I were different and more "normal."

6. **Forgetting about Aspergers**. I joke with myself sometimes. I think if I write enough and share enough, I will process the Aspergers right out of me. (Sir Brain and LV are hovering in the corner beneath a magenta blanket, terrified.) Some silly part of me believes I'll wake up and be "cured" of my Aspergers traits, and if not cured, then much better able to function. The truth is I don't need to be cured. I am not sick, or ill, or broken. I was born with a brain that is different from most of the general population. If society were different I would be responding differently. But society isn't different. I have tried ad nauseam to change myself, to try to fit in, and to try to function. And the more I try, the more I find I am battling the same resistance. What I have found that works is contact with other people who understand me. I feel safe with most people who are neurodivergent, and to a degree safe with people who would classify themselves as "artsy," "quirky," or "shy." I fit nicely with the "oddballs" and "misfits." I don't need to let go of Aspergers. I need to let go of isolation and thinking there is something wrong with me to begin with. The more I meet individuals with brains wired like mine, the more I learn to appreciate my uniqueness and beauty, and the more I recognize the depth of my own intelligence and empathy. I was created differently, but different is not wrong and need not be terrible. (LV and Sir Brain high-fiving) With the right balance of release and acceptance, and with the right connection with like minds, I am learning to navigate myself in this world. Where I used to believe I was dropped down on the wrong planet, I now believe that I am right where I am supposed to be.

86. NOTE TO PRETEEN SELF

I sometimes think if I could go back in time to meet my preteen self, I wouldn't. Mainly because of the whole butterfly effect and my inner dread of somehow erasing my own children, or possibly my own self. With that said, if I were able to travel back in time and actually be triple pinky promised by the Big Man in the Sky Himself that nothing would change in my life when I returned, and that my entire memory of the event would be wiped out, and that the girl (that is little me) would not be negatively affected in any way whatsoever or have her life altered drastically, and I could verify I was really talking to God, and get the archangels, all the great gurus, and talking trees to back Him up, then, and only then, would I maybe consider traveling back in time. I'd want an insurance contract, too, that guaranteed I wouldn't explode on impact, and I'd likely ask for a cute doctor of some sort to come along.

In meeting the younger me there are several things I'd want to say. Beyond the initial greetings, saturation of love, information about men and safe dating, lessons on proper etiquette and manners, the reassurance that all would turn out all right, and much more, I'd definitely want to set myself straight on the whole hygiene and puberty thing. I'd probably put the pertinent information into a list form, specifically explaining things I was relatively clueless about. The list would look something like this:

1) Brush the back of your hair. I went until my early forties not realizing that just because I cannot see the back of my head does not mean that everyone else cannot.

2) Look at your toenails every once in a while. Try to get into the habit of cutting them and cleaning them. Despite what you were once told, in an attempt to get you to cut your nails, you will not get nor die of toe fungus. Never. Stop obsessing. You'll always forget to cut your children's toenails, so teach them young or else they will look like little hobbits.

3) Remember that food gets stuck between your teeth. I know you don't like smiling in the mirror. Eventually your chipped, discolored, and dying

front tooth, and your extreme overbite, will entirely vanish. Look in the mirror, open your mouth, check in between your teeth, and floss. If you don't have floss, you can use a piece of your hair. If you learn this before you are a senior in high school, your boyfriend's older sister will not have to teach you these things in a public restroom.

4) Scrub your hair with your nails when you shampoo. Suds up the soap and scrub all over. Scrub hard and only use a dab of shampoo. The chemical shampoos will cause an allergic reaction. Start saving up now for the expensive natural alternatives.

5) I know you don't like washcloths. Even so, try to scrub behind your ears. You will discover in your forties that dirt collects there.

6) You don't need to go to the dermatologist at all the first four-plus decades of your life. The spot on your eyeball is a freckle. It will not kill you. It will not grow. It will not change. You only have like five dark freckles on your entire body, and the doctor will not consider that a concern or a lot. The red spots are red freckles. There is nothing they can do about the dark patches you got from pregnancy on your forehead and along your jawline except offer expensive laser treatment. Just wear a hat and sunscreen in the summer. When you move to the dreary Northwest, you'll be too pale most of the seasons to notice. (By the way, you will get every pregnancy side effect imaginable. Don't panic. You will be fine.)

After answering hygiene questions, I'd sit myself down and tackle the topic of puberty. Then I'd leave my little self a reference letter:

Those pictorial sexual-education books Mother gave us in third grade aren't going to help you in most areas. I know the nude beaches were creepy, but wait until you watch those movies in that Human Sexuality class you take during your first year of college. Maybe prepare a bit for that. Your bodily changes at age twelve will totally freak you out. Hair is supposed to grow in those places. Please, please, please try not to kiss so many boys. Perhaps fixate on a movie star and write him letters—a much better choice than boy chasing. Do not, I repeat, do not tell your friends everything. Do not tell anyone about kissing boys, your body, or fantasies. Write it out and don't show anyone. Keep it under lock and key. Try very, very, very hard to share nothing private with ANYONE. Remember we spent an entire day together, you and me, discussing the concept of PRIVATE. Do not under any circumstances draw pictures of boys' private parts, or the diagrams will get passed around middle school. I guarantee you will regret it. It's funny when you are thirty but so not worth it! The entire "here comes the period" drama . . . you are not bleeding to death. That terrible feels-like-your-guts-are-being-eaten-by-a-mutant-hamster-clan, those are called cramps. Take some pain reliever. It will improve after you have babies. Don't wait four months to tell your mother. The toilet paper won't work. Give Mom a note, if you are afraid to speak to her. And talk to her years before the event, so you can fill up an entire walk-in closet with supplies. Huge warning: Do not take the free samples of supersize expandable tampons that the PE teacher gives out in gym class! That should be illegal. But if you do by mistake, whatever you do, DO NOT USE THEM. Also, do not look too closely at that baby-birthing area after your first child. Your insides are not on the outside. I totally promise. The resulting emergency examination by your family doctor caused by your full-on panic freak-out episode will result in the same level of humiliation as the penis pictures in middle school. And goodness, use soap and water or shaving cream when you first shave, unless you want a scar atop the shinbone area of your leg the rest of your life. Oh, and don't announce to the other seventh graders standing in the lunch line, "Look, I got a new training bra." That circles back to the whole privacy thing.

87. NOTE TO THE LITTLE ONE

My wounded one, I see you. I see you there crying alone. I see you with your hands pressed against your fragile skin; your endless wonderment less chariot than dungeon, your blizzard mind a target for jagged daggers. Though you are fearful and doubled down with fear, though you are strangled, the agony rising and choking dragon from within, I see you; I see you there crying alone. I see you with your heart set out for all, freshly pierced and bled out upon your sleeve. Your efforts ignored, your desires stifled, your wishes buried with the agony and trembles. Your dreams trampled, your journey unknown, the light dimming and dimming. Though the isolation suffocates and pulls you further inward. Though the ground sinks beneath, trapping you in what can only be hell, I see you; I see you there crying alone. I see you, the streaks of your past spread across the room and painted black on each wall. Your moment passed, your joy forgotten, your answers diminished, a sunrise never set, your sense of isolation churning and twisting, your path unknown in its familiar confusion. Though the images of the future be blurred and joy feels beyond reach. Though the exhaustion breathes alive and misery claims you as chained companion, I see you; I see you there crying alone. I see you, your swollen eyes, your swollen love, your swollen wants and needs. Your sadness pouring and pounding out in waves, your veins split open and pouring hurt, your flesh a painful reminder of who you are and who you are not. Though you are crushed and beaten, bombarded by questions and uncertainty. Though abandonment seems certain and slumber your necessary avenue of escape, I see you; I see you there crying alone. I see you my sibling of this strange land, captive to the unknown hauntings. Your strength burdened with heaviness, your view one of bleakness and doom. Your begging a desperation born into being, your emptiness still empty. Though you be an injurious child, nailed to what appears to be destiny. Though you be a fallen star, burned out and spread upon the masses as aged ash, I see you; I see you there crying alone. I see you my precious earth traveler, your shoes worn, your feet bruised. Your image I hold, as I hold the most cherished of nature's treasures. Your journey I behold, as I behold the purifying waters of a revisited well. Though we be apart, I recognize you as my equal warrior. Though we be separate, I recognize you as my equal healer, for I see you; I see you there crying alone. I see you there calling out in the whispers of your silent ache, your beauty penetrating the deepest portion of my own existence, your strength fueling the carved-out substance of life that has surrendered. Though you feel blinded, your gift of being grants me the capacity to carry on. Though you feel unworthy, your gift of being grants me the capacity to see my light, I see you; I see you there crying alone. Your heart as my heart, your soul as my soul, your pain as my pain, your fear as my fear. Though we be temporarily burned within the flame of all-consuming mystery, though we be masked in a disguise of imprisoned misery, I see you; I see you there crying alone.

88. Imaginary Lines and Empathy

Recently there has been talk of people on the autism spectrum lacking a form of empathy—*cognitive empathy*. Before that there was talk of Aspergerians lacking empathy in general. Lacking in cognitive empathy implies a person cannot read between the lines of communication. While this might be a true experience for some people on the spectrum, and this theory might help some on their journey to self-discovery and understanding, and even in connecting with others, I do not believe I lack any type of empathy.

I am not lacking. I am not lacking in anything. In my world the word *lacking* does not exist. In my world *lack* is a manifestation of judgment, for I cannot lack without being compared to a *norm* or a *standard*. I cannot lack anything without being diminished in my worth and character. I adamantly claim I do not lack anything, and neither do you.

This world longs to classify and compartmentalize; yet, I know I am mystery beyond classification. In this knowing I have seen what divides us, the one from the other. At the base of all division is fear. I recognize that in claiming my true self and having no secrets that my own actions diminish fear.

Perhaps if I am lacking, I am lacking the ability to partake in imaginary games. I observe the rules and social customs—most, if not all, seemingly built to hide a part of self. I observe the whispers that speak, "If you are you in completion then you shall be hurt." I am an observer who knows the risks. And despite the claims of experts, I have learned to read between the lines. I have learned to read between the lines of pretending and falsehoods and lies and manipulations. I have learned that one word is replaced for another based on fear. I have learned that we are sometimes so afraid of being hurt or hurting another that human communication is a dance of avoidance.

We are told to embrace our individual selves. Only there exists this underlying message: "Be yourself, but don't make me uncomfortable in your being. Be yourself, but make yourself squeeze into my guidelines." These are the messages I find in between the lines. "Be, but not in totality."

I do not understand these lines that have been drawn and why they have been drawn. I do not understand why there are so many rules. I do not understand why others do not speak from their deepest self. I do not understand what everyone is hiding from. I am honest. I carry no manipulation. I have no intention to harm. I continually release anger and judgment. I recognize my humanness. I recognize my frailties. I pray for humility. I pray to recognize self in others. I state my own need for love and connection. I work my best to implement boundaries. I am gently assertive in nature. I practice coming from a place of acceptance and compassion. I believe people are doing their best. I forgive. And I forgive again. In this way there is nothing I have to hide.

Coming from a place of transparency, I question when one is hiding. I question what it is he or she is afraid I might see. Perhaps it is the very essence of me being real that stirs fear in another and makes him scream *lacking*. For what am I lacking beyond my incapacity to be none other than self?

89. BREATHE INTO ME

Let me not suffer for self alone. Let me suffer for all. In my own suffering may I find release in the reckoning that my suffering be not in waste, and not of need of rescue or refinement, only fortified by your wishes and every movement, blended with your glory and honor, and slaughtered out in division of whole as bounty for the wolves. Let me be the bait for the miserly and enticed ones; let me be the horror that the others seek in self, so I might find the avenue of retreat beyond the hauntings that no longer exist beneath your sheltered wings. Let me cry out to the world, loudly; make my own piercing deafen the silence that besets me. The silence of where I once stood in knowing. Whisper me back into the place of forgiveness. Speak me into being. Beyond the valley of your goodness, carry me home. Breathe into me. I beseech you. Breathe into me your goodness. Erase all that is flawed and forge all that is forgotten. Breathe into me. Awaken, refueled and renewed, a star child no less bright than the dimmest star existing in your painted sky of eternity. Feed me from the misery I pour out; turn what is wasteland into purity, the soils rich with your own bounty and making.

Dim me once and then again. Smother me so I might sit in the darkening nowhere. Dim me so I may not know my own face, my own ways, my own words. Dim me into the doom of doom, so that I might awaken rebirthed again in your glory.

For it is not the darkness I fear. And it is neither the wolves nor the shield of fear that carries me back. It is thy own self, wrapped in the misery of others before me and beyond. It is my own wishing, my own doing, my own bending, turning me round and round to the place from whence I came. Turning me over to see that what is beneath is also about, beyond, and within. For here is my sword of truth, turned sideways in fashion, with fear begetting the emptiness from which it came. Here is my sword, positioned without cause or pretense. Dripping out the substance of nothing upon nothing until vanishing in the banquet of your coming.

90. Vignette, Entering Father's House, Age 18

Though I was deemed a full-fledged adult by all societal standards, the summer day I strolled into my father's quaint suburban home, hauling a Hefty bag of weathered stuffed animals and plastic piggy banks, I was still very much a child. In the previous years, had I been afforded ample time with my father, I might very well have exuded a glowing aura of self-confidence and formidable strength, instead of the bubble of palpable vulnerability I steadily emanated. Then again, unless Father had somehow discovered his capacity to face his own inner demons, then regardless of the time Father and I had spent together, the inherent benefits I hoped to gain from a fatherly presence most likely would never have materialized.

Entering Father's house, I was far from the ideal daughter. Selfish in many ways—lost in my own mind and my own thoughts. Broken. Frightened. Naïve. "Spoiled," without ever having truly been spoiled. A child turned woman, incapable of moving beyond her all-encompassing trepidations. An eager-to-please daughter unable to determine how exactly an offspring ought to act around a parent that was practically a stranger, and how to contribute productively to a household that was foreign.

With only a frail shell of adulthood, covering a far greater mass of innocence, I'd had as much chance of maturing in fortitude as an unborn chick beyond the protection of an incubator. Had the heat of a father's attention warmed me, certainly I would have hatched; but with Father's adoration absent, seemingly lost and unaccounted for, I was exposed and out in the open, incapable of breaking out of the shell that both entrapped and protected me.

Most days, Father was absent. He could be sitting there, right beside me, and still exist millions of miles away. And his hobbies, too, were his means of escaping, one interest bleeding into the next. In watching Father interact as he did, I could find no particular blame. The fridge was piled high with food, the house was clean, the bills were organized and paid, and there was a tangible stability and routine to every day. Everything was in order. Everything organized. Everything in place and accounted for.

He was a brilliant and well-built man, capable of astounding mental concentrations, feats of physical endurance, and mastery of studies. Though, it seemed none of my doings could gain Father's interest or approval. I always managed to disappoint him in one way or another. All our conversations usually centered on his accomplishments, all compliments sent his direction, and all criticism aimed at me.

Father had never truly wanted to be a father, is how I saw it; to him, I was the making of my mother—someone he eminently longed to forget. Being there, after mostly being separated for fifteen years, I'd longed for that final reprieve, the cherished prize at the end of childhood—the answer to my waking prayers. To be held, to be praised, to be catered to, and made to feel special, and if not special, at least seen. In my eyes, he was still that gallant caretaker treading me across the hospital wing into the safety beyond the threshold. He was still that lionheart who would swoop down at any moment to the rescue.

In time, I'd see what before I could not, and finding Father dressed in nothing more than a childhood-imagined cloak of heroism, I'd observe his naked flaws with discerning eyes. I'd take in his hurtful words. I'd watch him depart again and again. And I'd understand I had lost my father before I'd ever found him. This would leave me terribly twisted inside. I would reason, in my moments of self-doubt and in my moments of trial, if I were only prettier, or smarter, or more noteworthy, Father would love me. And in this way, I grew into a woman who believed if she only tried a little bit harder, she would finally be worthy of love.

91. Super Bowl Blunders

I have to say at a recent Super Bowl gathering, one in which I only broke out in one hive, I was totally myself. So much so that I had to private message a new friend after the party to say, "I am sorry I talked so much. I usually do that when I like someone. I am not very good at parties." Fortunately, she messaged right back saying, "I like you, too." I felt like such a grade schooler.

I don't want you to think in the past couple days I have been depressed; I have not been. My vitamin-D levels are freakishly low, and that adds to my pool of spurts of melancholy, but all in all I am doing quite well.

Miraculously, I walked through a valley of darkness, being plucked by vultures, and came out unscathed and rather well lifted in faith. As of late, I have been pouring my heart out to my higher power, which I choose to call Jesus (and choose to not push on anyone else). I'm not sure what's up with all my prophetic and spiritual writing. Though I seem to be tapping into something, and my God seems to be the conduit. It is remarkable, scary, and satisfying all at once—like a gigantic ball of chocolate flying through the air at dart speed.

Back to that party. Something funny happened. There was a lady there, a mother of the hostess (never did get her name, forgot to ask). We sat near each other a good stretch of the game, particularly during the game's power outage (super-boring-sportscasters-don't-know-what-they-are-doing part). We were chatting a bit. Well, I was mostly giggling and cracking myself up, as is my protocol at first-time gatherings—that and stuffing my face with food. Anyhow, we were talking about the Super Bowl commercials when I said something to the tune of, "So far the best commercial is the one with the older people." I was careful how I worded my sentence. I didn't want to say "senior citizens" because there was one sitting right next to me. I looked over after I made my statement, feeling relieved I'd dodged a bullet. Then I kind of blabbered. Not being able to stop myself, I added, "Did you notice how I didn't use the words 'senior citizens'?" I paused to giggle. Then more poured out to substantiate what had already leaked out. "I was careful, as you are sitting here." I blushed. Time to regroup and repair, I added more, "Two of my best friends are senior citizens. I like senior citizens. I really do."

But nooooo, that wasn't enough. I laughed, again. "Oh, man," I said, my face aflame. "That sounded so bad. Like saying, 'I like black people, two of my best friends are black.'" The senior citizen, well she just started busting up. Me, in the meantime, I'm wondering who the heck is controlling the mechanism between my brain, thought, and speech. After that mishap, I set about to chat my new friend's ear off. I think I basically told her every ghost encounter and psychic experience I had ever had in my entire life! And boy, I really didn't know I had enough eerie moments to fill up over an hour! Luckily, when this oh-so-patient and kind lady messaged me back later that night, she also added, "It's nice to talk to someone who doesn't think I'm weird."

92. MY ASPIE FRIEND ROCKS

I love weird people. They are typically so dang interesting. My favorite weird person (and that is a high-ranking compliment from the planet she comes from) would have to be my super fabulous friend Alienhippy. We met through blogging. I checked her out and studied her blog before I started mine. I don't know if she knows that I used her as a prototype. Don't think I've told her that, yet. That said, I've pretty much told her everything else. We talk every single day. I love her immensely; so much that my husband just said, "Looks like our next family trip will have to be to England." Of course, I adamantly concurred and set about to wonder how I'd feasibly survive that flight.

Alienhippy (that's not her real name, in case you are that one percent wondering) is a dynamo of a friend. And this is why:

1. She never says: "I am fine" or "I am okay." When I ask her how she is feeling, she tells me straight up how she is, inside and out, how her physical body feels, her spirit, and her mind. I don't have to wonder, or guess, or pry, and there is such freedom in the realness of the experience of knowing. I won't get into details, but I even know about her bowel movements!

2. She always, without fail, tells me she loves me so much. She used to say she loves me too much, but I told her that wasn't healthy, as I be who I be. And now she just says she loves me so much and just enough. She tells me over and over, almost each time we touch base. She loves me so much that I feel this syrupy liquid of protective jell all about all day long.

3. She has no hidden motives and is real. She just tells me her heart and her soul. She tells me of her faith, her trials, her children, her life. She doesn't hold back anything. Any subject is open for discussion—and I mean anything! You name it, and we've probably talked about it. I never feel embarrassed or ashamed or stupid for sharing. She gives me the freedom to be completely me because she is completely herself. We laugh so hard and have invented our own secret code words. We make up names for each other. I like to call her "banana slug." Don't ask me why, because I have no idea.

4. She loves me no matter what. She would love me if I were green and slimy; she said so. I would love her no matter what size or shape, no matter what species, no matter what! She is just the bee's knees. Her heart is as big as the universe and my heart fits right inside hers. I tease her that if she had a "package" I would totally own her. You see, we can talk like that.

5. She doesn't lie. She's like me—lying feels like we are dying inside. We have no choice but to spill our beans and be truthful, and because of this we have this unbreakable trust. We know we are what you see. We know we have no curtains hiding secrets. We know we won't tell, won't shame, and won't break each other's trust. We have an unspoken truce. We have a code of honor.

6. She reads me. She can tell when I am holding back and not saying everything. She can tell when I am sad, broken, or lost. And she not only reads me, she helps me. She gets me. She knows my pains and understands how it feels. That's how she can read me. She knows when to ask, "Are you okay?" She knows when to say, "You are beautiful inside and out." She even knows how to comfort me when I am looping in my head.

7. She is a reflection of me. She is so dang beautiful that I just feel very lucky to be her friend, and she loves me so much that I know I must be that dang beautiful. I am very honored to know her. The compassion she carries for others is out of this world. She wears her heart on her sleeve. She is the best mother and an honest wife. We like to tease about our husbands; they are alike in their ways. Even her son shares the same name as my middle son and has Aspergers.

8. She gets my brain! Praise the heavens. I don't have to explain anything to her. She understands my fixations, my breakdowns, my panic attacks, my insecurities, my passions, my obsessions. She's been there and done that, and is still doing it. I don't feel like I'm a loner traveling through a strange planet anymore. In her, I found my people!

9. She is so smart, it's scary. Oh my goodness. I've never met a wiser woman in my life. The things that come out of her mouth, you'd think she was a senior citizen, a super smart one who has been around the block and inside the mind of brilliance. She just knows how to untangle things and find new angles and read between the lines. Her analytical mind coupled with her heart is amazing.

10. She is unique. In all her "Aspieness," she is still a uniquely divine and gifted woman. Her Aspie qualities just enhance who she already is—a gift to this world and me. She has longed for a friendship like ours and I have longed for a connection like I have with her. God matched us up, her and me, to show us our inherent goodness; I am her forever friend, the one she would swing with under the big tree in her childhood dreams and she is my earth angel. In fact, I know she is my angel because last week when I was crying and at the end of my rope, I pleaded up to God, and I asked, "Why have you given me so much without assistance, without a sign, without hope?" And he adamantly replied, in a curt and matter-of-fact way that only my God can, "I gave you Alienhippy, didn't I?"

93. Pass Me the Port, Please

I am extremely analytical, acutely self-aware, and live in a heightened state of sensory awareness, but I often forget that the majority of the mainstream isn't like me! I forget that most people do not respond to their surroundings like I do. For instance, there are moments when I feel as if I am being sliced and diced (Ninja Turtle video game flashback) and dissected visually by another, only because when I spot a person I generally have to take each piece of a person apart and put the features back together in order to make sense of what I am seeing. I try to take apart another person and piece him or her back together without being judgmental. In other words, if a big nose is the first thing I see, I remind myself that *big* is a judgment and based on my limited perception and biased collective experiences, while understanding that societal norms determine the essence of beauty for most folks.

Thusly, as I'm beholding another's appearance and trying to make sense of what I am seeing, in regard to features and taking in the whole picture, I am also simultaneously reminding myself that the individual's features are not right or wrong, good or bad, or striking or dull—they just are. And beneath this linear thinking of releasing judgment (based on the indoctrination of societal norms), in the same juxtaposition I am trying to remind myself that this other person and I do not even exist as separate entities (according to certain spiritual practices). All of these thoughts come to pass just as I am glancing at another: the release of judgment, the reminder of the limitless of the illusion of the universe, and the fact that I am entirely analytical when it comes to viewing another, added to the fact that I know way too much for my own good (and would apparently make a good sitcom character).

With all of my thought processing, I become distracted and don't realize that the other person I am analyzing is more than likely not viewing me in the same manner as I am viewing him or her. While my mind is racing at a million miles per second, the other person has probably just thought, *Nice red sweater* or *There's a brunette middle-aged woman*. But I forget this. Somewhere between wondering if my fly is open, my teeth are flossed, my nose is big, my hair is brushed, and my socks are matched, and wondering what the other person is dissecting about me, and what conclusion the bystander has drawn, and how he or she has categorized and judged me to fit me into his or her comfort level of classification, I turn into a tailspin of panic, fearing that the other person is not only doing to me what I am doing to him or her, through dissection and examination of part, but also reaching conclusions based on the accumulated data.

Ultimately, when all is said and done, in the midst of my boggling analysis of said other person, I am fearing the conclusion the other person has reached, whether it be *red sweater* or *big-breasted tart*; I am wanting to huddle into a corner and make myself entirely invisible and inaccessible to onlookers. Whereas if I lived in a world where I was masked and cloaked (and perhaps entirely invisible), I think my anxiety and resulting depletion of energy would be drastically reduced. However, since I live in a world where I am seen, I am also faced with the reality that I am judged and categorized based on my appearance. (It's no wonder my Aspie son refuses to wear anything other than plain clothes—no designs, no images, no nothing.)

In the meantime, I am having a miniature debate in my mind about how the release of fear and the release of worrying about whatever people think is optimal for my state of well-being and reciting the random quote that says, *What people think of me is none of my business*, while holding back an entire dam of dialogue that I long to thrust upon the person returning my glance, in order that I might attempt to accurately describe my spirit behind this cloak of humanness.

By the end, all of these processed thoughts (including the deductions of reasoning circling around the unbeneficial and detrimental effects a fear-based outlook has on spirit, mind, and body) have left me wiped out and wondering how it is that up until this point in my life I have not become dependent on the port wine I savor some evenings, or at least a stiff shot of cough syrup. For my brain is such a grand uniform of thought that even a sergeant general, marked with the stoic stars and stripes, could not maneuver his troops inside to find the potential threat of enemy.

And then, with the coming of more and more rushing thoughts, I begin to chuckle, realizing again that more than likely the stranger is not analyzing my distinct features. Now the sadness settles in—the reckoning that I am different and likely a different species of human altogether.

While battling all the aforementioned jumbled thoughts, I am also involved in a game of connect-the-dots, bringing all the facial features of the bystander back together to make a collective whole. Then there is always the lingering notion that this is all much ado about nothing, given that if I were ever to see this person again, I wouldn't recognize the individual because I cannot retain visual images of faces in my memory banks. By this time, when my thoughts have run full course into a state of exhaustion (Sir Brain riding a unicycle, swirling upside down on a looped ramp), the person I was with has either moved on and out of my view or has moved on in conversation. Nonetheless, the little voice in my head (LV) is having a full-on monologue,

Through all the analysis piled upon rhetoric and philosophical jargon, added to the process of scaffolding current information with past information and connecting other to self, and the tangent of strings my mind travels, I am left literally spent, my pockets of reserve penniless, and my wallet flung open for the taking. Pass me the port, please.

94. THE DEAN

I awoke in the early hours of the morn hacking like a hairball-ridden feline. I'd apparently choked on my own saliva. I was still mostly asleep, pacing the bedroom while gasping for air. My throat was parched from what had to have been an up chuck of bile. Out of breath and slit-eyed, I made my way upstairs and sat in the cold living room under the light of a singular lamp, contemplating my death. LV (little voice in my head) was wide awake panting and pacing in a pure state of panic, entirely convinced that at any moment the coconspirators of spit and throat would rebel and squeeze the last breath from me. Sir Brain refused to ever sleep again and started counting on his webbed digits all the ways a human could feasibly expire. Me? I passed out on the couch while bargaining with the gods.

Now I have a taste in my mouth like some Keebler elves were up late lacquering my teeth with pond slime. My chest hurts from choking, and my throat . . . from that good-for-nothing chopped walnut going down my pipe the wrong way—a direct consequence of swallowing (downing) frozen cheesecake a couple days ago. My legs, and basically every part of my body, ache from starting back up with my evil exercise regime. Oh yes, and my headache came back like black magic, right when the dean of education called.

The dean is heading to China. She gave me a quick ring-a-ding. I will get reimbursed thousands of dollars, it seems. Her advice, to set the final part of the plan in motion, was to write a very short, ambiguous email explaining to the vice president of the university that I had to withdraw from the college because of my *disability*. With that, all of the sudden anger (which I can only assume had been held hostage), came barging out full-force, trumpets and all. I had a thing or two to say to the dean. And actually sounded quite intelligent. First off, I reminded her that I would not lie and that I was not leaving the university because I had Aspergers! In truth I was leaving because of the way the professors had treated me. I added that in my last master's program, I had had no trouble whatsoever with the professors, and was in fact supported and well respected! (What a concept.)

After my romp, the dean was rather quiet. When she spoke again, she still said the same thing. "A brief email would be best." A few minutes later and I got to the bottom of the situation. (That's a hard phrase for me to use because I picture naked butts.) I discovered that the dean had no qualms about anything that I had said when I met with her in her office. In fact, she commiserated with many of my misgivings regarding my experience with the counseling department. With some careful questioning, I came to realize the she wanted me to write a brief email to ensure I'd receive my tuition back. The brevity would avoid the potential of my tuition reimbursement request going into the long, drawn out appeal process. She also concurred, quite nicely, that after I had the money in hand, I might consider sending a letter to the vice president explaining the truth of the events.

95. Chameleon

As chameleon I have perfected several degrees of metamorphosis. I do this by mimicking someone else (real), a character (television), or the stereotypical characteristics of a specific role (a detective's mannerisms in a movie). I'm quite good at imitation. I can pretty much take on any role to perfection. It's like a hidden talent—a type of skill that seems like it would come in handy, like double-agent-Jacquelyn-Smith-from-*Charlie's-Angels* handy. But it doesn't. It just pretty much sucks.

Case in point, when I first moved to the state of Washington, I met a spiritual teacher I admired. Bingo! Bingo! Bingo! Some part of my subconscious brain screamed, and then (without telling the rest of me), some part of me set about to transform. Not to be that teacher exactly. I mean I didn't want to live in her house or steal her husband; that's kind of loony. But a piece of me did want to clone her. Hmmmmm. As for this one woman, I learned how to mimic her voice, how to dress like her, and then studied to become a spiritual counselor, just like her! Surprise. Turns out I make a darn good spiritual counselor.

I think this discovery of acting out a role that is not actually my true self has to be one of the oddest sensations known to mankind. And you can't really debate me unless you've experienced this; and if you have experienced this (the taking on of roles without your conscious knowledge), then I am certain you would agree with me about the oddness factor. For all you non-chameleon types, the *presto-chango* experience is akin to being possessed by another life form or like being in a drunken spell for several months, and then sobering up and wondering what you did during those blackout moments. Only you never black out completely, just a part of your awareness does. Maybe it's like waking up and finding out you have had a third hand for a few months but didn't even see it or realize you were using it.

How, with my keen observational and analytical skills, I could not notice I was doing something so brazenly obvious baffles me. I imagine that some-where inside of my subconscious is a tug-of-war where the participants are fighting. This way—be like her, be like her! No this way—be like her, be like her!

96. THE BOX

I am an unopened box;
I sit sealed;
I am also outside of the box.

When the box is opened,
I emerge,
I am nothing;
I am the box itself.

In opening the box,
I see again
Another self,
Staring at another box—unopened.

But who is it that sees?
Who is it that opens?
And who will be,
The last to find nothing?

97. PROBABLE THEORIES OF WHERE I COME FROM

Audacious Spirit: Before I was shot down to Earth by the spiritual beings (who guard the hall of records in another realm), I met before a board of angel guides that had agreed to help me in this life. I jumped up and down and was extremely excited about my list of goals I wanted to accomplish here on Earth. Being headstrong and determined, I did not heed the warnings of the master experts, the ones with a thousand more lifetimes under their belts than me. I am one of those ambitious youngsters who thinks she is *all that*—the type the elders laugh at with such intensity that the skies of heaven thunder. Of course, I was clueless to my hubris and audacity, and thought myself brilliant. I recited a long list. Essentially, I wanted to learn all the life lessons possible in eighty-eight years. At half-life I would metamorphose. I wanted to see in all ways—to know through multiple senses. I wanted to experience extreme agony, displacement, heartache, rejection, abandonment, physical pain, and so forth. *Just bring it on*, was my attitude. I had no clue how long earth lives were; I had never been a human before. I was a dolphin. Now I am stuck down here with this master plan and I can't change it. I dream of water constantly and get uncanny cravings for fish. The good news is half of my life is over.

Dropped Down: I come from a planet where chocolate is the staple nutrient for life forms and no one eats animals or animal products. Actually no one eats anything beyond air, energy, and chocolate. There are twice as many trees and the trees talk and sing. They are the only ones that talk. The rest of us speak telepathically; thusly, there is no need to shift through the multiple variables of words to express the multiple variables of thought. Thought just arises in images and picture form. Beings are conscious about their intentions. And there is little fear; nothing is hidden. Nothing can be hidden. Faces change based on experience and emotion and one's energy. There is nothing that is stagnant. We see the energy of the world spinning and multiple worlds within everything. Beings have soul mates, intense soul connections, kinship, and a knowing of peace and serenity. I was dropped down here on Earth by accident. And it sucks.

The Woman's Wisdom: I was a male sage in my past life, something akin to a buddha, but not quite. I was considered enlightened by all who encountered me and all who heard my name. But then this scrawny, two-faced hermit lady, who lived in the deep caves of some forgotten place, she came and she cursed me with her wisdom. She said, "You are a man in form in this lifetime. You are not truly enlightened, in the complete sense, unless you come back to this realm as a woman, and as a woman in form you live through the following: the extreme emotional and physical confusion of hormonal cycling (PMS is a blast), the pain of giving birth (and most of the complications that can arise while pregnant, including the agony of inducement), the challenges of marrying and living with a man (as a woman you will see the male gender in an entirely new light), raising children (and let's add children who never nap, don't sleep through the night, have chronic health conditions in their early years, fight for the first ten years . . . nonstop), the experience of Aspergers (You will not recognize this fact until half of your life is over; but that's okay, because with Aspergers you'll have the capacity to fixate and obsess to such a mind-blowing degree that you'll figure yourself out in no time.), the pressures society places on women to look beautiful (you can rock that whole half-front-tooth-that-turns-dead thing), the cattiness of women turning against you, predators, and a chronic pain condition that has no explanation and no cure. Hmmmm. (She smiled her toothless smile and raised a boney, crooked finger.) And let's add that whole mother-in-law dynamic bit. Of course, female or not, you can still be endowed with all the gifts from this world: prophecy, precognition, seeing, sensing, empathy, revelations, etc. You can take all you need with you that you've gained from this life of a man. But I am telling you now, it shall not be enough! Do all this and come back at the end of the lifetime; then you will be ready to teach me!"

I concurred and naively agreed. After my nod, she quickly inserted, "And, just for fun, let's give you voluptuous curves which you are entirely uncomfortable with, and the mind of a prudish, but lustful, nun!" And with that I was born.

98. BODILY CHANGES

Bodily changes freak me out to the point that I don't want to change out of my nightclothes and I don't want to leave the house. I wig. I spaz. I obsess. My aches and pains become my fixation—the new growth mark, the burn in my throat, the boil. I hate being me right now. I am cranky, bloated, short-tempered, and FAT. My amazing superpower jeans, which normally tolerate fluctuating weight changes, don't even fit. My hair seems ghastly thin. I would pay someone to transport me ahead five years, preferably (unaged in appearance) to post-menopause.

Recently, I concluded, after much Google God research, the pig hormone I was ingesting during the last eight months (under doctor's orders for suspected hypothyroid) was causing fluctuations of my body's progesterone levels, a reaction that led to various hormonal mayhem. The low-dose thyroid pill (the lowest possible dosage, cut in half), I believe affected the hormones associated with the muscles in my tongue (during sleep hours), particularly progesterone; this led to frequent early-morning sore throats, which led to full-blown, week-long head colds, every month for six months! The colds typically occurred the two days before my menstrual cycle, accompanied by the dreaded adult cystic acne, a.k.a. face boils. I soon recognized reoccurring head colds and boils every consecutive month around the same time of the month meant something was going on internally. Who wouldn't? Plus historically, I'd only been sick once every one to two years. In researching, I concluded the colds and the boils were a definite result of the pig hormones. Even though I listed fifty quotes from others who cited specific hormonal changes and cystic acne for the FIRST time after starting thyroid meds, my prescribing doctor didn't believe my anecdotal proof; however, my gynecologist did. Needless to say, I am off the hormone meds and praying my body will adjust naturally.

It sucks that I am this sensitive to medication. I can't even take over-the-counter allergy medicine without getting depressed and anxious. An eighth (yes, an eighth—a tiny blue crumb in your thumbnail) of a low-dose anxiety pill (I've tried various brands under doctor supervision) causes me to have hallucinations, fogginess, disorientation, a rapid heartbeat, or suicidal thoughts! Prescribed painkillers, I don't even go there; they bring on freakishly realistic, nonstop nightmares. Lately, even animal products (such as cheese; I don't eat meat) make me sad—like I am energetically connected to the animals' suffering. Oh, bother! I wish I lived in a body that could tolerate certain types of medication—just to get a little release at some point.

99. HOSTESS WITH THE MOSTEST

A few weeks ago I hosted a party, and I was entirely wasted before the guests arrived. This marks the second potluck in Washington my husband and I have hosted since moving here, almost three years ago. The event was a big deal to me, and I loaded my grocery cart to the max to ensure plenty of booze and munchies. The last time I threw a party for my neighbors (which was also the first time), I was politely informed that there wasn't enough alcohol. One of my neighbors actually left and brought back four bottles of wine from his house. This time I was prepared. I bought the hugest bottles of rum and tequila I could find and several bottles of wine. I am not a big drinker. No, sir! Never have been and doubt I ever will be. Before this last year, I probably averaged between two and three glasses a year! Since finding out I am Aspie, the intake may have increased a wee bit. My reasons for not drinking are multifaceted; like everything else in my life, nothing I do is simple. I focus a lot of thought on the right path. Even though I recently have come to terms with the fact there is no frickin' right path, I still have that old "right path" mentality, much like a gag reflex.

Not doing the right thing feels like a recent ordeal I underwent at the orthodontist's office when I was being fitted for a new retainer device. (The diagnostic x-ray revealed that I have unusually large sinus cavities; no big deal or of special interest. I only make mention just in case you are collecting random data about me.) At the orthodontist the lady worker gently shoved a metal contraption filled with cold, grainy cement goop atop the roof of my mouth to take impressions for my new retainers. As she pressed the banana-flavored, pink goop into my mouth she said, "Remember, breathe slowly through your nose." While my mouth airways were obstructed, I kept saying to myself, "You aren't going to die. You aren't going to die. You aren't going to die."

That's how I feel if I don't follow the right path, or rules, or guidelines. I feel like I am being gagged, out of breath, and will die. Makes no logical sense. I know this. But my brain has "follow the rules" tattooed around its frontal lobe. I am still working on the removal process of this tattoo; it's slow going.

On the day of the party, the right path meant temperance—a word I had latched onto and deciphered, and longed to apply in my life. *Temperance* meant no indulgences and no drinking alcohol. The party would be the perfect stage to practice my temperance and do the "right" thing, at least according to the recent rules I was applying. The gods laughed, for by the time the first guests arrived, I had downed three glasses of port wine. Trust me, I had good reason!

In the end it all turned out fine, except for the time the one guest mentioned how her memory is bad, and then she laughed in jest, saying, "It's because I'm a genius." Totally joking she was. And then I, being so very much beyond tipsy, blurted out, "The funny thing is, I am a *gifted genius*. A professional psychologist just recently verified this." And then, after slapping my knee and elaborating about my big brain and Aspieness, I went into a full confession about how I was trying to release ego and be filled with humility. I ended this, I think, with telling a woman I barely see anymore, "You know you want to take walks with me now; a gifted, published genius I be." I'd thrown in the whole publishing story in there somewhere, I suppose.

I don't drink much. I am an extreme lightweight. A half glass of hard pear cider at the local pub and I am yelling, "That guy is checking out my butt." I try to curb my alcohol intake, not so much for the constant records that play when I am drinking—destroying liver, destroying liver, destroying liver, and/or you'll become an alcoholic—but because I become a dang fool. I really do. I lose all inhibition and feel like I am freeeeee.

One of my (drunk) relatives once got onto my aunt's electric wheelchair and flew up the freeway onramp to take a ride on the freeway. And I think that's me. I think when I drink I take a ride on the freeway! Weeeeeee. So I don't drink much.

But that evening, an hour before the guests arrived, right after I put the freshly made salsa into a pitcher, my hands began to burn. At first I didn't notice. I just kept rinsing my hands under water, thinking the burn would pass. But no! The burn did not pass. It grew increasingly worse, like my hands were in the snow without gloves and the frostbite was setting in; it was a deep, unreachable burn, penetrating and erupting from the inside of every finger. The guests were to arrive in less than an hour!

My husband was not home and I was terror-stricken. I rationalized and reasoned, and then concluded the culprit was the serrano peppers! I had used my bare hands to not only cut the hot peppers for the salsa, but, when my food processor had stopped working (all electronics like to malfunction around me), I had dipped my hands in the freshly ground peppers to scoop out the remains and transfer the mixture to the blender. Oh, my gosh! I had soaked my hands in hot pepper oil!

I quickly went to the Internet for help. Google God to the rescue. I soon found other people who had been as equally dimwitted. The remarks were reassuring. There were some helpful tips to end the horrific pain. Eventually I tried everything listed as remedies: butter, milk, yogurt, sugar scrub with olive oil, etc. But nothing decreased the agony. I thought for certain my flesh was going to peel off. I was going to have fleshless fingers! The pain intensified. At this point, my feet broke out in hives from the stress. Yes, with the guests arriving in less than a half hour, I had burning flesh hands and hived-up feet. Glorious!

When my husband returned home with some cortisone cream that the local pharmacist said would stop the pain, I shook my head NO. My husband insisted, and I gave in. Soon I was screaming at a high pitch and downing wine as fast as I could. The cream had only served to intensify the burn. Dumb pharmacist. My husband at this point is saying, "You are like Lucy from *I Love Lucy*, you know?" That didn't help. At last I found the answer in one of the comments online: "Called ER (emergency room); there is nothing they can do. The pain will last four to six hours." Really? No one could say that from the start?

What should have come up on the top of the comment section was: "You are so screwed!"

And that's how it began, how I began slurping the port wine. The pain reliever I took did nothing. The wine really didn't decrease the pain much either, but by the time the first patrons arrived, I didn't really care. And eventually the margarita helped to ease the ordeal to a hilarious event.

As our first friends arrived, I confessed, "I am already drunk. Let me tell you a story . . ." And at the start of the party, to another couple I said, "I am not rinsing my hands under cold water every minute because of OCD, just so you know, let me tell you a story . . ." And by the end of the night, three hours of hand rinsing later, shortly after my gifted-genius, I-am-Zen-and-egoless spill, I said, "And you know what the best part about being drunk before any of you arrived is, and especially about being in so much pain?!" I paused, dipping my hands further into a bowl of ice-cold water. "I really honestly don't care what you think of me." And that was that.

100. To the Professional

Take away the notepad and paper. Take away whatever you are about to write on. I am more concerned with what you are writing and thinking than about my own self. I am uncomfortable looking at you. I probably don't like your office for one reason or another. Maybe you are messy or maybe too clean. It might smell in an offensive way or be too dark and cluttered. Then again, the sunlight might be seeping through and displaying the dancing dust and pulling me into thoughts of germs and uncleanliness. If you cleaned, I am hoping you didn't use toxins. I am wondering how many people have sat in this chair before, and how they sit—how they position themselves.

I am wondering with each syllable I utter what you think and if I have answered in an appropriate manner to meet your expectations and intentions. I can guess half of what you will say and how you will say it, because I have studied you from the moment we met. And I have studied those like you before. I know more about the human language and the nuances and gestures and games than you can likely imagine. I can feel your energy and I can feel how your opinion of me switches. I can feel you weighing in on me and feel my words balanced against your thoughts.

I am uncomfortable in all ways and trying to present myself as comfortable. You are watching me, as if in watching I will grow in security and trust. But I won't. I will feel for you what I feel for everyone. I will either like you instantly or want to run. With the liking I will analyze the whys, and if my conclusion is valid. I will linger here a short while, especially contemplating if I want to run. If I want to run, my thoughts will circle around you for a favorable amount of time. If I distrust you, I will likely always distrust you. This may be nothing you have ever said or done; this is my natural instinct. I have been preyed upon by predators and sought out by experts. I have been probed and prodded and measured one too many times. I do not like the way you measure me. Not one bit, and I want this time to end. I also want to like you, and if I don't, I fear my own rejection;

I fear the dialogue that will reach into the contours of my mind and debate the hows and whys of my own inclinations.

I will listen to you as best I can, but don't count on me hearing all of what you say. One word will set me adrift into another place, one unusual sound or one ordinary sound from you, or from the room that seems silent. I will hear what you do not hear. I will hear the quietness. I will hear the pauses in your monologue and I will question your expertise. I will wonder if you like me, and then I will wonder why I even care, and why it is important that you do like me. I will want to be your friend and a part of me will still love you, an adoration akin to that of a pup rescued from a cold alley. I will seek harbor and refuge in this space you have provided, knowing I am paying, or someone is paying, for this form of companionship that frightens me.

I will question your degrees, your education, your protocols, your knowledge, your book smarts, and your conclusions. And all this I will do as you sit there scratching away notes about me. I will have compiled a list a volume thick in the time you have taken for me to answer a few questions. Simultaneously, I will have composed my own representation of self to you, pulling out what is expected and what might make you comfortable. Playing the game, in order that you might take in a version of me and not be swooped away by the *real* me that is locked away behind this worn curtain of self.

You can't reach in, as hard as you try, unless I know you recognize me. I won't let you past, unless I know you are real—that you have felt the deepest pains and angst—that you, too, have been in the shadowed darkness weeping for reprieve—that you have been abandoned, ostracized, left for nothing, created into something others wanted you to be. I will not let you near, unless I know your heart has grown in the depths of the dark valley.

Entirely, I sit. Entirely, I am. And I understand beyond measure what grips you and shakes you and what makes you spin. I can tell in your eyes when you are complimented you are lit, and when you are unsure you falter. I see you, like a master watching a child; I see your discomfort, your wavering, your questions. But mostly, I see straight into the core.

So please don't waste my time with man-invented games and manmade questionnaires that nibble away at my character and personhood. I am beyond this—this guessing and marks, this test to prove something that needs no proving. I am human in need of being seen. I am not a test subject, nor am I confused. I am a unique and special individual born out of the ashes into the phoenix. Do not look past the secrets in my eyes to check off the boxes of your own design. Seek first in me the wisdom I carry, the answers, the knowledge. See what I have to say. Hear what my world is like—for unless you have lived inside of this *me*, then you are the one that remains alien.

Present to me your own self—the deepest part of you. Take off your mask and meet me beyond the playing field. Do not strip me of the very armor that sews my seams. Uplift my attributes and charm, the gentle grace that illuminates from the spirit I am. Do not think that because you have a title or name that you are therefore any more than the others. You are still garbed in your fashions and mystery. Undress, strip down, bare your nakedness, and show me your frailty. That is the only reason I am here. Not to teach you how to help me. Not to teach you how to change me. My way is not wrong. Nor is my mind hindered. My way is the one of the child of authenticity; and until you understand that what I carry is no less damaged than the stars in the sky and no less worthy than your very own heart, than you cannot reach me. If you want to help me, if you want to truly help, then become my student, so I can become yours. Meet me as one.

101. LOST COLORS

I was standing in front of a variety of buckets of paint. I dipped myself in paint after paint. I was in search of answers. Soon I was multicolored and dripping in knowledge. I dipped and dipped more, and a brilliant rainbow blossomed. I dipped and dipped, covering every inch of me, until the colors all merged. Then, and only then, I was the color of black. But it did not bother me—this guise, this dark, this black. For I knew all the other colors were still there, still with me, and now in me.

But then the "experts" and "professionals" entered the room where I stood dripping black. And they observed—their clipboards and furrowed brows moving in an unwanted rhythm. The dance of them entering my mind and hurting my being. And they looked and looked where I stood, noting this black shroud upon me. And I knew then that they were blind, that they could not see all the colors. They only saw black.

They were quick to form theories about this "black." And they were quick to find words, and labels, and meaning. They assumed since I was garbed in black that I liked black, and only black. They assumed what they saw was the truth. The only truth. They couldn't see. They couldn't see that just as black was my companion, so was every other color. Colors they had never imagined.

I couldn't explain the colors to them. I couldn't go back and show them where I'd been. I didn't know how. I didn't know the words. I was blind to their words just as they were blind to my colors. To them I needed black. To them I was black. To them this end product of black was everything. They didn't know that black was merely the mixing of everywhere I'd searched and everything I'd questioned. They didn't know that black was not the end. There were still many more colors to find. Still more colors to be. Only when they looked at me, they only saw black.

They gathered their boxes next. They needed boxes like I needed colors. I understood that we both craved things that the other did not see or comprehend. Though somehow I was supposed to accept and understand their boxes. Even though they do not attempt to see my colors. This made me cry inside. This disconnection. Soon the black grew darker, thicker, and coated— a darkness that stopped the colors from seeping through altogether. And stopped me from dipping and dripping. Stopped me from being. I was placed in their box of black. And from there I watched them scribble their words of who I was.

102. Navigating the Female Aspergerian Mind

As a result of under diagnoses, a large majority of females on the autism spectrum are reaching adulthood as survivors of multiple emotional and physical traumas. Because limited resources and tools are available for working with female clients with Aspergers, professionals sometimes fall back on what has worked with clients who do not have Asperger's Syndrome (AS). More often than not the practitioner treats the symptoms and not the condition, focusing on the obvious challenges, such as depression and anxiety, without full consideration dedicated to the whole of the person, in particular the fact that he is working with an individual who views the world somewhat differently from the mainstream client.

Considering the sensitive nature of the female with Aspergers condition, an individual who has likely found herself a subject of alienation, ridicule, suspicion, doubt, and abuse, it is vital for the professional to understand the power she holds to make or break her client. Especially the client's feasible outlook on seeking out further assistance as pertains to her emotional well-being. For example, females on the autism spectrum develop both conscious and subconscious strategies in their attempt to function effectively in a world that appears unpredictable and potentially volatile. Oftentimes, an Aspergerian female is using all of her mental and emotional resources to merely survive and navigate the social world. In response she is fatigued and overtaxed. If a female with Asperger's Syndrome is partaking in mental health therapy, and the therapist suggests to her that she change or adjust some of her coping mechanisms (for example, seeking out strategies to decrease verbal processing), the suggestion itself has the potential to create increased anxiety and, feasibly, shutdown.

In understanding that the female's (with AS) mindset is uniquely different from the majority of mainstream society, including her capacity for complexity of thoughts, intense mental connections/scaffolding, and advanced logical sequencing, and taking into account the potential effects of a lifetime of repeated humiliation and abuse, it is advisable for the professional to consider the client's trauma may reach far beyond what is considered the typical depths of post-traumatic stress. Add this to her tendencies for sensory overload, and the (AS) female will likely exhibit an instinctual fight-or-flight response to any new situation, especially those pertaining to vulnerability and emotional intimacy. Other factors hindering the benefits of therapy include the client's ability to recreate her self-presentation based on how she perceives the professional is viewing her. Often a master actress, the female with AS has developed a toolbox of masks enabling her to move in the world undetectable to the untrained eye. Here in the client-practitioner relationship, the client is likely to mold herself into the persona that she believes best fits the comfort level of the professional, moving within the room of therapy just as she moves in the exterior symbolic rooms of her life. A professional who is unstudied in the elements of the female condition of Asperger's Syndrome is apt to miss the nuances of a given client's chameleon qualities, overlooking the client's subtle changes in representation of self or wrongfully assuming the client is resorting to trickery and sabotage.

The female with Asperger's Syndrome may exhibit continual emotional fragility. In some cases, this is hidden behind emotionally detached humor or within the guise of a persona she is currently portraying, e.g., she may imitate a character on television. Though she is emotionally vulnerable, she is capable of hiding herself from other people. Given her nature and character, one word or mannerism from the practitioner may be overanalyzed and/or perceived by the client as a threat or criticism.

Misinterpretations, distrust, or a number of other variables can lead the client to shut down (emotional withdrawal), melt down (emotional outburst), retreat into imagination or fantasy, recreate the presentation of self, and/or switch from a state of emotional presence to logical analysis. When the client is triggered by the professional and responds accordingly, the quality of the therapeutic relationship is adversely affected. Unlike the mainstream client, an Aspergerian woman may never trust a professional once she believes she has been misinterpreted and/or criticized.

103. REVISITING DOOR THREE

Today before the sun rose, I wept. I revisited my time at the local university, the place I chose to leave based on the way I was treated for briefly mentioning I had Asperger's Syndrome. I revisited it all, the whole of it—unraveling emotions, illness brought on by the stress, the mourning process, the desire to prove my side of the event and expose the injustice, the sob-filled telling to my counselor and her concurring I had been the victim of appalling behavior on said professor's part, the humiliation of being set up in a mediation that wasn't a mediation . . . and on and on.

I reread an email—a blunt note one of *those* professors sent to me in response to my non-accusatory change-of-grade request. (Before I sent the professor my email, I had two people review my words to ensure it was logical and professional in manner, and not emotional in presentation.) I knew beyond a doubt this professor had not kept accurate records of student work; in fact, I had been the one to kindly remind her to take class attendance, since she informed her students that a large portion of our grade was based on just showing up. I was also the one who read every single extra-credit reading assignment (three books), assisted my classmates, created a video presentation, and received top scores on all my assignments. But for some reason, my final grade in her course didn't reflect my efforts. This was the adjunct professor, the one with no previous teaching experience, who often shared intimate details about the lives of her mental health patients—individuals she had only just counseled that same week.

Despite her multiple teaching "flaws," my email was straightforward, factual, and void of criticism—businesslike, to say the least. I focused on my experience, only listing reasons why I believed I had earned a solid grade A.

Her response back was far from supportive. She wrote: ". . . another faculty concern is tone and professionalism when communicating conflict. This is very important when requests are made both here in school and in your future work. You yourself, if you become a counselor, will need to remain calm and non-defensive in dealing with many clients who are upset and *dysregulated.*"

She prefaced this email with the assumption that since I had told her I had Asperger's Syndrome that she assumed I was open to her professional communication advice. Later she changed my grade to a solid A, blaming her initial error on some computer glitch and her delay in response on a power outage.

That email kept replaying in my head most of yesterday, alongside with what the dean of the university had said to me when I sought out her assistance: ". . . that group of professors tend to have 'their views,' but their views don't represent everyone's, of course . . . Based on everything you have told me I think it is best you don't continue in the program . . . It is probably best if you don't tell any professionals you work with in the future that you have Aspergers. It's not the appropriate environment. *They aren't your therapists.*"

How dare they, I thought. And then I circled in my mind, pulling up the evidence—including the telling emails from the witness who at the time of mediation froze up and remembered nothing. I dug up so much old stuff. I thought back to the high marks I received as an educator. Always the highest marks. How my master-level college classes previously, before this university, had been a place of safety. How the professors had appreciated my input and intelligence. At times how I became the exemplary one or the teacher's pet. I remembered how with every endeavor I'd set out to do, I had excelled, even exceeded others' expectations. And here, in the span of little over a semester, with the hearing of the word "Aspergers," the others, a group who were supposed to be my mentors, painted me with their own muted blacks into something I was not and am not. Suddenly, all of me became *Aspergers.*

104. Vignette, The Fig, Age 9

In some ways during the first year at our duplex, our home served as a transitional stopping point for strangers—a person would arrive and rent out our spare bedroom, and then, as if they'd landed on the jail space on the board game of Monopoly, after a few rolls of the dice, they'd move on. Our first roommate, kindly Jeff, a man in his early twenties, arrived a few months after Mother and I had moved in. Sprouting a fantastic full head of cherry-red clown hair, Jeff was entirely intriguing. He had gigantic gold-rimmed glasses and a smooth glass eye with an iris-blue center that he'd pop out from time to time and let me examine up close in my hand. Jeff also had a puttering VW bug that jerked and spat and carried us to fancy places, like the local Taco Bell and the red-boxed television booth at the corner Lucky grocery store where I could watch Woody Woodpecker cartoons. Sometimes, my favorite sometimes, Jeff carried home his rectangular-shaped work case, much like a fishing box, laden with the grocery store price numbers, each type housed in its own tiny pull-out drawer. They were a hard, flexible plastic, nothing I'd seen or touched before. These clear drawers, and the miniature treasures inside, far surpassed any old dollhouse.

For a very short while, an eccentric, plump puppeteer with wiry white hair lived in our home. She also had a case, but a much more impressive wooden one which housed her enormous stringed puppets. Though the puppeteer wasn't with us long, I fondly recall her performing puppet shows out on the high front porch with her life-sized floppy marionettes. Unlike frizzy-haired Jeff and the plump puppeteer, the next roommate in the line of strangers, Ruth, did not bring any sort of portable case with her.

From the start I avoided Ruth, except for the times she watched me when Mother was away. Those days I was made to be at her side. She hurt me—her pale, freckled skin and blubbery lips. If my brain had been a holding case for hornets of worries, Ruth's presence alone had quadrupled the hornet population. Even when I rearranged my bedroom knickknacks and organized my stuffed animals, I could not erase the buzzing. To comfort myself I talked to Buddy One, a transparent teenage ghost. In looking back, I had always planned for a Buddy Two to come along—mainly because no one, besides Mother, seemed to stay in my life for very long. Buddy One performed all types of tricks. He enjoyed the rooftop the best. One time a friend and I were snuggled on our couch watching *The Donny and Marie Osmond Show* when we heard a sawing sound above us on the roof. Expecting the ceiling was about to collapse, we escaped through the front door. But as soon as we stepped foot outdoors, the sawing noise abruptly stopped. Confused, we returned to the living room and settled back down. Yet just as we did, the creepy sawing noise would begin again.

Buddy One was also partial to knocking on the front door or turning on the bathroom faucet full blast. Late at night he'd turn on my mother's record player. Once, Buddy One saved me after I'd reached up to grab a container of red vinegar off of the top kitchen shelf. The glass bottle came tumbling toward my head, and it was Buddy One who stepped in, switching the course of the fall in midair, in the shape of an upside-down L, and landing the bottle upright on the counter without so much as a plop. Buddy One was fond of everyone—my friends, my mom, even my dog Justice—everyone but Ruth.

In late October, right before Ruth left for good, I played the role of the wicked witch in a community play. Mother made the black costume by hand, and I was so proud of it that I dressed up as a witch for three Halloweens in a row—even after the costume had shrunk up far above my knees and I could barely tie the backside. The role of the witch was my debut performance, a one-minute act basically limited to me and two other clone witches sinking down in slow motion, moaning in painful defeat, and disappearing under a dusty, black stage curtain. I still remember thinking it was downright silly to have three wicked witches. My debut performance as a child actress was to be my last. Mother had this odd way of signing me up for classes—art, theater, tap dance, ballet, gymnastics—and then yanking me out right when I was getting the hang of it. Tap ended right after I'd learned the *heel-toe, heel-toe, slide, slide, slide,* ballet after I'd been late to my first performance, gymnastics when the leotard split down the side, and art when I'd run out of paints.

Soon any memories of Ruth faded in my mind, much the same as I had on stage, slowly sinking down and disappearing behind a thick, dark curtain. Eventually, I only knew that in the spare bedroom there had once been someone, a woman, Mother's friend, a roommate. The rest I had forgotten, as a person might want to forget the sight of a mangled cat on the side of the road. I only remembered a fig. How I could peel one open and lick out the insides with my tongue. And I remembered the shower, how I could no longer face the stream of water rushing down for fear I would drown. The other memories of Ruth were somewhere else.

105. LOVE AND FEAR

For decades I carried fear, as if fear were my only shield. Indeed, oftentimes I mistook fear as a friend. Looking back, I understand I chose fear and *he* did not choose me. I chose fear because at the time fear seemed the only thing I could comprehend. Fear was my feeling. Encompassing fear— virtually sprouting off of his imagined edges—were his dynamo of legions, his mutant henchmen, cloaked in garbs of abandonment, not enough, isolation, ugly, stupid, crazy, and so on.

People could sense this about me—my fear. What I thought was evidence of my love—e.g., smothering with attention, caretaking, continually checking in, oversharing, creating, placating, agreeing, giving, being there regardless, etc.—was in actuality not love. My love for another did not exist. My love for others could not exist because my love for self did not exist. And as I had no love for myself, the only thing I could find was fear, and the only thing I could give was fear.

Today I am only beginning to understand the concept of love because I am only just beginning to accept and love myself in completion. The more I accept who I am, the more I step away from fear. The removal of self from fear resembles the removal of residue from a glass window. I spray the film with love, and the love washes away the fear, revealing the beauty of existence. Fear is more so a drug to me now than a partner. He is enticing and familiar. However, I recognize the dangers. I lose myself in fear. When with fear, my energy is not my own and I become unhealthy in behaviors. I feed off the fear by attempting to suck up the love from others, perhaps in the form of approval. I feed off the fear by taking myself out of the picture and focusing on what is outside of myself. Inside the realm of fear someone or something is wrong. Whether this wrong is assumed to be in a behavior, a projected outcome, a circumstance, or in self makes no difference, for regardless, illusion exists. In attaching onto fear, something neutral turns to something beyond neutral. In applying fear, I judge.

106. PMDD

Just yesterday I was able to slip out of a depression brought on by Premenstrual Dysphoric Disorder (PMDD), a hormonal condition similar to Premenstrual Syndrome (PMS) that I am finding is common with some women on the autism spectrum. Through reading my past writings I can clearly see how I become sad following a cycle of hope. I am recognizing that the first twenty days following my menstrual cycle, I typically (barring an emotional trigger or health flare-up) have energy, renewed hope, and an abundance of joy and confidence in my journey. But soon following, during the last ten days of the cycle after ovulation, I sink day by day into a greater degree of pain and disheartenment. Knowing I am part of the 3 to 9 percent of the population who feel an increased sensitivity to hormone levels makes complete sense. To some degree, this knowing has led me to several aha moments. During my PMDD cycle, my strength in who I am falters. I can see this in photographs of myself where I am bloated and appear discouraged. I now understand, why for some thirty years, I have struggled monthly with a feeling of being lost to myself. To a degree, I have been. For during these hormonal shifts I develop a skewered view of my physical body, and I actually believe that I am extremely fat, ugly, disproportionately put together wrong, unworthy of recognition, and shouldn't leave the house. I essentially hide from the world. This PMDD (possibly a result of a variant enzyme), this makes sense!

107. Why I Am Smiling

I am forever twelve. I have the passion, innocence, spirit, and love of a child. I always will. I love people and animals. I see the best in people. I wouldn't change a thing about my innate nature and my heart. I cannot imagine being any less of a person than who I am. I wouldn't decrease or increase me in any way. I lack much capacity for lies. I might lie, but when I do I feel terrible. Supposedly, many people lie throughout their day; falsehoods are just a part of life. This *lying way* doesn't make sense to me, and I don't think I want lies to make sense. I don't want to understand lying and I don't want to understand deceit. If I am called *naïve*, *gullible*, or even *unaware*, that is okay because I know who I am. I know that the person I present to the world is the same person deep inside. I don't have to wade through layers and choose alternate personas for different events; nor do I have to placate, please, or impress. I am just me. And I would rather be loved by one who loves me for my authentic self than by hundreds who admire a façade of who I am.

I know my calling. I know why I am here. I want to serve, give, love, share, create, and make the world a better place. I conversely know why I am not here—I am not here to judge, hurt, put down, discourage, rage, blame, lie, steal, cheat, take, or destroy. I have clarity about my mission. And I feel my calling. I understand the temporary and quickly fading sense of accomplishment. I understand the long-lasting sting of failure. And I choose to attach to neither accomplishment nor failure. I choose to not classify by right and wrong, by good or bad, by beneficial or unbeneficial. Whatever happens, happens. Much like in nature, I have learned to flow with the circle of life and ever-changing seasons. Nothing is stagnant—not my mind, not my body, not my world. I am filled with trillions of microorganisms and my imagination is infinite. I am mostly water affected by the moon and I am mostly space affected by something I cannot begin to explain. I am made of a molecular structure that moves in accordance to thought. I know these things and I accept them. And at the same time, I accept I know nothing and that I may change my mind at any given moment. I listen to my body and to my intuition. And I question authority. I question the rules and the logic. And I especially question those who believe they have found the way, the truth, or the answers. I know enough to know there isn't one way, one path, or one direction.

I know I am a good friend. I have confidence in myself, in my abilities, in my intelligence, in my loyalty, and in my kindness. I have confidence in my capacity to lift others up. I know my character traits in all lights. I have done massive soul-searching and looked deeply at myself and my behaviors and thoughts. I understand that even my perceived "faults" are part of my uniqueness and enhance my capacity to connect with others. I understand I am being the best person I can be and try my best not to judge or persecute myself. I accept me in all my phases and stages.

I am comfortable being autistic. My brain is magnificent. I am in good company. I have no shame. I have seen how magnificently brilliant my Aspie son is; and in watching him, I have been able to embrace aspects of myself. Whatever name I am called makes no difference. I don't care about the labels or the words used to classify and quantify. If a word can bring me closer to people who understand and want to know me, and if that same word can bring me closer to the uniqueness of others, then so be it. I know one word doesn't define who I am and never will. I choose not to make any words my enemy, as I choose not to make any people my enemy.

I am an awesome mom. I don't put pressure on my children. They get to be who they want to be. I don't invent rigid rules and create an environment of rigid structure. I don't continually force them to do things they don't want to do. I also don't base my self-esteem on my children. They are not an extension of me. Their school grades and talents are not my accomplishments. I love them for who they are, not for what they can prove or show the world. My esteem does not fluctuate based on their behavior. I try my best not to criticize. I don't hurt intentionally. I don't manipulate. I don't talk superficial talk. I ask my boys straight out, "How are you feeling today? Are you sad about anything? Anything I can do to make your life easier? Are you overall happy?" I admit my mistakes and explain why I acted a certain way. I hug them when they are mad and hold them in a space of love when they are frustrated. I try my best not to take their actions personally. I know their opinions of me are not who I am. I know my opinion of them is not who they are. I don't pretend around them. Never have and never will. I don't depend on them for my emotional support, but I don't hide my emotions. My world is open to them. I protect them from harm because I am their mother. I don't expect them to be a mini version of me; I don't expect them to believe in the same faith, the same truths, or to like the same things as me. I know that I can teach by example. That if they see I am at peace with self, they will naturally desire to understand this; if not today, then another day. I also know they are above all else my teachers. They teach me more than any book or guru could. I simply watch how I respond and react to them. I watch how I feel when I am with them. I watch them with keen curiosity and I embrace them with unconditional love. I tell them they can do anything with their lives and I will love them the same. I know they will figure life out in their own time and in their own way. Since I was a young child, I prayed to raise children that were happy, secure, and confident. I know these attributes are produced from love, honesty, predictability, stability, and acceptance. I told this to my eldest, who is approaching sixteen, and he responded with, "Yay, Mom. You did it." And I said, "Yay, God!" And we both shared a chuckle. I am the mom that is loyal, dependable, and speaks the truth. I am the mom I choose to be. Much like I am the person I choose to be. And that is why I smile.

108. TRUE EMPATHY

I am a complex individual deciphering large amounts of random information at multiple levels, and classifying this information into categories to better make sense of my immediate surroundings. When I hit a roadblock and don't understand something, I decipher and categorize and attempt to locate a prior experience so that I might better relate. I do this by searching back into my memory banks and bringing up that which would best serve to connect to the current experience.

In regard to feeling empathy, I am unable to demonstrate empathy when I am unable to find a reference point from my past that relates back to a current situation. In example, if a man is upset his winning sports team has lost, and I am not a sports fan or a man, I will have difficulty bringing up something from my past to relate to what this man is experiencing. Regardless, no matter how I process another's situation, I still will have a form of what is clearly *empathy*. When I come in contact with a person, I attempt to sort out how his or her experience is akin to an experience I might have had. This is how my brain works. I can see no other feasible way of relating to someone without doing this.

I would suggest that what mainstream calls "showing empathy" is not the same as *feeling* empathy. An action does not equate an emotion. I would furthermore suggest that there is a blurred line between what society deems as *having* empathy and *showing* empathy. In my view, the capacity for another to empathize is not related to what he or she says or does. In other words, a person's internal degree of empathy, or ability to empathize, cannot be determined by actions or words. Furthermore, the capacity for empathy should not be based on how an individual responds to another on the spot or how quickly or "accurately" he or she reacts to a given situation.

Herein is where some get caught up: in concluding that the person's behavior alone, in and of itself, is a direct reflection of empathy. This is a false view. For empathy is much more than an action or behavior, and it is not something that can be evaluated based on specific statements or response time. Yet this is what many do. True empathy is indeed a connection reveled beneath the layers of presentation. Underneath what is spoken and done. Most people can fake empathy but that does not make them empathetic; however, false actions and words pass as *having* empathy. I observe what passes as empathy in daily interactions—the ritual nodding, habitual back-patting, the common, "It will be okay;" however, if one observes closely, there aren't always feelings or a sense of connection behind the actions and words—though these aforementioned mannerisms somehow always pass as *having* empathy.

Many are trapped in the notion of believing what one says and does is truth, when oftentimes another's spoken words do not accurately reflect their underlying feelings and fears. As is such, I believe true empathy is found in the emotions and the thoughts beneath the actions—not in the actions themselves.

109. YOU

You know everything. You were brought here and formed in pure perfection to shine your light upon the world; in our darkest hours you shall rise up and be the bright star that births beginnings and awareness. You are none other than universal life itself, beating to the rhythmic pulse of the magical web of life, your every string a vibrating tune that resonates goodness and righteousness.

You are the essence of Mother Earth's womb and the kindling burned by Father Moon, bringing forth a warmth to the inhabitants that radiates endless joy with the capacity to heal. There is nothing you can do to remove this joy from the center of your heart, or the pain from the center of your mind, beyond recognizing no mind exists and only heart beats true.

In recognition, you shall go forth and conquer fear, and in freeing self, free the multitudes. You are loved with an endless passion, created in the image of pure beauty, no less perfect than the one you hold most beautiful or the one you hold least special. Lift up all, and in turn you lift up yourself. There is no one and nothing that can touch you, for you are infinite in your grace and essence, a star seed set down to grow in the space of emptiness.

You have rooted your spirit in the likeness of me, and in so doing blessed me with abundance of opportunity. Everything about you—the way you move, the way you speak, your mannerisms, your substance—is pure honey. I could search eternity for your love and find nothing in comparison, for you carry a divine uniqueness that is entirely you, a blueprint spread out that carves your life into my life and sets us both on the path of mystery and newness. Your brain is a superpower of radiating virtues, capable of deciphering the deepest puzzles and coming up from the depth of wisdom with the knowledge of the ancient ones. You have the direct capacity to tap into supernovas, to spinning planets, to the world beyond worlds, to the infiniteness of your own being. Inside of you are so many answers waiting to spill out and cleanse the world like healing waters. You only need open the gate, the circular lid of closure; just lift and let your beauty flow.

You are these waters, and your time has come to embrace the loveliness of you. Nothing you do or say reduces this loveliness, as nothing maximizes the girth, for you are innately and substantially enough—no holes, no fixing, no nothing about you that needs forgiveness or retribution. You are guiltless in your passion to do good will, in your capacity to heal, to serve, and to dive into the sorrows of the worlds. You were given the birthmark of healer and potential warrior of good, and every path you carve out is blessed with gratitude and freedom. You are a freedom maker. You will divide the truth from the falsehoods and show truth in the light of your waking.

I am firm in my belief in you and everything about you. For I have made you, created you, and molded you in my goodness. How can one part of me be any less than the whole; how can one part of you be any less than me? I am your savior, your righteous one, your demon, and your forger. I am anything you make me. I am your shadow speaker, your sage, your guru. I am the truth and the light, or I am naught. For I exist not outside the illusion you create and the aspect of love.

I am the endless cycle of love, stirring the stars in heaven so you may rest your head beneath my twilight. I am none other than your father, your mother, your sister, your brother; I am all, and I am none. You paint me with your visions, and your visions surrender onto themselves, dripping out the substance of truth, like raindrops dropping through the green to the brown earth. Droplets of knowledge seeped through the healing energy of towering love, the very love that enables you to breathe. Call me Spirit or call me Mystery, call me by any name this man of man chooses, but call me first and utmost: You.

110. How Do I Exist without Existing?

Something is happening. Miraculous healings. I have no doubt about this, but I cannot and will not manifest my role into a Catholic mystical icon. I tried the Buddha route, and that was hard enough, but at least Buddhists keep their childlike joy and lightheartedness. Too much diving into the lives of saints and I feel stifled and dragged down, like the very life of me is being siphoned out as a sacrificial lamb. I am afraid (the only fear I possess right now) to study any more religions or spiritual practices, for I have jolted my capacity to morph into any way of living I study. I don't want to live like a saint. I still want to make jokes about poop and sex and about other people. What am I to do? Crap! Every role I take on, or persona I think I am, makes me eventually strangle in the rules and rigidness of said "type." Despite the fact there are truly no rules, they still lasso me, as if the rules themselves are my dark virtue, trapping me at every turn.

How do I exist without feeling a need to be all I can be? How do I exist without doubting if I am my true self? And what if I am now so empty in the result of recognizing my own invisibility and illusion of self that I morph into anyone I am with—become who they think me to be, become a part of the observer?

What if I am slipping through these pages as a sage of sorts revealing the aspects of the ever-changing, complex mind of Aspergers primarily because of my capacity to change roles and cling to rules? If in truth my suffering through Aspergers is serving the world in some way, then should I continue to suffer just to carry on my duty? Or is it that even this Aspergers is something I created to serve as a carrier of sorts to bring me from one edge of the river of self to the other? And if so, what was I when I set out across the water, at the start, and what will I be when I step down on the other side? What if the waters are safer and my mind itself the murderer of serenity? How can I be anything when I can see the complexity of everything and dissect myself enough to bare no untruths or falsehoods? How can I exist so readily spread out to the world—open, honest, and true—when the rest watch in bewilderment? Surely I am some creature not of this earth, not made for earthly ways, and made to suffer through the maze of never-ending questions. How to turn off this mind long enough to be me without finding a rigid way to do so—whether this be misery, melancholy, creation, or taking on the role of someone or some purpose. How do I exist without existing?

111. BUBBLED LAYERS

Recently, I explained to my husband that I was confused by most of mankind's behavior and that I felt alone and isolated. During our conversation several things occurred to me. I was reminded that people frequently judge and categorize other people, and that I tend to think differently than the average person. I also realized the following: I pick up on others' energies and emotions; I still long to belong and be seen; some people seem less aware of self than me; just because some claim they adhere to certain principles doesn't mean they do; and people lump collective thoughts into a theory and then generalize about a set of people.

During the discussion, my husband took some time to explain some of the NT (neurotypical, e.g., non-autistic, alternative to *normal*) behavior. He was actually quite good in his description. He gave this great analogy. He said that he believes most NTs (himself included) walk around in these bubbled layers of walls. There are several, at least three. (News to me.) And that when they first meet another person their bubbles kind of touch each other, and that this is their "line of defense." They (some of the NTs) like to bump and meet several times before letting down the first bubble wall. Therefore they talk about things that aren't personal or don't seem risky at all (safe, boring, surface-level stuff). They do this to make sure the person is safe, not a threat, not someone to fear, or someone who is after them; and also, to see if they share common interests and viewpoints.

By this point, I had interrupted several times and drifted in and out of my imagination, because the bubbles were fun to picture, and my husband is very used to me "interjecting." Here are some of the things I asked: (1) Why? (2) What do you talk about? (3) Isn't it boring? (4) What is in the last bubble? (5) What are people hiding? (6) What are people afraid of?

Here are the corresponding answers from my *bubble* NT husband . . .

1. **Why?** We have been trained not to trust. Think of all the messages you hear. For example: *You let him into your house? You told him what? You let him do what? You gave him money? He is just going to buy drugs with it* . . . The fact is, people basically don't trust other people.

2. **What do you talk about?** I don't know. Basic stuff.
3. **Isn't it boring?** No. I think we enjoy it.
4. **What is the last bubble?** Probably our deepest self that we think is unworthy; fear.
5. **What are people hiding?** Their deep, dark secrets.
6. **What are people afraid of?** Being found out. Being hurt, basically fear.

During our discussion, I kept saying, for quite a long while, "But what are you afraid of? What is there to fear?" We went round and round for quite a bit, and it came down to the fact that most humans have an innate distrust for other humans and most humans think at a core level they are inadequate; and some people do things they think are terrible and could never share or have had things done to them that they feel ashamed about. There was also some discussion about the "dark side" that people hide. I couldn't understand what the dark side was, and what people were hiding and why they were hiding it. I tried.

I asked, "What is my dark side?" My husband said, "I haven't found one yet, and I hope I never do." That seemed silly to me. I don't hide anything and have no places of hiding, and no bubbles, so there isn't any place the dark side can live. But the other stuff, it started to make sense.

Soon I asked, "Well then, if there are two different types of people, some that are honest, don't manipulate, don't hold back, don't have these bubbles, but are trusting and loving and completely open, and try to see the best in others, and there is another group who lies, manipulates, and plays games to protect an inner fear that stems from someplace about something they are unsure about, then it makes more sense to me that the group that lie and are in fear try to adapt and be more like the ones that trust and are open, instead of reverse; don't you think?" This is when we can really clap for my husband—for having lived with the sincere challenges I sometimes offer out in a relationship, he still had the honesty and sweetness to say, "That's why I think at times that Aspergers is a new race of people come to help the world." Then he chuckled and added he'd been watching too much sci-fi. I took this as an NT immediately putting up a bubble, and I understood.

112. I SCARE PEOPLE

"Why is it when I am authentic and true and real, and entirely me, I scare people?" I asked my husband, and he replied with several suitable answers, all of which made sense, but still baffled me.

He said: "You scare people because people don't trust people. So when you are honest, kind, and sweet, they question your interior motive, your genuineness, and your truthfulness. People don't feel comfortable having someone spill out their whole self all at once. It is too much and over-whelming. They don't know how to respond, what to say, or why you are that way. They are confronted with their own inability to not be authentic and real, and this reminds them of their own secrets and feelings of unworthiness and lack of confidence at the center. They also wonder what you are hiding, for surely there must be all these layers you are hiding; and if you are hiding, then why are you faking authenticity?"

This saddened me and intrigued me, all at once. I responded, "Some Aspies love the company of other Aspies because we are real and some non-autistics like the company of other non-autistics because they are pretending instead of being completely real at first." My husband explained that many people like to spend a lot of time together until they trust. They build trust. And he noted that I don't need to do that; I love instantly, share instantly, and trust instantly. I didn't understand the need to build up trust.

This brought me back to a local church event. One of the speakers, a well-spoken woman of faith, who was trying hard to do her best, explained that everyone's intimacy with God takes time, just like our everyday rela-tionships. That we share our deepest secrets with people we've known a long time, not just a few days, and that in this same way one must spend a long time with God to build intimacy. I found this entirely wrong and stopped myself from saying so. I don't need time with my friends to build trust. I trust in reverse. I give the benefit of the doubt ahead of time. God gets that. And He is good with that.

113. MY PEN NAME

A few days ago, during a small group discussion at a local venue, someone asked me about my pen name *Samantha Craft*. I explained *Craft* was the last name that belonged to a woman who was like a mother to me, who was a strong woman of faith, and who took me under her wing. I added she had died of a brain tumor at the age of fifty and that I had chosen her name to honor her gentle and kind spirit. Everyone, the nine women sitting in the circle, wore solemn and supportive expressions while I shared. Then I heard, "And what about the name *Samantha?*" At that point the little girl in me, she popped up, twitched her nose, and said giddily, "The witch from the television show *Bewitched!*"

This sums up why I confuse people. After hearing my last response, the group members' faces scrunched up in the same way my kindergarten classmates' tiny faces did when I was a youngster and I announced my favorite color was *magenta*. (WTF?) That is why I shall never earn my wings. I am much like the angel in the Christmas classic *It's a Wonderful Life* (best movie on earth)—I confuse people because I have this deep, prophetic spirit that is filled with catacombs of endless love. And then I also have this little girl inside who totally wants to be a nose-wiggling magical witch from a popular sitcom. People can't figure out who or what I am, so they judge me to ease their own minds.

114. Vignette, The Broken Board, Age 11

A bunion of a gal leaned on a century-old redwood tree picking at a quarter-sized scab on her elbow. She was unsightly and red all over with flakes of dead skin saluting the wind. When I thought about cousin Debbie, I visualized a witch hunched over a littered kitchen table yanking on the blue ligaments of a cold chicken leg with her silver-crowned, tobacco-stained teeth. I couldn't help myself. Debbie was hatched from a disorderly clan, the type I would purposely cross the street to avoid in later life. I wished to bleach out my days with her relatives, erase them from my memory completely, or at the very least fast-forward through the events like I did with the songs I didn't like on my portable cassette player.

Debbie's Aunt Marge jiggled across the campsite with her signature loopy hair, loopy walk, and loopy smile. Spotting her at full speed I went rigid and shot invisible armor up every side of my body. But it was of no use. I was soon smeared in snail trails of sticky orange lipstick. Jane, Marge's crystal-blue-eyed daughter, my camping buddy ever since I could remember, approached next and draped her thin arm around my waist. "What took you so long?" she asked, handing me a miniature box of Lucky Charms cereal. Her little sister stood at her side trying to weasel the other box of cereal from Jane's clasped hand. "Scram, stupid!" Jane barked.

By noon, Mother, her boyfriend Ben, and a dozen of their camping buddies loaded atop the highest level of a double-decker tourist bus while Jane and I waved good-bye. As the blue bus puffed around the high pine trees and the last of the exhaust fumes cleared the air, a woman sporting yellow high heels and a visor wobbled up a nearby hill, jogging after a porky dog that looked identical to my grandmother's ottoman. Giggling, Jane and I teetered up and down on a board we'd propped up on a rock. Cousin Debbie sat on a picnic table, cracking her knuckles.

"Thirteen," I said. "That's thirteen times!"

Jane bent her knees low and then shot up, springing me into the clean mountain air. Debbie grumbled something, flapped up a piece of her choppy red hair, and shriveled her face into an unappealing scowl. Then, she eased herself up off the bench—bent toothpick, frayed towel, and all— and flip-flopped forward. Upon reaching us, she slammed her freckled fist on our makeshift teeter-totter. I held my breath.

"Give me that board before you bust it up!" she demanded, with a flick of her toothpick. I set my eyes on the settling dust and counted. "I was told to look after you. So don't be acting stupid," she continued.

Jane got up off of the board and skirted around. She was always more direct than I was. She had a boldness I could not compete with. Staring up surely at Debbie, Jane hollered, "Don't tell us what to do! You're not our boss. Leave us alone!"

I opened my mouth and breathed in and out, repeatedly, reminding myself that Debbie was nothing more than an overfed teenager with nothing better to do than terrorize a couple of little kids.

"We won't play on it anymore. I promise," I said.

With my words, the cousin's petulant expression settled. "Fine, just don't do it again," she said, and then made a grunt, before flopping away.

I glanced over at Jane and shrugged my shoulders. In response Jane shook her head in obvious disapproval. We stayed away from our board a good hour before we were drawn back to the forbidden. And just as mean cousin Deb predicted, after we'd teetered a few more times, the board snapped right in half. The sudden break sent Jane and I tumbling backward, the dirt covering us from head to toe like powdered donuts.

Hearing the commotion, Debbie's tall sister Bev poked her narrow face out of a green tent and stepped out, her brassy, blond curls waving in the breeze. A clove cigarette dangled from her mouth. Bev approached at a slow pace, her eyebrows squeezing together in a caterpillar-like style and her blue eyes settling down on the broken board.

Jane and I stood together holding hands, while Bev folded her arms across her flat chest and flicked the ash of her cigarette. She spoke down to Jane. "Now, look at what you've done." With one hand, she lifted up half of the splintered board. "Now, what are we going to do?" Redheaded Debbie approached, leaving a trail of dust. Jane squeezed my hand and blurted out, "It wasn't us. It was my little sister. We didn't do it!" Jane's scrawny sibling was nowhere in sight.

I examined the sisters' mirrored grimaces and knew at once we were in trouble. I wished Jane had kept her mouth shut. I would have much preferred the cowardly apologetic approach. We could have bartered. I would have offered to sweep their tent or to buy them a bag of barbeque chips at the campground market. I would have given them the fifty cents in my short's pocket. But it was too late. I leaned back on the picnic table, catching a splinter under the nail of my thumb, and bit my lip. I had already pushed open a corner of my mind and was thinking back on the leather belt, the black one on the hook in Jane's father's closet. I didn't get through a spring vacation or my birthday week without at least one swipe of the belt. During my visits, Jane's dad would order Jane and me to climb up on top of his water bed— the tall type with the mirrored bookshelves and drawers beneath—and there on the waving mattress we'd pull down our pants. When I got hit with one or two lashings across the butt I cried, but Jane, she always remained stoic, just staring back at her dad with eyes of ice. Sometimes he would whip her once more just to spite her attitude.

These cousins could not be as strong as Jane's dad. They were not liable to hurt us. I reasoned at this point I had better tell the truth and save us a far worse punishment. I blurted out, "Jane and I broke the board. We didn't mean to. We won't do it again. I promise."

Jane retaliated, "We didn't break it!"

My stomach buckled over. Debbie smacked her puffy, chapped lips together. "You idiots! Why'd you have to go and do a backward-ass thing like this? What were you thinking? Then on top of it all you have to lie to us. Why'd you have to lie?" She stopped to smash the butt of her clove cigarette in the knot of the table. "Come on. Let's get this over with."

Above us a bluebird perched himself on an overhead branch and cocked his head, as if he had paid admission to observe us. Bev ran her tongue across her lips and leaned toward Jane. She ran her nail-bitten fingers through Jane's long strands of hair and then gave me a severe stare. "You first."

Moments later my wobbly knees somehow managed to carry me to the tent.

Tall Bev was the last to duck inside. After flicking dirt from under her nails, she tied the tent door flap behind us. I could stand upright inside the tent and the stout cousin could too, only the lean one had to bend a bit.

"Get up here," Bev ordered. She tapped her hand on the cot and her smile vaporized. I visualized a frog-green haze rising from beneath the canvas floor and the faces of repulsive witches materializing as the cousins peeled away their human latex masks. I slid down, faceup on the cot.

"Turn over," the fat cousin ordered. She smacked a piece of gum in her mouth, an old wad she collected from her pocket, and blew a pathetic bubble. I turned over and pushed my blushing face into a dusty sleeping bag.

"Pull your pants down!"

I squeezed my lids closed, much like I did when anticipating a vaccination shot, and tugged down my pants and underwear. I remembered I hadn't changed my underwear in four days and hoped they wouldn't tease me. I could smell lotion and dust but nothing more. Seconds after my pants were down a coarse object crashed down on the back of my bare thigh. The intense burning began at my upper legs and shot down to my shins. *What was that?* And then there was another harder smack. The same pain again. Smack. Again a hit came, first to the left a bit lower, then to the right a bit higher, and then to the right again, just above my waist. I lost count. Smack. Smack. Smack. Too fast to count.

When the beating stopped, long after the tears began, I unclenched my hands from the top slate of the cot and clicked my jaw, stretching my mouth and reassuring myself that I could still take in air. Bev dropped the board onto the tent floor and the porky redhead announced, "Since you told the truth, you're all finished." She cracked her neck to the side. "You're lucky. Jane, she's in big trouble. For every hit you got, she's getting double."

All I could think about was that it was my fault that Jane was in trouble. I'd ratted on my best friend and now she would have to pay the price. I waited at the picnic table and through my tears watched Jane disappear into the army-green tent. A fire was trying to push up from under my skin. I searched the empty campground for any sign of Mother and then stared out into nothingness. Gales of laughter flittered out from the tent and then Jane stumbled back outdoors—her thin legs marked up and down with the beginnings of bruises. I was thankful they were finished with us.

We were both speechless as I hobbled with lowered head behind Jane up a dirt trail to the public bathroom. In the bathroom mirror the blue of Jane's eyes, the beautiful Tahoe blue that changed with the light of the day, was glossed over. But where I expected to find her tears, I saw only a faraway stare. Jane took in a deep breath and blew out through her flaring nostrils. A lady with wavy black hair walked into the bathroom.

"Hello," she said. She looked down at the back of our legs. "Girls what happened to you? How? Who did this to you?" The stranger quickly grabbed a stack of paper towels and wet them under the faucet. "Here, wrap these around your thighs." I accepted the coolness of the towels and smiled softly, keeping my eyes set on the molding grout framing the cracked floor tiles. Jane stared forward in the mirror. The woman ran her fingers through Jane's bangs. "Despicable," she whispered, before she disappeared.

At sunset the sky splintered into prisms of brilliant red. Under a canopy of trees, the campfire illuminated Jane's solemn face, as she twisted a long stick out from the flames and blew on her burnt marshmallow. The whites of the marshmallow's insides busted through the crusted black. Up high on the trail leading down to the camp, Mother was the leader of a group of women, an engine in a long line of slugging boxcars. The pain of the beatings still hurt worse than any sunburn. I feared I could die of the bruises—bleed internally by morning. I forced myself to focus on the uncomfortable stickiness of the marshmallow between my fingers and the frothed-out beer bottles littered on the ground. Mother settled down amongst the clan, finding a spot on the log. She was a lone sapphire intermixed within a cauldron of plastic rhinestones.

"I love you, beautiful," she said. "Did you have a good time?"

Feeling emotionally cornered, I fought back tears. I knew if I lied and said I had a good time, Mother would smile and relax. However, if I told the truth, Mother would demand to know what had happened and I would have to mull over the board-beating details, and risk being called a liar. I thought back to my English teacher and pictured myself as a character in a novel. This would be the brave me. The scared me I could save for another page.

115. At Last I Am Me

I have been able to alleviate most of my fear about everyone and everything. Including death and illness. This is the first time in my life I remember feeling this way for an extended period of time. As a young girl I had many moments of carefree wonderment, but since my teenage years I have been prone to bouts of depression and, to put it mildly, emotional suffering. I don't know exactly what is different now except that I have accepted a part of myself that I previously pushed down. I have been afforded the opportunity of remarkable realizations regarding self, Aspergers, and my spiritual life. If one ventures back through my philosophical prose, it is evident that some profound creation has been forged through me. My husband has noticed what he would call *astounding* and *mind-altering* changes. What I am seeing in reflection is that I had a core base of fear. I had to learn, above all, how to love myself and to love other people unconditionally. This was a huge undertaking. I took a hard, honest look at all aspects of myself that I could feasibly find and used an audience as a sounding board for further discovery.

I don't think my healing would have advanced had I not had a potential audience to read my works and share in my journey. Journals and diaries never worked for me because they were short-lasting special interests. Having an audience was appealing because I could put on stage the part of myself undergoing excavation and (unknowingly) slip into a role or alternate persona. This process of taking on a role is similar to the times I was an actress on a real stage or a cheerleader in high school, where I was able to exist and interact with others because I wasn't fully me. Whoever I was inside (the real me) during this time was lost. I know that now. Who I was at the core, behind all the personas and roles, got lost in the process of trying to fit in.

I have a natural ability to step outside of myself and view self. In doing so, in stepping back and observing this other me (the roles I took on), I had ample opportunity to find out how I moved in the world through observation of self. When I adapted this new role of "person-healing self" to an audience,

I was able to observe that *person*. It seems for most of my life I have had the lost me (who is hidden and out of sight), the role me (who fluctuates), and then the observer me (who steps back and watches the transitions and progressions). Interestingly, the observer has never changed, the role me has always changed, and the real me has always hidden—until now.

I have been able to reclaim the lost me. She has come out of hiding and replaced the role me. And the role me appears to have gone. Observer is still here to a heightened degree. Now I (as the observer) am able to watch the real me who was in hiding for decades and help her through aspects of life. Before, the observer could not help the *real me* much because she was unavailable—lost behind the always-changing *role me*.

When I was in a role, I was not *me*. I thought, at the time, I was *me*, but I always changed, lessened, increased, or vanished. I became a chameleon without conscious choice. There was no willingness involved in changing roles. It just happened. And I didn't know it had happened until they (the personas I had taken on) were leaving. For instance, I might take on the role of a college student or a spiritual teacher, and that would become my entire identity and focus. All would be centered about this new self that I finally believed I was.

This time is different. A new role hasn't surfaced. I have resurfaced. I feel like I have reached back in time and reconnected with the little girl lost. And I love her. I adore her and want to share her with the world. I have relatively little to no fear introducing her to people, as she is *me*.

This is huge, in the dynamic, life-shifting sense. I believe that I was only able to retrieve my little girl because I relived all she had suffered, gave it recognition, let her be seen, and then released her through the act of forgiveness. I understood ultimately she was an innocent and pure one. All shame vanished and all blame. This came about after I spent years writing and forgiving people in my life. After my total clearing house of forgiveness occurred, more room inside was available for healing. Here is when something entered me, which seems to have been akin to dramatic self-love, self-respect, reassurance, and inner knowing. Also, I believe that Spirit began to take hold.

116. SERENITY

Where I once lived my every day with constant thoughts of analysis and processing, especially loops of fixations, now I have a profound silence in my mind. I am observing as the little girl and all appears magic and beautiful again. I am filled with joy and able to navigate the world with a fresh and innocent perspective instead of a fear-based one. When I am in conversation, I am sometimes able to behold the person with a silence in my mind. If I feel a worry about what I said or how I said something, observer comes and helps me clear out the fear. I have no need for outcomes in conversation, for defense, to prove a point, to fix, or to prove anything. I just am, with no intention but being. I don't worry as much anymore about what another is thinking about me.

I no longer categorize people. This process of not sorting others began a couple of months ago. Everywhere I went I started redirecting my thoughts. If I saw another, I would tell myself, "This is all an illusion. She is another living being of light and nothing more." I would then repeat something easy to my mind that didn't hurt, as sometimes certain types of thinking hurt. I simply said: *beautiful, beautiful, beautiful* or *love, love, love*. I still could see the labels, but eventually the labels were replaced by silence. If the labels come now, observer steps in and gently removes them.

For most of my life I had honed in on others and used a highly intuitive and logical ability to analyze people. This happened through nonverbal and verbal cues, and what seemed to be the energy of the person. Recently I realized I was choosing to see the negativity in others. And just because I could didn't mean I had to. I prayed about wanting this released. I wanted to see the light in everyone and nothing more. Within two days following my prayer, my ability to see what other people lacked was replaced with the ability to see immeasurable beauty.

This process of analyzing others seems to have been a survival skill from the start. Something I depended upon to navigate through the world, particularly the world of communication. I understand now that I saw myself as negative, wrong and flawed, and as a result projected my own self-image onto other people. I was choosing always to see what I wanted to see, even though I thought I was detecting these hidden mysteries. This was a game I invented, thinking if I could figure people out I would stay one step ahead of them and avoid potential harm. The key to release this dependency on seeing the "negative" was in loving myself and realizing no one's words or energy can harm me. They just can't. Once I accepted this, love became my new truth.

For years I had been perpetually holding myself prisoner. I firmly believe this. Today I am free. In choosing to see the good of people, more and more good is coming to me. By good, I mean aspects of beauty and awareness, because ultimately, in my belief system, nothing is good or bad. I no longer see myself as separate. I seem to blend in with everyone else. I see their beauty reflected in me and my beauty reflected in them. I love them. I love people. And everyplace I go is like a parade of violet-blue butterflies. I imagine this is how the world looks when one is still a young child, before the trust is lost and before the heart gets broken.

I realize now I can choose to recreate my own life outlook. Presently, I am able to understand that the world is a safe place. I was taught and shown the world was unsafe, repeatedly. But the world is safe. If I choose to live with no fear, the world is very safe. Matter of fact, no amount of worry and anxiety and planning and reasoning is going to prepare me for all the imagined dangers. I don't need to live my life as if pending danger is looming around every corner. I recognize that isn't living.

I have been able to use the observer to comfort the child in me. Now the observer is my watcher. If I (the real me) start to fear, then the observer steps in and reminds me that fear is false. With Spirit's help I can recognize every emotion beyond love as a false entity spawned from fear. Fear has so many faces, but I recognize him quickly. If I feel anger, resentment, urgency, anxiety, or anything that disrupts my peace, I say *hello* to fear. He has gotten to the point where he actually speaks and says, "Shucks. You caught me, again." Then I release him. And *poof!* Back to serenity.

117. STATE OF LA-LA

Here is what my sons said from the back seat of the van, each contributing their not-so-discreet two cents worth:

Son 1: "Mom, You are always nice and kind. You are uncommonly good to people."

Son 2: "Yeah, but it's creepy, Mom, really creepy. I mean who is so nice?"

Son 3: "Yeah, I mean how do we know you're not a sociopath or something? Because based on your characteristics, it's quite feasible . . ." (My Aspie son—first few lines of what turned out to be an analytical dissertation about my behavior.)

Lately, I've been in a grand state of la-la-land happiness. I am that magical little girl I used to be. I love her. She is so fun and sweet and terribly kind. On my walk a few days ago I found a twig with sea-green moss attached and a natural loop on the top, and I pretended it was my elven princess wand. I kept knighting my little black Labradoodle the name *Sir Princess Violet*, until I poked her in the eye. Then after that she smelled this really cute mutt's butt, and I said, "See what good fortune you have after I knighted you?" My little black dog has crazy white facial fur that looks like Einstein eyebrows, and when I am in my little-girl mood she raises them often, as if to question if she'll get the bed to herself when I go to the nuthouse. On our walk we stopped and took turns looking through the wooden-looped wand. Every once in a while I pretended to change people into other things. I have this new game I play. When I see someone, I attach random words to the person. I say *sack of potatoes*, or *tow truck*, or *peacock butt*. I just make up any random name to teach myself that nothing I have learned before is real—just all names someone made up at one time or another. I like to do this to keep things straight in my head. Nobody needs to be labeled *fat, shortie, dirty, stinky, ugly*, etc. So I like to turn people into things before my mind can catch up. So far my favorite was the *turnip*.

On our walk we sang, "We're off to see the wizard, the wonderful wizard of Oz, because, because, because, because" . . . (long pause) . . . (and start song again.) That's how we sing it because I have a terrible memory for song lyrics and my dog Violet never saw the movie.

118. WOVEN KNIGHT

You are the ever-gladness of my everglades, my gratitude lifted from the waters of greenery, the etching of my soul made new. In you I see eternity, your eyes the light of my lantern, the cave to my longing. To glance but once is to see the distance song awoken, the beat of my heart renewed, the pavement marked with the blood of footprints, red.

I follow, and I follow more. Your steps, my steps; your way, my way; and reach to anchor what is me into what is you, forging through the sun-swept grasses to lead my soul within the trappings of kindness. If I could ascend, I would; my foot, my hand, like the climber upon the stronghold of rock, lingered there at the sandy grip between my limbs; how I long to dive and slip into the places you are made, into the very start of your beginning; to see you form and bend in completion, to watch as witness as the light of my world is first sparked.

How glorious, if I could be your maiden and set each braided dream upon your lap, as you, like the purest of daylight, move past my flesh, and penetrate with the grandest of sweetness. I cannot but imagine how dreams become answer, how I become found, without the drumming of your castle, calling me forward, a lone soldier centered and marked, inching her way to the trumpets of your name.

I awake to the morning day, and yours is the face I see. I dance in the starlight, and yours is the wish I make. I mend my own existence with the remnants of your memory, waiting beyond the blindness of what can only be such bitter spell. My darling enveloped babe, I cannot hope but to be anything less than your maiden, my kisses upon thy cheeks, thy lips, thy buried chest of grandeur. To whittle my fingers into bare bone, to make my flesh peel asunder, my eyes leap, my scars each burst renewed in the aching. For I would die for you a thousand deaths upon a thousand more, and ring my life around the circumference of your calling.

Take me as sweet river, my beckoning, the one that rushes through the caverns of my heart, rupturing like the gold dust glitters upon the landing.

Am I but this remainder, this fragile broken shell, scattered on the endless shore, glistening in the break of day; my pieces fallen from the lost sky, my tears hidden in the lines of the encasement? Or am I true, the one formed with your first breath, moved by your ocean, chaliced view rendered through the breaking of bread of two; for you, my darling, my eternal lover of the ever-time, have with first step, with first entrance, with the ancient tumbling of my name, awakened the angel who slept in the shadowed swell. You, in your mercy, in your truth, in your direction, have laid way for the dawn of passion so deep that the carving of universe would do no justice.

Can you not see how I love you? Can you not see how I wait within the waiting? How each day that grows becomes centuries spent? Each second a reminder of your destined departure? Can you not see me here, cradling you in your own goodness, lathering you in the light turned and aged as fruit rendered wine? How I carry you through the meadow beyond meadow, in the space of pure joy, and await your coming. For you are my mystery unborn, my dream unawakened, my precious feathered dove gently set upon my threshold; and though you hear me not, as I cry from the hallowed space of light, I shall guard thee in the blanketed folds of eternity, my wishing heart made whole, with the needle that threads through the layers of my woven knight.

119. Vignette, Screaming for Justice, Age 12

If I had to choose this wouldn't be the place I would have wanted to lose my dog. But in life as I know now, and as I discovered then, I don't get to choose how my losses play out. Without a doubt, going back in time I would have preferred to have seen my dog Justice live to a ripe old age and to have watched him pass in my arms beside the protective watch of my mother and my father. Though by then my father was barely visible in my life and Mother needed my protection more than I received hers. Nonetheless, I wished sometimes to go back and rewrite Justice's end—to claim my right and his right to a formal departing embrace. To have never received the phone call that confirmed my worst fear.

On a memorable Fourth of July, I found myself once again at my friend Jane's house—some couple hundred miles away from our home in the bay area. That morning I settled myself into a matinee of half smiles and cigarette smoke at a cluttered kitchen table, while Justice—a coal-black ball of raggedy fur—nestled nervously at my feet. Jane's mother Marge, Mother's best friend since before I was born, wobbled about her space in a peach robe looking a bit on the raunchy side. She yawned, exposing a tongue covered in a dense layer of white. I thought back to my recent orthodontist experience, in preparation for my braces: how the x-ray tech's breath had haunted me for months.

Mother was behind somewhere, drifting about much like a newly birthed butterfly—an imago burst from chrysalis—damp, fragile, withdrawn. She was much absorbed into her own world; sucked up like water into a cotton ball, so in essence she was still there, yet her form was masked by something else.

Sitting there in the dimly lit kitchen, with Jane's family members hustling all about, I thought back to Shara—my little friend. She had been kidnapped many months prior by strangers that her mother had hired; stolen from her father when she was snatched up and hidden in a van. Shara was somewhere faraway now. I missed my friend like I missed my stepfamily, like I missed my two canaries that had recently been murdered by cats. And I wished more than ever that I had a sister or brother.

I thought back further in time to the first time I had slept at Shara's house—a bare rental lacking most of the necessities that made a home a home. I remembered her dropping the red brick on her big toe, her toe turning a purple-black, and her toenail eventually popping off, and how she'd had to take baths with her tiny leg flopped over the side of the blue tub. I remembered having to stretch out on some daybed in the outer corner of Shara's house, made to sleep in the strange-smelling place with all the creeping sounds. I was terrified of most places by then, as Mother had made it very clear that our fifteen-century German cabinet was haunted and required a blessing with holy water by the local priest. I was scared of most places by then because I always sensed something lurking somewhere.

I recalled that first night at Shara's, waking up mortified to discover I had peed my pants because I'd been too frightened to search for the bathroom in the unfamiliar dark. And I remembered slinking into Shara's bedroom, harboring myself into the safety of her proximity, taking my place on the floor next to her makeshift bed—several blankets sprawled out on bulky floor pillows. And I thought back to the sad moment when Shara set up on our couch, with quivering lips, and informed Mother, Mother's boyfriend, and I that her mother was going to take her away and never bring her back.

One of the last times I ever held Shara's hand was at the Santa Cruz Beach and Boardwalk—her chubby-cheeked face glistening in the lights of the swirling rides. We'd sat there together atop a steep flight of sandy stairs, my thoughts tethered to a distant buoy, hers to the discarded candy apple abandoned before its time. Clumps of sand were in her tight curls. It was dark, with the tourists pouring in from all directions to gather their towels and belongings—trekking up the walkways, one passerby after the next. Mother was nowhere in sight, and neither was Ben, Shara's father.

I patted Shara on the top of her head and made up a story, and later tickled her plump little tummy. (She had an outie belly button. I had an innie.) She poked me back and giggled, before sighing her deep familiar sigh. I clamped my front teeth down on my chapped bottom lip. The thoughts were coming quickly, like they always did when I was nervous. I figured Mother would eventually return, like the time after I had stepped off the PSA smiling plane (after a week-long stay with Jane and a two-day stay with Father) to find Mother wasn't there. I had waited, ended up in the airport "lost and found" with the unwanted luggage and an uppity airline attendant. Mother had eventually found me.

Shara tapped my shoulder and asked, "Can we go now?" I let out a deep breath and thought of my mother's familiar phrase: "Things could always be worse." I reasoned that was the case. At least we weren't at the nude beach, again. Another siren rang out. Someone up above was a winner. Shara began to cry, the tears sliding across her brown cheeks.

"Hi, ladies," Ben, Mother's lover, called out from the distance.

My body tightened. Shara sprung up and charged her father, wrapping her arms around his hairy legs. Mother and Ben grinned. I stopped picking at the sand in my scalp. I grabbed the stair railing to pull myself up. Mother rubbed her clammy hand across my cheek. "I told you we'd be right back," she said.

I stared out blankly.

"What are those sad eyes for?" Mother asked. Her breath smelled of vodka. She walked back toward Ben with a staggering gait and extended the cigarette pack toward my direction. I was overly aware of the strangers passing.

Ben spoke up. "Let's go." He then mumbled something about "a damn tourist trap" and led Mother by the hand across the causeway underneath the dark wooden rafters. Shara pitter-pattered in their footsteps, seemingly oblivious to everything. Ben picked at his butt through his shorts. "Can't people find better ways to spend their time?"

I followed in silence counting the wooden boards above. Mother belched, politely.

I could not feel my expression. I examined the two grown-ups as they strolled further down the boardwalk. There was no space between them. Sometimes when a man and woman walk together there is a bit of light that seeps through the gap where their bodies touch, but with Ben and Mother there was nothing.

Back at Jane's house, pale-faced cousin Betty donned in the same clothes as yesterday—all white, all stained, all wrinkly—kept tugging on her short-shorts in an attempt to cover the dime-sized bruises on her goose-pimpled thighs; no doubt the brand marks of a hanger beating. Sitting there that dry summer morning, I felt acutely aware of Betty's pain. It was ever present. I had a brief impulse to reach out to her in some way or another, to show a bit of compassion, but knew any attempt would be pointless. Sadly, when I tried to converse with Betty, it was like throwing a rubber ball hard up against a playground wall—nothing came back, except what I threw out.

Approaching the age of thirteen, I had no desire whatsoever to be in Jane's kitchen. None whatsoever. No desire to be in the house either, for that matter, no desire to be in this hot suburban town, except perchance to spend a couple nights with Father.

Regardless of my qualms, I understood why Mother visited. There was some value in these people. Certainly, there were aspects that brought cause for liking. Jane's mother Marge was a cheerful person, often chuckling. And she had enough genuine spunk to draw anyone out of dismal thoughts. She also instinctively knew how to both nurture and humor my mother. As sad as my mom often was, I understood she needed Marge, much as I understood how I needed Justice. I was never angry with Mother for bringing me along, nor was I disappointed; instead, I felt rather disheartened and homesick.

That hot, hot summer I lost Justice—some one hundred and ten degrees of sweltering heat—I partook in one of Jane's family's Fourth of July traditions. As the sun slinked behind the valley hills and the evening sky turned a hazy velvet pink, twelve of us piled into the bed of a rusted, yellow Ford pickup. Slender Mother, dressed in her halter blouse and frayed cutoff jean shorts, was one of the last to board. She sat gleefully in the shadows; her bronze skin in striking contrast to pasty Betty, who took a seat to my left and balanced her generous backside on an ice cooler. That evening Betty was smirking as she peeled back the wrapping of the white taffy candy she had stolen from my suitcase. I took my place in the back of the rusting bed, alongside Jane. From the rear of the truck, a beer bottle clanged against the side of the metal bed and then rolled back tapping the tip of my tight shoes, an old hand-me-down pair that were a size too small—Grandma's red-striped Nikes. Up above, bottle rockets flared through the air, arching like flamed rainbows.

As night moved further in, the puttering truck carried us up a steep suburban hill, bringing with it a sharp mixture of stale ale, cigarette smoke, car exhaust, and hints of moist heat escaping the cooling asphalt. Soon the height of the tradition began. We banged and clanged pots and pans. We howled, "Happy Fourth of July!"

Bumping and cheering along, I was trapped between a sensation of elation and trepidation, until a sudden panic took over. It was then I recalled a recent nightmare. The noise was my signal—the banging of objects, the crackling of fireworks, the ear-piercing hollers. Just seven days prior I'd told Mother I'd had a dreadful dream of loud noises, of banging and clanging, of a tall wooden backyard fence, of singed summer grass, of my fearful dog, of a car . . . and then of Justice—stiff and listless on an unfamiliar road.

In that moment of reckoning I knew my Justice was gone. Lost were the days of romping pirates, bubble baths, and dives under the coffee table. Lost, his curly dark fur, hot breath, tickling tongue, cold wet nose, and the depths of amber eyes. Back at Jane's, I approached the backyard. I was the first to escape the night's noise into the frightful silence. There alone, I wrestled through the shrubbery and searched the yard. Justice was nowhere to be found. I sobbed and sobbed again, screaming for Justice. "Justice! Justice! Justice!" But Justice never came.

120. Ten Ways to Spot an Aspie Girl

1. Deep, soulful eyes, which perhaps dip down slightly and/or are very distinguished and large. There is someone in there with a story. There is truth.

2. An uncomfortable smile that cannot find a home, which fluctuates between a chiseled, serious frown and the most amazing genuine smile, wherein the whole self and soul lights up—a childlike expression, too pure to be mistaken for anything other than authenticity.

3. Continual statements of second-guessing, checking for understanding, clarifying self, and offering out extra information in an attempt to be understood. Indications of never reaching a full conclusion, as there are limitless possibilities. Questioning self, harvesting advice, and then tossing everything out and starting anew. Having the kindling of multiple thoughts about multiple directions, all at the same time.

4. Fleeting, atypical eye contact that is intense, attempting to linger, and constantly moved about to find an object of focus. Unusual gestures whilst conversing and seemingly never being fully engaged in the speaker unless strongly intrigued; and even then the imagination takes over and causes a drifting appearance. Unless overtaken with a special topic of interest, then all mannerisms and ways of being become forgotten, and all that exists is the spoken word.

5. Eyebrows that raise up when a smile is formed or a distinct maneuvering of the facial features, as if to represent who they are, even when smiling, in effort to not distort a truth.

6. Unnatural-appearing stances and movements. Presenting as never quite comfortable moving in body unless preoccupied and/or in the midst of strong emotions or a special topic of interest.

7. A sweetness that isn't outgrown that is entangled with an enchanting childlike nature and naiveté. Swirling within a constant flux of varying emotions and heavily influenced by the happenings of everything and everyone.

8. An undeniable, unique way of self-expression in all forms: in thought, in writing, in art. All is an extension of the greater self. Spread out with an openness lacking self-need and wanting, and instead represented by an honest soul in search of connection.

9. A flowing nature with undercurrents of stability and predictability. At first glance, she may seem unstable, but with careful observation she follows the ebbs and flows of life, much like the tides to the moon, and the flowers to seasons. She rises and falls. She opens and closes. She is a manifestation of the greater good of cosmic unity, of togetherness, of the interwoven web of us.

10. Her deep reflective state, no matter the topic or situation. The way in which intensity is brought into the room, even as a lightness of being remains. There is a quandary of sorts, an advanced duality, in which she is powerful yet she is meek, she is substantial yet she is invisible, she is love yet she is fear. She carries the badge of courage in her heart, the white dove of humility in her hands, and everywhere she goes she is either touched or touches down, leaving a trail of fairy dust, or a slough of mud, either way, the path altered.

121. STILL NOTHING

Most of the nightmares in my life transpire in my thoughts of what-ifs—all the grasping strings that loop and latch onto anything remotely tangible—offsprings of my fear-induced imaginings. It's as if I have some superhuman capacity to see the infinite ways in which chaos might occur. I battle within, the voices of fear and the voices of reason, all enmeshed in a wild osmosis-like parade. Wherein many living beings have the likeness of a simple version of reasoning, mine—the way in which thoughts enter and stay, one hosting the other in their terrible overestablished party—has the capacity to produce an unreasonable amount of possibilities, all in one colossal moment. In this manner, the present becomes not only unbearable, but a circus unto itself: each way in which I attempt to look springing forth a ridiculously overdressed and overindulged showpiece giving its all, in hopes of fair bidding for eventual attention.

I am grateful for my mind, and yet, at times, I am disappointed with the way in which it wallows in its own self and pins me to the corner regions where I shake alone, clutching my legs and edging into the bloated corners of existence. I am in a dark place without hope when the thoughts inch forward one by one, each with a minion of sorts attached to its back—some evil knapsacks piled atop the crawling creatures, each housing an unlimited theory of possibilities.

To say the worst of it is the thoughts is to not tell the full truth. For the worst of the matter is the thoughts behind the thoughts behind the thoughts. Given the overcapacity to evaluate and process, I experience multiple levels of reasoning in one swoop—a sea bird of recourse taking in with wounded swallow the million molecular creatures of the ocean. The trick in saving self is to not listen. To close the ears to the luring voices when the parade begins. To ignore the outreaching temptations of stone after stone unturned. To recognize nothing exists in the promises. To understand each promissory note of victory need be only deception and trickery. Yes, I am made victim to the makings this mind hemorrhages. Yet further away exists this eternal hope. Somewhere there is another voice that doesn't require hearing. That doesn't hurt when entering. That has no desire, no demands, no hints, and no requests or expectations.

122. How to Create a Female with Aspergers

Gather unworldly ingredients selected from the finest of giving spirits. Place the all into a one-of-a-kind crystal bowl of beauty. Sprinkle in lots and lots and lots of unconditional love. Add a dash of spunk and assertiveness. Blend in gigantic masses of insight, perspective, energy, and focus. Layer in aspects of divinity, forethought, accomplishment, and inner truth. Add sliced and diced reality. Stir in heightened awareness with a spoon smothered in wholesome goodness. Taste for the pure sweetness. Crack open the shell of authentic being and let the light drip into the blessed mixture. Whisk with wit and wisdom. Inhale the aroma of tenderhearted empathy. Embrace the healing sunshine in soothing hands. Form into cute balls of reasonable gratitude, generosity, and forgiveness. Let the happiness of service and angel kisses tickle the senses. Peek at the forming essence of angelic eyes of knowing. Watch the dough rise with the delicate rays of understanding, freedom, and creativity. Bring into the creation the nurturing warmth of spirit. Divide and blend into the form of one cherished being. Baste with opportunity, benefit, and connection. Cook until tender but firm in belief, integrity, and strength. Set wings upon her hopes and dreams. Place her on the window of soul-knowledge. And in joyous celebration let her flight be a light to the world.

123. VIGNETTE, TORNADO, AGE 13

Mother strolled into my room with a confident air and found me absorbed in my sticker collection book, categorizing each sticker by theme. I was on the butterfly page. There were thirty-three butterflies—one more butterfly than fairies. Mother had a faraway look, a deep and distant gaze that made me think she was traveling with the angels in the sky or the dolphins in the sea. I knew innately from all my years with her that she was happy; and so I also knew she wasn't going to tell me her boyfriend Ben was finally leaving. Still, I held onto the hope, even though all the signs pointed in the opposite direction.

If she did leave him, I had thought, if she threw him out on a whim, I would be there for her. I would comfort her and reassure her that everything would turn out all right in the end. Just like she'd done for me when some chatty girl at school found my drawings of different-size parts of the male anatomy, labeled with schoolboys' names, and then circulated my detailed, full-color illustrations around the middle school. Mother had pressed me tightly to her chest that evening as I was crying in embarrassment. She let me know all would be forgotten in a few days' time, and that in the future, when I was an adult, I'd laugh and laugh about my penis pictures. That is how I would be with Mother, I had decided. If by chance she broke the news of her impending breakup with Ben, I would tell her someday she would laugh and laugh, even though the day might be far away.

Mother leaned the weight of her body against my bedroom wall and eyed me. "I have something important to tell you," she said. The word "important" caught my attention. I knew important meant more than the bills and my grilled-cheese sandwich on the kitchen table downstairs. "Important" wasn't a word Mother used often. Like the paprika she sprinkled on deviled eggs, mother only took out the word "important" on important occasions.

"Well," she said, treading forward at half speed.

I tried to whistle. I don't know why, but I tried just the same. I wasn't much of a whistler.

Mother redirected her eyes away from the wall poster of Rod Stewart. She brushed a hand across my purple comforter. Her magenta fingernail polish was chipped. I glanced down at my splitting nails, never able to grow without breaking apart—odd how Mother's nails were so gorgeously lengthy and mine so brittle-broken.

Ben's footsteps padded up the stairs. A blur of his figure swept by my open door—a tomcat passing through an alley. For a second Mother's face was expressionless. I thought she was at a loss for words, until her mouth opened, and from that moment on everything was in slow motion. The pace was similar to the time Jane's cousins had taken us kids on a bike ride along the Sacramento river, when I was the last in line of a dozen children, pedaling my heart out on a bike with a rusted chain and under-inflated tires. As hard as I had pedaled I remained the last in the row, moving nowhere fast. That is how the minutes moved while I listened to Mother: nowhere fast.

"We're going to move to the East Coast with Ben," she announced. I focused on the way she twitched her eyes, not on the words. I didn't want the words. They felt gigantic. I ducked, pulling the covers up and hoping, with all hopes, the words would bounce off the wall, instead of pummeling into my head. But it was of no use. They came and they smacked like a ruler to the knuckles.

"What?" I yelled out, the question escaping me.

Mother continued like a well-rehearsed game show hostess who was pointing to the green and orange, numbered curtains and explaining what was inside. I used to watch those shows, like *Let's Make a Deal*, and imagine my reaction if the host were to call me up on stage. I'd always planned on picking the number three curtain. I thought about what Mother was saying and realized she was choosing the curtain for me. I wasn't going to get to choose. I looked up at her with an angry glare.

Mother went on. We would move across the United States to the East Coast. We would live in Connecticut. Everything would work out just fine. And then she said the words: "Think of it as an adventure."

"An adventure?" I echoed an octave higher and an octave meaner. "An adventure? You've got to be kidding me." By now my eyes were too sad to look across the room. They were too sad to look anywhere. This was no adventure, unless Mother was talking about the type of adventure where the passengers take a three-hour trip and end up on some deserted island, and spend the rest of their days and nights wishing only to return home again. That was the type of adventure Mother was offering. This was pure and utter crap, the thick kind that spoils under the outhouse.

I ducked under the covers and shouted, "Leave me alone!" and forced back my tears, holding them in reserve, just long enough for Mother to step out of the room. Hours later, I emerged wet-faced and whimpering with a look of disorientation, like a child climbing up from her basement stairs after a tornado to find the whole of her world flattened.

124. MONEY IN THE METER

On my way to see the doctor this afternoon, I left a message on a stranger's voicemail. She'd placed her business card on my van. Stuck it beneath a windshield wiper—a random act of kindness. The back of the card read: "I wanted to let you know I saved you from an $18 parking ticket." I held onto her words and gesture, while I sat at the doctor's office, struggling to please. "Aspergers" was listed on my medical chart under "conditions."

As it happened, the doctor at the urgent care center lost his patience with me. I have this tongue thing, like a gag-reflex tongue I suppose, and a super long tongue at that, and my tongue never cooperates, especially with dental x-rays and the like. It truly has a mind of its own. No kidding. The doc, well, he tried all different ways to get a culture of the tiny white patch at the back of my throat with this long Q-tip thing. But my tongue kept blocking the pokey stick like it was sparring. I was embarrassed, to say the least. The doctor threw the stick away and huffed. Quietly and professionally, but the frustration was obvious.

Me, being my nervous, giggly self, offered, "Are there any tricks? Something you can teach me to help?"

I think he was fed up with the tips he'd already offered throughout the procedure. He kind of snapped, "Tricks? No, I don't have any tricks." I felt all of twelve.

My demeanor makes me come across as a stupid head sometimes: the posture, the anxious laughter, the inflection of my voice. And I fumble with words, as my voice squeaks in all of its youngness. You'd think I had the IQ of a horsefly. My unkempt hair and sloppy attire of the day likely didn't help to set the mood of "got-it-together woman." I was wishing at this point I'd dressed up for the doctor, at least had my hair up and not all straggly in my face.

Regardless, seeming a bit perturbed, the doc concluded I likely didn't have strep throat anyhow. The chances were very unlikely: no fever, no swollen glands, etc. But I knew I was feeling big-time lousy. I knew when my cheeks had flushed bright red earlier in the day that I'd had a fever and I knew I couldn't risk getting sicker. I had to know. The anxiety grew. He left the room without telling me anything, except to explain it was basically a sore throat and to gargle with salt. I opened the door and asked a nurse if I could go. I don't think the doctor appreciated that. He seemed bothered when he explained the procedure of when I could exit. At this point my resources of Zen were all but empty. I had a lot on my plate and felt like crap.

I don't remember the particulars, though somehow the subject of tricks surfaced again. And the doctor said, very bluntly, "I know tricks for kids. I teach kids tricks. I don't teach adults tricks. Adults should know."

Man, that wasn't nice. I swallowed and felt my little heart race. I retorted, "I have to disagree. I have autism and my son has autism. And sometimes adults need tricks too, because our bodies work differently." He kind of gave a glance, and that kind of made me feel worse.

He then said, in a demeaning tone, "Have you ever heard of the phrase 'Where there's a will, there's a way'?" He then asked if I wanted to try again.

I said, "Yes," already doubting, coaching myself with the silent *you can do it*, and feeling terribly inadequate. While the doctor prepared another culture test, I offered kindly, "The reason I want to rule this out and take care of it right away is because I have to travel a long distance in a few days."

The doctor approached with the long thing. This time, after several more minutes of "ahhhhs" and "Look up at the corner," and "No, stick your tongue back in your mouth," and much more, the doctor sighed, saying he'd likely gotten something, hopefully. Again the sense of not enough.

Somewhere in the timeline, after something or another, which I can't recall now, I lost my equilibrium. I don't know if it was one final shrug or sigh on his part, or my urge to speak my mind, but I kind of unraveled in a calm but definitely I've-had-enough-of-this way.

Exhausted, I asked, "Do you not know what Aspergers means and how it affects people?"

He responded, "No."

I said, "I write for a psychology journal. Would you like me to leave a copy at the front desk, so you can learn?"

He kind of looked either perplexed or bothered or preoccupied—I couldn't tell. He said something that indicated agreement.

I said, "You know you were kind of rude. You didn't treat me well." His back was still mostly to my chair. He was staring down at the culture. I was thinking this guy was definitely an undiagnosed Aspie. I explained, "You sounded like you were belittling me." I was on a roll then, like when you finally get the ketchup in the bottle unstuck, after that final hiccupping glob, and the rest of the red comes pouring out swiftly. I continued, "When you talked about not having to teach adults tricks, and you asked if I knew what 'where there's a will, there's a way' meant, you sounded like you were mocking me. And who doesn't know what that means? You insulted my intelligence. Did you have a bad day or something? I mean the way you were . . . oh, I don't know what you were. You just weren't nice."

I felt a bit like I was in *Gone with the Wind* in an important scene. Only I was in old blue jeans and wearing socks with my sandals.

He mumbled, "Well, I've never had an adult who could not do a culture."

I said, with a rising voice, "Well, do you think I was doing it on purpose?" He probably wasn't too keen on being in a room with me at this point. Poor man. I should have given him my husband's number so they could commiserate. The doctor left. I had some time to wiggle and squirm and text a friend about my experience.

When the doc returned, indeed it was strep throat. He handed over some stick and started to explain about the red line. I said, "It looks like a pregnancy stick." Now he was nice. He was smiling. He was more relaxed. He was finally sitting and looking my direction. He seemed like a different person. He actually seemed genuine and concerned. I could have sat with this person for hours. He was much changed. I remained there hunched with a blank stare contemplating the reasons for his demeanor. I was thinking: (1) He realizes I wasn't a moron because I told him I write for a magazine, (2) he is feeling kind of wrong for assuming I wasn't sick, (3) he is realizing he was a boob, (4) he has no idea what else to do but to give in, (5) he thinks I am nuts, or (6) he is so happy I am about to leave.

Before my departure, regarding my strep-throat confirmation, I said, "Yes, I thought so. I usually can tell stuff about myself and my health." I imagined I would have talked more and more if he hadn't been ushering me out the door. I was fine then. He was like my newfound friend. I'd forgotten all about the rest—the stuff before he smiled. He'd been kind and that's all I'd needed.

I remembered back to the stranger, to the business card on my van's windshield, to the voicemail message I'd left the stranger earlier: "I was out of sorts when you left your card because I'd just returned from the airport. I was dropping off my husband. And now I am headed to the urgent care doctor because I think I have strep throat. Your random act of kindness kept me from feasibly having that last straw. My mother-in-law died this morning. I thought you should know you made a difference."

125. FOURTEEN MONTHS, SHIT!

It's been fourteen months since I started writing, and I am a flutter of blossoming self. No longer clinging to fixations, rapid thinking, complex worries, and obsessive anxieties, I find I have an overabundance of creative juices. When I first started this writing journey, I was afraid of judgment, of evaluation, of being seen and not being seen. I longed for validation and approval. Up to that point, I truly thought I was an unconditional giver. Now I realize I had set many expectations on others, held onto projected outcomes, and lived on a roller coaster ride of being built up (for a very fleeting second) and then torn down (for torturous hours of misery). I dissected others' comments and instinctually found the tiniest bit of objection, insult, or incongruity. I was a victim through and through, fantastically gifted at highlighting my flaws.

I am pleased to report that's not part of my mode of action anymore. I am not easily offended these days—nor am I brought off balance or quick to judge myself based on another person's opinion of me. Swear words don't even make me quiver anymore! Shit! That's crazy healing right there. I see my "faults" as humanness. I see my "gifts" as part of the collective. I fluctuate now between a state of inner peace and moments of "Crap, I am in pain." When I am in physical pain (or have PMDD) I tend to get melancholic. However, I am learning to live with the melancholy and accept myself as I am. I went through a brief phase of aspiring to be an ideal Buddhist, semi-saint, or what have you, and telling myself I could never complain or say one thing negative. I realized, shortly after I adapted this way of being, that as long as I am human I will continue to have periods of time I need to *be human*. What a concept!

I have since learned that the intention behind my words is what matters and that the intention affects the outcome. If my intention is to be the best person I can be, then when there are times that I am struggling emotionally, then that's okay. My low times allow others to witness my humanness and assist me. I am not above or beyond receiving help. I don't want to be. I want to be on equal ground with others. I smile often now. I am still frank and to the point, but I am much quieter. There is this stillness inside that feels divine. At moments, I think I am glowing. I do miss aspects of prior Sam. I miss her wild humor in which she would ramble on and on, sometimes with no point at all. I miss her brain energy, particularly Sir Brain, and the seemingly unlimited ability to write and write. I miss her constant stat tracking, organizing binges, and the way her mind could leap from one cliff to another. I mourn her some. I truly do. However, those aspects of self have transformed.

126. Things Not to Say or Do When I Am Sad

1. **Don't ask me to explain or reason my way out.** When I am sad I have already evaluated everything to death. I have looked at the pros and cons of my own life and my own suffering. I am no dummy. In fact, part of the reason I am so sad is because I am so dang smart. I am my worst criticizer and have evaluated all the benefits of not being sad versus being happy. I cannot reason myself out of the sadness.

2. **Don't tell me I need a pharmaceutical drug.** Chances are that I've done my research or tried the medication before. My body is so sensitive that any and all chemicals I ingest have adverse reactions. I get the so-called "side effects." I am that less than one percent. I am the canary in the coalmine. I am the one you read about who gets the suicidal thoughts from antidepressants and the one who has bizarre things happening to her body when she ingests foreign substances. I am already affected by the environmental pollutants, the toxins in our water and food, the hormones injected into products, and the chemicals that seep out of most homes. Truth is, I likely would be far happier if I lived in a world that didn't reek of destruction.

3. **Don't tell me you know the reason for my sadness.** More than likely, if it's not my PMDD or the result of an autoimmune disorder, or a variant enzyme, an allergic reaction, a virus or illness, or something or another that is deficient or out of whack (perhaps in my intestines or stomach), then it is situational. And not just the typical situations, like a bad day at work or a letdown. I have learned not to let "bad" days affect me. I have "bad" moments each and every hour; I have "bad" moments, and I choose to spend my day grasping onto the light and the goodness. Only sometimes I get tired of reaching and trying. My life is a struggle to fit in, to appear "normal," to follow the rules, and *understand* the rules. I am exhausted. I am a warrior who wakes up every day with the past day erased,

all the previous trials conquered—gone. And then I have to start from square one to try to make sense of a world in which I do not feel I belong.

4. **Don't give me advice.** You, more than likely, have no advice I have not heard, read, seen, felt, or experienced. One way or another I have studied what you will say. I have studied others' emotions through films, music, literature, and even in nonsensical jokes and in animal behavior. I understand emotions and I understand my sadness. I read to understand myself, and I even study you to understand myself. I know more than you think. I may not understand the root cause, but I know that there isn't an answer you have that I don't have within myself. Your suggestions of correct verbiage, positive thoughts, rest, fresh air, exercise, meditation, visualization, diet, supplements, and the lot do nothing more than boggle my brain and make me think you care more about your role as a wannabe helper than you do about my pain. I can't be the object of your fixing. I don't want to be, and refuse to take on that role. I am not less than you in my sadness and you do not have the secret key I need. I did not express I was sad because I look to you for answers. I told you of my sorrow because I just long to feel less alone.

5. **Don't tell me what I have to be grateful for.** Don't suggest I make a list. That is crap. To me I am grateful for the tiniest of thoughts, gifts, and actions—that most people take for granted. The near sight of the dew on the majestic grass, the soft smell of the fire-painted lily, the brilliance of a child's laugh, the comfort of my favorite blanket or favorite song. All these lift me. Much of the world lifts me. Many moments I travel in an extraordinary world filled with magic. Many days I am thankful for my mere existence. My list of what I am grateful for is not divided into good and bad things I stopped judging right from wrong, the just from the unjust, a long time ago. I live in the space in between the extremes of yes and no, and laugh at the ones who think their view is the only view. I can't see making a list of all that is good without classifying at the same time, in invisible ink, what is bad—or worse, what others are lacking. I am no less and no more grateful than the homeless man on the street. If he is happy, I am happy. If he is sad, I am sad. To even make a list seems pompous and unjust; to single out how lucky I am in such a world of misfortune makes no sense, unless I hold

greed as a virtue. Unless I single out what is entirely missing from another to satisfy my own growing need for satisfaction. I know to let go and let my higher source lead. But when I am very, very sad, sometimes I forget how to release. I forget how to let go of the clinging of suffering. I forget I am not alone unto myself.

6. **Don't tell me how wonderful I am**. I know who I am. I know through and through. I know I am kind, gentle, sweet, generous, forgiving, genuine, giving, smart, keen, and many other positive attributes. I am not sad because I have lost sight of why I am enough. I know I am enough. I am sad because the world has lost sight of me. Because I long to reach out and connect, but when I do I often feel nothing reaching back. To touch another fully is all I want. To touch in full extreme without pretention, want, need, expectation, goal, or outcome. To just touch. I, as I wait in my own self-created exile, as I wait without the sense of feeling another, grow in sadness.

7. **Don't tell me that this too shall pass**. I know the sayings and tons of other random words collected to form reprieve. I am an avid reader and collector of quotes. I am a philosopher, an artist, and a creator. I have the heart of a lover, the mind of a composer, and the spirit of a warrior. I am brilliant in my creation, and I understand the ebbs and flows of life. I move like the sea with the moon. I move like the willow with the wind. I am affected by the give and take of the world, by nature, by weather, by other people, events, and tragedy. I dream things. I see things. I experience emotions in extremes and sometimes cannot tell if I am carrying my own pain or the pain of another. People find me. I don't know how, but they do. I am a vessel of sorts, harboring the lonely through the storm. They crawl in with their tears and woes, and their aches leak through, crushing me to the core. I know everything will pass. I know that life is a cycle, and like the seasons, my sorrow will come again. Do not attempt to help me to look forward to the end of my pain, help me to go through my pain.

8. **Don't criticize or mock me**. Do not call me "overboard," "too much," "too intense," or the like. I cannot help that I am the way I am. I can often control my behaviors and be the best person I can be, and I do this daily. However, my emotions sometimes take over. I don't know how or why, beyond conjecture, but they do. And the more I fight the wave of

pain, the more the pain comes. Sometimes I need to submit—to be in the turmoil—to wait for the tunnel to evaporate and the light to come again. I fret over the tiniest of perceived imperfections. I judge myself for not being caring enough, attentive enough, or loving enough. I cannot lie without deep remorse. I cannot name enemies. I cannot even hate. I know not this emotion *hate* beyond the emotion of anger turned deep sadness. All is huge from my perspective. There isn't a small suffering. I hurt for the tiny spider as much as the buffalo. I feel and take in such extreme happenings and know not where to lay my burden down. Just as I spend all day contemplating how to maneuver in a world that remains unfamiliar, I spend my inches of time trying to figure out how to once again release my burden—where, this time, to bury my woe. Shall it be in words, in rhythm, in rhyme, in the deep wilderness real, or the serenity of my imagination? Will I get lost again in my escaping? Where shall I take this misery and when will I have my fill? Do not criticize me and do not tease me. Do not laugh your way into a stream of mockery. I do not do what I do for attention or purpose. I do not do what I do because I want to. I do not do what I do because I am made wrong. I am perfect in my being. I am just sad. I am sad. I am sad.

9. **Don't abandon me.** Do not leave my side, if I need you there. Do not hang up the phone, if I am crying. Do not say you will return, and then not. Don't say something and not mean it. Don't lie to try to make me feel better. Tell me straight what you think. You covering up only make things worse. I need you to be safe. I need your word to be strong. I need your integrity, your honesty, your truth. I need you to prove again you are here and I am not alone.

10. **Don't perceive me as something I am not.** Try not to label me or to find the answer that brings you closure. It is not my job in life to fit neatly into a box for your comfort. My moods are my moods; my pain, my pain. I don't expect anything from you in your pain and sorrow, so please don't expect anything from me. I need you to try to accept and forgive me, to love me in completion.

127. THE ISOLATION OF ASPERGERS

Sometimes Aspergers is the scariest thing in the world—not the name, or label, or stigmatism the word brings, not even the essence of autism itself, only what it represents in my soul. No matter how many friends I have, or people I confide in, no matter how far I go in my search of self or how many ways I accomplish goals for relief, I end up back at the starting line. Facing forward with the force of the world against me. Only someone on the autism spectrum will know what I mean. People that are not will think they can understand. They will look at their own depth, take in what they know, decipher their inventory. Though, with all of me I know, it is impossible to understand the pain of Aspergers unless you have directly experienced it.

There is nothing more isolating than knowing myself completely, understanding fully the mind and the way in which I act and respond, and still being helpless to alter how I am. It's not that I want to change, but I do long for relief and a mild form of adaptation, minor assimilation—something that makes me feel I have made progress, even as I know I have nothing to progress from.

I am entirely an anomaly in all ways and in all forms. Indeed, I am beginning to think I am the essence, the exact symbolism for yin and yang. For I cannot go out to one extreme of the pendulum without going full swing to the other side, in regard to emotions, experience, outlook, opinion, even circumstances. To know so much is disheartening. It's maddening to see so much, to be able to pick apart my mind piece by piece and understand my inner workings, and still remain seemingly helpless. I can't cease to think nor stop my methods of multifaceted interpretation. My mind is some giant mechanism that grinds and grates to piece things together, including complex analysis of my own thoughts, emotions, and renderings.

Everything I am and everything I do is adamantly dissected without choice, including everything I watch, like some intertwined web spinning past my mind's eye. It appears at times I am thinking three times over—that my mind is somehow capable of deciphering the immediate now, the effects of the immediate now, the thought processes of the two previous aforementioned, and even the predictable outcome and by-product of the thinking process itself.

I cannot help but become overtaken and mind-boggled, drowning in a perplexity of images and thoughts, some speaking over the other, some repeating, some making complete sense, and some the markings of a crazed woman. Add this to the noise inside my head of all the rules I have been taught (or more so taken in as truth) and I become cluttered with an endless echo of noise: my thoughts, my thoughts about thoughts, and their thoughts, as well as my analysis of all of these thoughts. I become lost in myself. And this is only the first layer of a multidimensional sponge cake of mayhem.

Next comes the bombardment of guilt. The ways I should be, should act, the tools I ought to use, the ways in which I "should" think. The world is full of norms for the neurotypical, even full of remedies and concoctions for recovery and sanity, all of which do not work on me. I know myself inside and out. I know my body inside and out. As a result of my intellectual and instinctual capacity, all the places people typically seek out for comfort do me no good. In the last four decades, I have sought out priests, reverends, psychologists, psychiatrists, spiritual healers, astrologists, herbalists, shamans, teachers, professors, energy workers, and the like. Over and over they saw in me what they wanted to see and nothing beyond. No one could penetrate me and get through to me. No one could truly see me. In the end, my search accentuated my isolation and only added to my fever for connection and knowing.

In this there is no relief. There is no refuge. There is ultimately nowhere to go. The only way is through it. Through the bleakness and drudgery. Through the hellish thoughts. Through and through, until I come out returned.

No friends can assist, definitely no foe. I don't need foes. I punish myself enough. I shall never be good enough, kind enough, or loving enough. It's not a matter of perfectionism. As I have said, the ways of the "typical" aren't my way. I am that dichotomy again: I know I am good, I know I am enough, I know I am love, but then I know naught. There is that perpetual swinging of self, from one view to the next. Belief systems, religions, rituals, magic, or what have you, those don't work either. Temporary bandages or bondages, considering the source, until I analyze them and their happenings to no end and find the loopholes, the questions, the reality behind the illusion. I often wish I were more blinded to the ways of world, a bit more oblivious, a bit less aware—that I believed there was a something or someone out there in which to seek refuge. This isn't to mean I don't have faith. The truth is I have a faith, a blind faith, and that is what leads me to write and teaches me that the vulnerability of truth heals. Still, there is an overbearing loneliness in the rawness of truth.

This post is dedicated to Pascal. We will miss you.

128. DEAR YOU

Please know you are not alone. I know at times it feels that way—really feels that way. So much so that even your own keen logic cannot convince you otherwise. The voices will tell you are unloving, unworthy, undesirable. But the voices are lies. You are love. You are worthy. You are desire. I have been in the dark place more times than I can count. It comes, the bleakness, spontaneously in huge, volcanic ruptures. The pain itself tears at my heart and my soul and leaves me breathless and weak. It is there in the black that I cannot find solutions, when I believe I have no one and that all about the world is my enemy. But that is not truth, as much as it may seem. It isn't. I know it isn't. I know because I have witnessed our beauty in the countless people I have encountered. Their truth and love are evident, their souls transparent. Please know that by being here that you are making a difference. You are making a difference to me. Your pain is my pain. Your story, my story, and we share a lifetime of similarities. I understand you. I truly do, just as you understand me. If we were to sit alone in a quiet place and talk, you would know me, and I, you. We are sisters and brothers. We are one in our quest for truth, justice, and love. I know how you suffer in your silence and how you suffer in your immeasurable thoughts. I know how you have to always balance what is inside with what you display on the outside. I know this extreme burden, the heaviness—the endless, weary mind. How exhausting that task remains, day in and day out, night after night, in what seems a thousand lifetimes wrapped into one. I understand how you see beyond the illusion of what is indoctrination and beyond the falsehoods of societal norms. I know. And I know what isolation comes from our being. I know what it is to be ostracized, questioned, blamed, persecuted, attacked, and victimized. I know. And I still stand tall, more so for you than for my own self. For I will not stop. I will remain whole in my determination to rise above the chaos that is this world. I will continue to seek out kindred souls. And I will be here waiting, always. No. You are not alone. Not anymore. Even as we suffer at times in our isolation, circles and circles of beings on the same path surround us. Please understand that I think of you daily. Please understand I am here rooting for you. Without you I wouldn't know where to stand or how to be. With you I remember my light. I remember me.

129. VIGNETTE, EVERYTHING WAS CLEAR, AGE 14

"There it is," Ben said, curling his lips into a satisfied grin and tapping his hands on the steering wheel to the beat of the song "Sexual Healing." From the back seat of a dented sedan, amongst a cluttering of mismatched suitcases, I drew in my breath and lifted my head in doleful resignation.

The car engine stopped. The music stopped. And Ben started. "Just take a look," he said, with an easy stroke to Mother's bare shoulder. "It's just like I told you. Look!"

Glancing forward and to the left a bit, I followed Ben's rounded back up, and then across and down the length of his burly arm to his stubby finger that pointed through the car window to a pathetic dwelling. There, outside atop a plateau, slept a muddy-brown structure—most of its windows draped in faded, tangerine-colored sheets—the worst house on the best street in town.

The place was in desperate need of paint, the yard weeping with neglect, and even the mailbox itself was a rusted clump of sadness. My soon-to-be new home, this place where I would slumber and eat, shower and dress, and partake in life in general was ironically misplaced, set out in front of the world in its crummiest garment and accessories.

Almost instinctively, I narrowed my eyes into a half squint and scanned the surface, alternating the image of the house from blurry to clear and back again to blurry. I'd looked at my reflection in the mirror in the same manner, after discovering by blurring my reverse self I was momentarily able to erase all visible flaws. Mother must have nodded or agreed. She'd muttered something. I hadn't bothered to listen. I had the gift of shutting my ears as easily as some could shut their mouths. And I could travel too—travel to faraway places without moving an inch.

I was hovering somewhere high above on the broken roof shingle when Mother, sitting erect in the front seat, summoned me with a quick clearing of her throat. With the sound of her vocal cords, my eyes popped open and once again everything was clear. Mother turned to the back seat, scanning my expression, evaluating me with probing eyes. I felt her inside poking around, and for a second, I was split in two, like a log from an axe.

Often unable to mind his own business when Mother and I were in the same space together, Ben remarked, flatly, "It looks great. Don't you think?"

There were few times I'd found Ben so eager to please. This was one of those rarities, those odd occurrences in life when what I expected to come out of Ben's mouth didn't. The hollowness of his eyes had been filled with a gleaming appeasement. He did want things to work out between us all. He did want a fresh start. That was clear. What wasn't clear was the fact that what I wanted just didn't matter.

"I think you'll like it," Ben said, giving one of those television-sitcom smiles, like the ones the dads give after they come home from a long day's work acting like they are full of optimistic energy. There was a tarnished genuineness to his smile. Still, it was a smile—an infrequent occurrence, since the kidnapping of Shara and subsequent heartbreak over the loss of his daughter.

Thwarted, and not wishing to even consider agreeing with Ben, I answered with a neutral half nod. "I guess."

Ben responded with a familiar furrowing of his brow. Still facing me from the driver's seat, he muttered in his native tongue. My palms grew hotter. Disappointed in myself for erasing his smile, I turned toward Mother, who was now rummaging through her purse for cigarettes. A drizzle of sweat found its way down the back of my neck.

Concluding I was cornered, I gave a plaintive sigh and offered, "It's sure big!" I remembered to flash my own painted grin—braces and all.

Unmarred and seemingly content, Ben turned back around to find Mother. And, much to my relief, together the two lovers rambled on in waves of elation before climbing out of the car into the hot midday sun. As we each emerged from the car, no better for the long drive, we each took our place: Mother beside the sedan, shielding her eyes from the sun; Ben leaning near the hood and letting loose a haughty chuckle; and me, waist high in dead crabgrass, searching up to a summer-blue sky of puffed white clouds. It had been a long two days, first the plane ride, and then a stop at Ben's friend's house in the nearby state of New York, where I was made to crash on some stranger's bed in the wee hours of the night. I hadn't bathed, changed my clothes, nor brushed my teeth in two full days, and just then had an overwhelming desire to stretch out on a bed and pass out.

I swallowed the air, sucked it in like I was getting ready to blow up a balloon, and then deflated my lungs in one long, even outburst. I searched out with my narrow stare, evaluating the scene. My eyes soared up to the rooftop, searched across and down to the attached garage, and then wrapped around the building in lamenting laps. There was so much to take in—too much, really. My homes had had many faces. But all of them had stood on California soil, all had breathed in the same air, and each had been surrounded by luxuriant foliage. Here, all about was an absence of luster, as if the colors and plenitude of life had been rubbed out and whitewashed into a dull, bland nothingness.

Following a few heavy clomps across the gravel drive and an open and slam of the car trunk, Ben proceeded to march up the driveway while fingering a wine bottle in one high hand. Mother, moving quicker than she had in months, made her way around the car and handed off the cat carrier to me. In no time she found her way to Ben and lathered him in giggles. Meanwhile I gathered myself, remembering to breathe and taking the time needed to calm my cat, who meowed anxiously from her plastic dungeon.

Once inside the house, I accepted the stale odor and dust. Wishing to honor Mother's traditional curse word, but feeling better suited for the lesser version, I let out a remarkably spiteful, "Shoot." Not knowing what to do with a cat suffering from post-traumatic flight syndrome, I set her loose in the dark, empty study to my left and shut the door, and then proceeded blindly up the stairs. On the upper level, to my left, the living room was devoid of furniture. I turned to my right and my footsteps found the first bare bedroom.

Mother shadowed me into the room, appearing from around the corner. "It's only temporary. We'll get you that new furniture I promised." I peered out the window to the rooftops beyond. And then, as if he'd tracked our scent, Ben entered the room, his face at ease. "Come. Let me show you the rest."

There wasn't much to see. The movers had come ahead of time, a few days prior, and dropped our boxed belongings and sparse furniture about in various corners of the house. I had my record player and my stuffed animals—the fifty or so plush toys I'd named. There was my small box of clothes, totaling two worn jeans and two shirts. I was wearing the only shoes I owned. Most of our belongings, like my childhood blue bookshelf and favorite mirrored dresser, Mother had previously sold at a garage sale to make room for the important items in the moving truck, like our once-possessed antique china cabinet.

In the days that followed, Ben would add a used portable, faux-leather bar stand with well-worn swivel chairs to the mix of furniture. He set the clunky thing smack down in the middle of our outdated, green-tiled kitchen. It would serve as our makeshift breakfast table. The rest of his contribution consisted of a couple of fringed floor pillows and a humongous glass tank filled with fish. There was one bug-eyed Oscar fish that caught my attention with his fanciful expression and wobbly mannerisms. In future times, I would sit upstairs alone in the dark, long after the rest of the house was asleep, and watch the fish swim back and forth in the tank. Ben made sure the tank was always clean and the fish were always well fed. Ben was good with fish.

Within a week I moved up in the hierarchy of bed allocation, and after happily discarding Ben's green sleeping bag, I inherited Ben's waterbed. I drained the vile water myself and then helped Ben carry the bed's wooden pieces down the stairs. Having slept upstairs near the master bedroom for more nights than I could tolerate, I now opted for the wooden-paneled study below—a dank and dismal, north-facing room.

The study was like the center of a musty maze and, with three doors leading outside of my bedroom, served as the heart of the thresholds. One narrow door on the back wall led to a cold room, a drafty space with no insulation that had probably long ago served as a potting room or workshop. This soon became my cat's retreat, pleasing her fine for her afternoon sunning and for a little graveyard for her hunting trophies. Another taller door to the far right of the study led to the two-car garage. In the evenings my bedroom served as a passageway for Ben and Mother arriving home from work. The main entrance to the study was located a few steps away from the front door of the house. When this main door was opened, the breeze from the entranceway would rush into my room.

But none of this mattered—the dark adjacent graveyard of small rodents, the passageway, the moving breeze. I even got used to Ben's stomping from up above and the fumes from the garage. Each of these were small sacrifices when faced with the wholly unfathomable alternative of being within hearing range of Ben's snoring and love groans.

Looking back, I continually see myself spinning around over and over in my dimly lit room while dancing to the music of Asia and Journey. I see myself obsessively playing Space Invaders, until I beat all the levels, and turning on the show *Three's Company* every afternoon, so as to not miss one single episode. These were the lights of my life: my music, my video games, my television shows. Since moving to the East Coast, I'd cut myself off from real people, at least for the last few weeks of summer. This was the first time I no longer wanted to venture outside. The first time I was afraid of what was beyond my bedroom. Sometimes I think I must have somehow known life would take a turn for the worse outside my three doors.

130. THE GIRL IN THE ALTERED STATE

My mind goes bungee jumping without my permission. It sees an avenue of escape and jumps. Boing! And I am left somewhere in between the launchpad and the landing ground, midstream in the air, flailing and screaming for rescue. My mind literally pours into multiple dimensions of jumping thoughts. The Energizer bunny overdosed on caffeine skydiving without a parachute. And what does my mind pour? Everything. All the data I have collected from being. Everything I have taken note of during my waking and sleeping hours: each person, each face, each smell, each droplet taken in by the senses, and even the liquid data beyond the common senses. Everything I have ever learned, seen, contemplated, deduced—all brought to the same overcrowded table for dinner, and each wanting a turn at conversation. It's loud. It's annoying. And it's uninvited company.

At times I enter an altered state. Inside my mind is a jumble of ideas edging their way through to exactness and refinement, entering a filter of dissection and biopsy, spit out onto a conveyer belt that feeds each piece with microscopic filaments of possibility. As my mind functions, much like a separate entity of its own, I get carried away in the potential outcomes, swept into immensely thick images and awakening. Often, in this altered state, I find retreat, a place of no unexpected upset, and instead a time of returning again and again to the predictable matter at hand. I can remain there, in this place, unaware of the happenings around me, the things occurring outside of my own thinking.

This serves me well, my thinking machine, particularly in times of deadlines, needed production, problem solving, and sorting. In this state, I have the capacity to debate both sides of an argument with ease, essentially seeing with expansive foresight the end trail of either course taken. Whether I am supporting myself or another's endeavors, I am more likely than not to find beneficial solutions and make beneficial progress with any given task. I am able to mass-produce with intensely focused concentration and powerful self-drive. Nothing is forced, induced, or made to happen; the output happens instinctually—the process akin to the effortlessness in which a flower unfolds. I am neither under pressure nor in a state of panic. More so, I find myself in a blissful alleyway of escape, with my troubles blocked out on one side and my worries blocked out on the other.

I have managed, in this manner, to slip past the mundaneness and challenges of life and bask in an inner state of creation. Here, I am blissfully working. Pouring out information in graphic and written form, what I visualize transmitted and then drafted—draft upon draft reassembled and reconstructed. In these moments, I can learn mass amounts of information in a short amount of time. Not because I am told to or want to, but because I am internally driven to fill my mind's vacant spaces with input. I am taking in what I crave like a body absorbing the exact required nutrients. I create with passion and fever, but not for the reasons others might suspect.

During other junctures, my mind takes off again, bound to creation with engines revved. Only this time I am digesting bits and pieces of data (typically emotions) that don't make sense. I become stuck on a loop: a conveyor belt that keeps recirculating with the same information. I keep misfiring, keep trying to solve the unsolvable, and inevitably end up disappointed and forlorn. I can step back while in this state and feel myself adrift, yet still unable to pull myself outside of the feeling of doom. Not one to dismiss possibilities or explanation, not setting aside feasible reasons, I keep forming hypotheses and testing theories through personal trial and error, digging myself deeper into confusion and darkness. During these times of reconstructing the same cyclic thoughts, I cling to my greatest fears. I climb into a storybook of sorts, living out alternate lives, wherein I am not the heroine, but the doomed sufferer—If not a storybook, then a vivid horror film in which the supporting characters all dissolve, and I am left alone in a sucking, suffocating darkness. In essence, the very tool I am endowed with that creates masterpieces is the exact same tool that creates my demise. In this way, the safety net I lack, that if available would prevent me from being funneled into the alley of reprieve, is the same item whose absence causes me to be sucked into crushing isolation.

131. WHAT IF I
DON'T HAVE ASPERGERS?

But what if I don't have Aspergers? What if this is just me clinging onto a thread in hopes of not being alone in this world? What if we are just aliens, empaths, sensitives, or advanced spiritual beings? What if I am a reincarnated sage? What if I am paying for previous karmic waves? What if I am truly crazy, self-inventing my own condition to feel more normal in claiming I am unique? What if Aspergers doesn't exist and this is just a human condition? What if this whole Aspergers thing is a trend and being over diagnosed? What if I am making this up in my head to fit in with a collective? What if I find out from an expert I have something else and not Aspergers? Am I smart enough to have Aspergers? Am I odd enough? Am I enough of anything?

Please stop! Who cares? Really? Get rid of the name. Call it *spaghetti monster*. Call it *pie in the face*. Call it *genius*. Call it *gifted*. Call it *loony*. I don't care! We found each other. And we have more in common than not, after years of feeling isolated and alone. I don't care what man-invented name based on a collective documented list of traits, based on the observation of some male behavior years ago was the reason we met. We met. And that's what Aspergers means to me: UNION.

We are together. We are no longer alone. Stop trying to analyze what we are and who we are and why we are, and accept that WE ARE. There is no you versus them. There is no us versus them. There is no separation. It is all just manmade games. We just managed to survive. To keep our heads above water. To see through the madness. To understand there are things, definite things, that need changing in this world. If we want to start focusing on self-awareness and self-acceptance, then yay us! I don't care how you get there—to that point where life starts to make sense and you start to realize you aren't alone and aren't imperfect and have much to give the world. I just want you to know YOU matter and YOU make a difference and YOU are never alone. Whatever you need to hold onto to build yourself up, after this world has attempted to break you down, is what you need and is your choice. Shine, shine, shine. It doesn't matter if you have Aspergers or don't, or if the word never exists again. Let go of the word and reasons. Just let go. Breathe. And be.

132. VIGNETTE, BLISTER SISTER, AGE 14

On a Monday, just past four in the afternoon, Mother, dressed in her secondhand dress and faux-leather heels, drove a little faster than normal—which was still relatively slow. I was seated in the front seat of Ben's battered sedan. Every few minutes a piercing pain drove up my left side causing me to let out a muffled moan, which gave Mother a reason to pat her hand on my shoulder and offer out a sympathetic smile.

This was an unusual ride, given the fact I was headed to the hospital and Mother's live-in lover, Ben, who was typically habitually attached to the front seat, was presently dutifully sulking in the back. I was so accustomed to seeing Ben's broad back hunched over in the front that upon spotting him there, behind me, sprawled out in excess of half the seat with his socked feet propped up on Mother's weather-beaten briefcase, I swore to myself I was dreaming.

Just before sundown, we stepped into the first wing of the hospital. In the waiting room I devoured Mother's attention. I needed it. I longed for it. And I was willing to pay the cost of pain. As we sat there together, Mother wasn't talking about herself or squabbling with Ben. She was with me. Always before, in the times we lived with my stepfather Drake, if I was ill, Mother was overly attentive to my needs, setting aside her tasks to bring medicine, hot fluids, and hugs. I still thought about her attentiveness each time I refused to drink apple juice, how she'd long ago dissolved the bitter aspirin in the juice as a remedy to lower my fever. I never imagined as a small child that when I grew older, and our circumstances changed, that my mother wouldn't be there whenever I needed her.

Once inside the second-floor hospital room—a small drab area with a thin pull curtain—I feared the worse. In situations concerning illness, my morbid thoughts take center stage. As I rested on the hospital bed clenching in pain and trying to subdue the bubbling pressure pulsating in my gut, the curtain of my mind opened to a melancholic first act. *Did I want an open casket? I ought to definitely be buried back in my hometown in California. Not here on the East Coast. Would Jeff, my freshman crush, come to the funeral?*

I would have continued, had my thoughts not been interrupted by Ben's shouts resounding down the corridor. "Why haven't you attended to her? Why are you taking so damn long?"

I supposed Ben's anger was his way of showing he cared, but his hollering, whether motivated from a good place or not, left me feeling terrible shame. Mother, on the other hand, seemed completely unmoved by Ben's remarks. Instead of pulling back in embarrassment, she remained steadfastly focused at my bedside, even so much as to make the effort to bring a cup of crushed ice. I was a bit uncomfortable, accepting the attention from my doting mother, a parent who had just the day before acted so aloof and distant, wrapped up in her own misgivings about her job and second-guessing her decision to move in with Ben, that she hadn't even remarked on my arriving home past the dinner curfew—a curfew which was quite ironic, since there was rarely any dinner prepared.

An attractive doctor entered the room, endowed with the looks of super combo order of Jimmy Stewart and the father from *Leave It to Beaver*. Mother, as I expected, sat upright, smiling fully. After a click of his wide jaw, the doctor scratched the center of his dimpled chin, and smiled. "We've finished most of the tests. We're just waiting for the x-ray technician. It should not be more than a few more minutes. How are you feeling?"

I answered, calmly, "The pains aren't too bad anymore." Just then, Ben, uncouth in appearance, with his white dress shirt unbuttoned midway exposing his undershirt and the top of his thick carpet of dark chest hair, barged in and stared down the doctor. "Might I suggest you find out what the hell is going on?"

The doctor, averting his eyes from Ben, looked at me. "Excuse me. I'll be back in a moment." The billowing tail of his hospital jacket floated past the foot of my bed and trailed out of the room.

Mother rolled her eyes to the ceiling, hesitated and hovered there a moment, and then focused back on me. Ben's look was incredulous. After kicking the foot of my bed, he backed away into the corner. There, lurking in the shadows like a chastised child, he fingered his wiry hair, setting down a mass of his cowlick before most of the strands sprung back up in greeting. Then he sneered in the direction of the door, sat down with a severe sigh, made a half stretch that flashed his sweat rings, and shot out a raunchy smell resembling earwax and bacon grease.

Blister sisters—that's what we had called each other, my childhood friend Jane and I. When we were seven years of age, after a day of swinging on the playground monkey bars, we had rubbed the opened raw blisters on the palms of our hands together and proclaimed an all-binding pact: "Blister Sisters Forever!" It was easy. It was painless. We didn't have to pierce our thumbs to draw blood like the *blood sisters* did. As *blister sisters*, whenever we were in trouble or worried, we had each other to lean on.

Atop the hospital bed, dreading the news the doctor was carrying inside the x-ray envelope, I thought about my Blister Sister. I pictured her with her Tahoe-blue eyes and golden-straw pigtails. And standing next to her was Ben's chubby little daughter Shara, holding my dog Justice. We'd been like close sisters for a few years, before Ben's former wife kidnapped her away. In the room, too, were my nana and nano. They were all in my hospital room smiling, surrounding my bed with their loving aura. Until, with the flash of the x-ray display board, they were gone.

The x-ray revealed a large mass on my lower left side. The doctor reported there were several ailments that could be causing the mass. He was concerned it might be cancer. On hearing the word, I went into a semi-state of shock. The room started spinning and I wanted to run back home. Wherever home was.

Ben stood up straight, his ears crimson, his voice hoarse. "Damn it! How dare you say that in front of a child! What are you thinking? Are you an idiot? What the hell is wrong with you?"

Now, although I was completely mortified and feeling the strong urge, despite my stomach cramping, to crawl under the hospital bed and never come out, I have to say, Ben impressed me. Not in the way a parent impresses you by throwing you a birthday party and inviting all of your friends over to stay the night, nor in the way a child feels proud when a parent attends the school's career day and knocks the socks of the classmates. No, it wasn't the type of impressive behavior that summons thoughts of coolness and grandiosity. Ben's behavior more so brought images of a fearsome bear standing on her hind legs with claws erected to protect her cub. It was a scary image, quite terrifying actually—though none could deny that somewhere deep inside the man who was set upon a blind rampage, huffing and puffing away at every hospital staff member within his path, that there was at least somewhere hidden a jewel of compassion.

It didn't take long for Ben to pack up my things, usher Mother and me out of the building, and drive thirty miles across the state to another hospital. Sadly for Ben, by then hospital visiting hours were over and the nurses insisted Ben and Mother leave. And thusly, I was made to stay in a strange place, miles from home, without a soul I knew, replaying in my head long into the night all the horrific ways in which my death might play out.

In the morning when I awoke, a lingering gait of worry crossed back and forth in my thoughts, like one of those rotating ducks at a carnival target booth. My heart pounded, my palms sweated, and I didn't seem to be taking in enough oxygen. After I'd practically hyperventilated and reviewed all the morbid ways I could die, a good dozen times each, a round nurse with a ruddy complexion entered the room and took my vitals. Sitting on the edge of the hospital bed, she met her eyes with mine.

"Well, honey," she said. "There isn't much we can do for you."

That was all I needed to hear. Now for certain I would die here on the East Coast, far away from my family and friends. My heart sank, a broken elevator crashing from the grand suite to the basement. This was the end, indeed.

Seconds later, disgruntled Ben sauntered into the room with two days' worth of black stubbles on his face. Mother followed at his side.

"Hello," the nurse said. "I was just telling your daughter . . ."

The room stopped for a moment. Well, not the room, but everything inside the room: the conversation, the noises, even the sunlight, everything went black. My heart raced. This was it. Mother would soon know I was dying.

The rest of the nurse's words came out at quarter speed, so much so that her mouth seemed to be stretched out and frozen in the shape of a contorted goose egg. She said, ". . . Everything . . . is . . . going . . . to . . . be . . . fine," in super slow motion.

What the heck? I looked over at the smiling nurse and arched my right brow.

The nurse rose off the hospital bed and scribbled some data on my medical chart. "What is happening is very simple," she continued, giving Ben an obvious larger proportion of her attention. "Your daughter is constipated and has a substantial amount of gas trapped in her intestines." The nurse held up a plastic bottle of some ghastly, purplish, chalky substance. "She can drink this down or try to go on her own." She turned her wide blue eyes to me. "It's up to you. Do you want to take this?"

I gulped. I looked out the window. My cheeks were on fire.

Most kids would have felt relieved to hear the news that they were not dying, but not me. I didn't know where to even begin in my disappointment. First off the nurse obviously thought Ben was my father; that fact alone panged me terribly. Then there was this unsettling feeling of grave disappointment, as if I'd failed everyone by not having something seriously wrong with me. And now three adults were all staring my direction and waiting for me to take a dump. I didn't even poop at school, or even at the house, when other people were in close proximity. I was screwed.

My eyes sideswiped the nurse, who was smiling patiently. Next, I glanced at mother, as she sighed in relief, and then I hovered my attention at the expressionless Ben. Waited to hear him scream, "What a loser!"

But there was no sound, no movement from anyone, only this unbearable silence.

133. CONFESSIONS OF AN ASPIE GIRL

1. I hate getting up in the morning. Why? It's not that I don't have the ability to like the day. I just don't want to have to get up and do it all over again. I mean, I just did the exact same thing the day before, e.g., showered, brushed teeth, chose clothes, discarded clothes, chose different clothes, stressed about my food intake, wondered if coffee is good for me, stressed over my next step—and man was it frickin' exhausting! By the first hour of thinking and mundane activity, I am smashed. Like a surfer punched smack off a surfboard and pounded into the jagged rocks. Theme music in the background: WIPE OUT. And then, lucky me, if I conquer the day, at least a portion of the day, say, 18.984 percent, then I get to retreat to the couch that has a permanent dent from my lounging hours, where I try to rest but end up, for the trillionth time, in some complex dialogue with a part of myself that really never learned to shut her mouth.

2. I like people, but they bug me. Actually, I adore lots and lots of people, but I see way too much. I see past the nuances and suggestions and idioms and babble, and I grow so weary. I am thinking and pondering about approximately one hundred things and tangents compared to each singular concept another brings up in conversation. I am distracted by the webbing style of my brain that largely resembles a graphic organizer big corporations use to plot out their schematics for the next decade. Trying to listen to a conversation in completion is an impossibility, unless I am in my Zen moment and steadily repeating each word said by my acquaintance back to myself while staring off with a tranquil demeanor. Even then, I am reviewing the rules of active listening and trying to recall at least a page of my Buddhist teachings. With the silence, I am baffled by all that my senses are taking in. I leap and run all over in my head, dissecting the molecular bits of a person. So much to chew off and digest that I am actually considering investing in a pair of dark glasses—so dark I can't see—that

way at least one of my senses is blocked. Then I only have to deal with the distraction of the bombardment of various noises, odors, textures, and bodily sensations. At least with glasses I won't be ice-skating about in thought, about to fall on my butt and shatter the ice, whilst distracted by the idiotic protruding mole on someone's face that is reaching out and wanting to form a conversation with me. "Hi, I am mole. I am big. I used to have a hair in me like a witch, but it was plucked out. Do you wonder why hairs grow faster on moles? Maybe you should Google it? What are the signs of irregular moles again? For a mole, I look healthy. Still ugly, though. I would have removed me. How much does it cost? I wonder if I have a soul, and where I would go if you burn me off. Hey, maybe you should listen to what the person who owns my face is saying."

3. Forming thoughts hurts, but forming sentences is far worse. I connect rules to words. Yes, each word is alive and a willing or unwilling participant. Some words deserve center stage, and some words . . . well, they deserve the malodorous secretions of a begrimed dungeon. I couldn't say the word "vagina" until I was in my early forties—which was another lifetime ago, because as you know I am effectually thirty-nine forever. And words like fu** and other connotations that suggest what my boys were watching two spiders (likely) do on our window last night (sidebar: I couldn't tell if the arachnids were eating each other or enjoying themselves) still make me feel like I am in a library with my hair in a bun wearing a prudish ruffled blouse. Think Mary in the altered life of George Bailey in *It's a Wonderful Life*. If you haven't seen the movie, that truly is the hugest mistake in your life. In constructing thoughts, I run into constant roadblocks and detours. Case in point, my steering off the road to discuss a movie you should have watched twenty times by now, if you have an ounce of good taste in your bones. See how I judged you? That's what I do with words. Is this one too provocative? Is this the best word choice? How does that word feel? He feels too fat, too heavy, too mundane, too cliché, too overused, and so on. It's not about perfection. The process is more akin to picking out the ground I want to walk on. The soles of my feet know that some foundations feel better than others. I mean I'd take clean laminate flooring over ten-year-old carpet any day, and I'd much rather risk the residue on green grass then the debris on

concrete, while shoeless. And I've gone off on a tangent again, visualizing all the ways in which my feet can travel and all the dangers flesh faces.

4. Life is frickin' scary! Life doesn't come with a guidebook or rulebook, or anything! And all these grown-ups are trying to figure out what direction to go, what to say, how to be, what to do, and are pointing fingers this way and that, and sporadically jumping from one idea to the next, clinging to this hope, and then moments or decades later, another hope. And it confuses the heck out of me. Slices me open like an overexposed, vulnerable fish with her guts hanging out and seagulls hankering about for a ripe piece. I know enough to know I know nothing, and to watch all this chaos wobbling about (like those weeble-wobble toys that don't fall down but get overwhelmingly annoying in their inability to go anywhere and do anything but remain stagnant) gets to the very bone of me. I feel nibbled upon and broken. I don't want to be told what to do or how to be, but at the same time I want some almighty guru, higher power (or at minimum Mother Nature's henchman), to come down and point out the *real* way. I am tired of people reinventing the right way and the wrong way, and proclaiming who is good and who is bad, and telling me what I can and cannot do— down to how I parent, who I spend time with, what I spend time doing, and worse, what I spend time ingesting spiritually and mentally and physically. In truth, at times I think humanity has reached an all-time low. People have left the concrete, physical examples of how to act and now are needling past the skin of others by dictating, preaching, and insinuating how people should form thoughts! I mean, talk about instilling further fear. Seems like a diabolical plan to me: "I know how to really inject terror. Teach people how their thoughts are bad. I mean, it's not enough to teach them that they are flawed, broken, and in need of repair. Let's indoctrinate them with how they are innately wired wrong in that their actual thoughts are imperfect. What a grand plan."

5. I don't know what religion I believe in. I just don't anymore. I have read and processed way too much. As a child I used to pray every night in an OCD-like manner: "Dear God. God bless my mom and my dad, my cousins and aunts and uncles, my friends, and my enemies, and everyone I can think of. And please include everyone I can't think of or that I am not

remembering . . ." I asked the Holy Spirit into my heart when I was twelve, primarily because I was sleeping with a rosary around my neck (and the lights on in my bedroom) every night, and warding off red, leathery-faced demons that were haunting me in my sleep. And fundamentally because life sucked to such a degree in its confusion, unpredictability, and lack of security that I needed the Big Guy to beam down and stand at the door to my heart. At least that way, when the aches of the world pounded on me, I had something or someone, imagined or not, to push back. Now that I have taken in massive amounts of spiritual clutter, I am left confused and spinning. I have a natural, instinctual desire to accept everyone and everything. Consequently, many religions don't fit me; that is to say, if the religion were a substance, it would feel, if ingested, like shards of glass, and if worn, like an oversized, sixty-pound cloak of fur—a heavy coat the absentminded shepherd of my flock forgot to shear. I just don't know anymore, and strongly think we need an Aspie prophet to develop a new religion— one that's not called a religion, of course, because religion is one of those words that munches at my eardrums.

6. I don't like me, but I love me. Yes, this is a concept similar to when you have a relative you can't stand to be around, and would never choose as a friend, and wish hadn't been born into your clan, yet all the same you have this unfounded instinctual love that keeps pulling you in because she or he (why don't we have a non-gender-specific word yet?) is your blood. But it's different, because I would choose me as a friend, and I do like to be around me, and I kind of think I am super cool at times. So that's not a super good example. But I like it anyhow. A better example might be when you love your dog, but she does stuff that really messes up your sense of serenity. I don't know, no names given, but let's say she piddles when she is anxious, or brings in dead surprises through the doggy door, or digs up dirt to find moles and comes in all muddy and tracks footprints through the house, or smells like last week's garbage left out in ninety-nine-degree weather; and you are way too tired and/or preoccupied to want to, yet again, deal with the fluffy ball of love's annoyances. That's more like it— how it feels to live with me—like I am my own best friend who annoys her own self to no end, but by nightfall is so warm and cuddly and loyal that I

can't help but overlook all the perceived failings and flaws and pain-in-the-butt doings. So really, let's erase the first sentences of this paragraph, at least from our memories (kind of like our self-worth has been erased from our memories by big-business schemes), and let's pretend the first sentence reads: "I love myself like I love my dog." I like to pretend.

7. I like my inner world more than my outer world. It's safe in my head, for the most part. Well, not really, especially when I am looping, spinning, panicking, or feeling like this time I really am dying. Feel my heartbeat! But still, with all the slippery slopes inside my mind, it still feels better than what's outside of me. I don't like all the judgment in the world. I don't like second-guessing. I don't like first-guessing or tenth-guessing. I just wish we all wore our hearts, integrity, and love on our sleeves. At least in my mind I know what to expect. Even if it's chaos, even if it's torture—at least it is predictable pain. Not unexpected hurts inflicted on me by a society I have yet to understand. At least in my mind there are moments of intense fantasy that take me to another place. At least inside of myself I can find the perfection, the love, the guidance, and the hope that the world keeps trying to dismiss or take away. I like it inside there. At least inside, the burden of the world isn't leaning up against me and I can hear the tender reassurance of a loving heart.

134. Bipolar Disorder or Asperger's Syndrome?

I was wrongly diagnosed with "rapid cycling" bipolar disorder, years back. The psychiatrist scratched his head, after I'd completed his brief psychiatric survey, and reported, "Well, you don't really fit the criteria for the disorder, but let's treat you with medication, just in case." I figured he was super close to earning his last pharmaceutical merit points toward that condo in the Bahamas.

After only a few weeks, I had to stop taking the medication my doctor prescribed, on a pharmacist's advice. (I had crushing chest pain and palpitations.) When I'd called the doctor's office to reschedule my follow up psychiatry appointment, and explained the situation, the snooty receptionist barked, "Well, we cannot treat you as a patient any longer. You stopped the medication and now are trying to reschedule. We have other patients who take priority, who listen to their doctor, and don't try to cause more hassle by rescheduling." That was the last time I ever went to a psychiatrist.

After my inaccurate mood disorder diagnosis, I spent a good two years asking my husband, weekly, if I seemed "moody" or "bipolar." I read up on the subject, and continually evaluated myself. Both my husband and I concur, to this day, that I am a very level person, despite my autistic traits.

Since finding out I am autistic, I now can recognize some distinct differences between bipolar disorder and my autism. First off, I am aware of my behavior, not some of the time but all of the time. I can watch myself get happy, and I can step back and analyze the direct reason, and even theorize when the happiness will end. My behavior is not unpredictable to me, especially considering what I now know about Asperger's Syndrome.

In retrospect, after I experience what might be a slight "high" or a "low" mood, I can always pinpoint a trigger; sometimes the trigger is as simple as something I ate (chocolate!) or someone who showed up at my door (stranger!). In addition, many of my feelings of "low," such as frustration, despondence, and discouragement, are directly related to my executive functioning ability: the way in which my brain organizes information or doesn't organize information. My executive functioning challenges can result in an inability to perform simple daily tasks, like showering, dressing, errands, phone calls, or cooking. And my sad feelings of "not enough" and "failure" are sometimes associated with what is called "autistic inertia"—an inability to do much of anything (theorized to be a response to executive functioning mayhem and sensory and emotional overload). My lack of ability to perform simple tasks will cause a sense of disappointment, a reaction that can easily spiral into a form of situational depression.

Usually, the mood I am in is a result of a response to my environment, my ability to function in that said environment, and my resulting thought processes. I am affected by people, foods, chemicals, the list of things I think I must do for the day, and my inability to cope with the overwhelming amount of information that I process. I might be triggered by my interpretation of another's words and my resulting confusion. Then I might spiral into a place that resembles depression; however, my state is actually more of a withdrawal from others, until my wounds are healed. There are times I can control my emotions and avoid a certain mood with self-talk, intervention from friends, and by employing a very strong will. Only I have to have energy to do this.

Similar to the moods of bipolar rapid cycling, my moods are fairly mild, and rarely extreme polar opposites. I am not super high and then super low. More so, I always have this silver lining inside of me: a mixture of hope and melancholy. And in all ways, I either have vast energy and the ability to accomplish a lot or a lack of energy and the ability to accomplish little. Yet even in my states of inertia, I am accomplishing something—I am recuperating from a period of high production and/or high intake.

In my opinion, living on two extremes of the spectrum of emotions is a trademark of the Aspergers condition. Arguably, the autistic extremes might be classified as a mood disorder, or not. Regardless, keeping the traits of autism in mind seems pertinent when establishing an effective and safe psychiatric method of protocol—especially when considering autistics are often prone to medication sensitivities. I've heard from a number of autistic individuals regarding the detrimental effects psychiatric drugs have had on them, e.g., suicidal thoughts, attempted suicide, manic episodes, depression. I myself became suicidal when treated with anti-depressants. Anecdotal or not, the evidence is worthy of professional consideration and the adaptation of extreme cautionary measures.

In my day-to-day living, I long to find the middle road. But I am typically, if not always, either in a state of one extreme or the other, energy wise. In example, I am hyper motivated, fixated, and a great accomplisher, or I am in state of reconfiguration of my emotional and intellectual well-being. I am similar in characteristics to a particular breed of nocturnal animal that needs to seek refuge in a dark, isolated space to rest for a season, until it's ready to go out and bear the elements. This is evident in all on the autistic spectrum, as far as I know. From an outsider's perspective, based on my productivity, or lack of productivity, it would seem I have extreme mood swings, but inside the moods don't seem that extreme.

All in all, I live in two polar places. I have two halves: the one who can do a lot in a short amount of time and the one that is immobile. But neither half is irrational or thinking thoughts that are grandiose, illogical, or the like. Neither one is risk taking, making detrimental choices, or extremely agitated. I don't lose sleep. I don't become overly hyper; I don't lose any aspect of clarity about my self, who I am, and where I am. If anything, I am overly aware of my mood because I feel off balance. And since I feel off balance a lot—I am often overly aware.

When I am in superwoman mode, I am aware of my thought processes, my actions, and my intentions. I am watching myself create and indulge. There is a high that comes as a result of creation and production and having finally accomplished things that I was unable to do before. The high is a huge relief, a euphoric sensation, of finally having the energy to produce and contribute. The high doesn't come first. Energy is given back to me, and I am happy and "high" because at last I am not couch bound, nor lost in an immobile state of over analysis of self.

Essentially I have been given two ways to live: one as a creative entity and one as the creative entity on pause. I am a computer that takes time out to reboot and clear up junk. I need time to take all the garbage and digest and restart myself. What might look to be manic is the creative me indulging in life and using the high intellect I have for a greater cause or good. What might look to be depression is the tired me, exhausted from creating, and on overload from a world burdened with too much information.

Note: The information provided is for informational purposes only and is not intended as a substitute for advice from a physician or other health-care professional. The information is not intended for diagnosis or treatment of any medical condition. It is not advisable to stop taking any medication without consulting a medical physician.

135. Emotion Ocean

When considering my emotions, things aren't always as they appear. My actions sometimes don't match what I am feeling. At times, when I am considering a new idea, interest, or project—I might come across as impulsive, overly opinionated, and impatient. When in actuality, I don't feel that way; I just seem that way. More than likely I am just excited. In other moments when I am anxious, I might not present as anxious. Instead, I might appear to be hyper, overconfident, overzealous, or even goofy. When I am nervous or "put on the spot," I tend to fumble for words, perhaps pulling out an exaggerated version of what I am feeling. Other times, stuttering or word confusion occurs. At any moment in my day, an unexpected and unfounded impatient voice or look could pop out from nowhere, or some awkward body movement, such as sighing and shrugging my shoulders. There are times that I wear a tight grin because I don't know what to say. And alas, there is always the resting bitch face—that lack of expression that others interpret as anger.

My frustration levels can be triggered by seemingly "small" things. I feel heightened levels of frustration when trying to retrieve a common item. I believe this has its basis in "object permanence." Object permanence is the ability to understand things still exist even when they cannot be readily observed through the senses (seen, heard, touched, etc.). My object permanence challenges add to my frustration with daily tasks and my insecurities surrounding relationships. I logically understand an item, or person, or concept (like a stable relationship) is likely there, and I can comprehend the probability of its existence; even so, there exists an underlying deficit of trust that the object, person, or concept remains. This distrust resurfaces even after I have rechecked (again) to reassure myself that something or someone is in its expected location. I might glance at a stack of piled papers and get a rush of panic, thinking the bill I set there, just yesterday, might not be there anymore. From there, my mind might lead me down multiple alleys of probable strategies to locate the bill, if it does come up missing.

Generally, I will avoid looking for certain items, particularly appointment cards, school notices, and bills, thinking my worst fear is true—that they are forever lost. Where do they all go? Who knows. My fear of not being able to trust something is there when it's out of immediate sight causes me to procrastinate. I sometimes miss an important event (theater tickets) or never call that person back (therapist).

I have no doubt that this "object permanence" ordeal leads to my insecurity in relationships. Just because someone told me ten times yesterday that he cared about me doesn't mean he does today. In essence, each time I leave a loved one I question if when I return the fondness a person had for me will remain.

My distrust of continuity can carry over into the workplace, wherein I question whether or not my job performance is up to par, even though my supervisor just informed me last week all was well. In actuality, I am surprised when something (or someone) is where it's supposed to be. This is likely why I get short-tempered when people don't follow through or aren't where they said they'd be. It's hard enough when they are! But when they aren't, it's doubly confusing. In the end, my immediate reaction to a found item or answered inquiry, or even a person's presence, can resemble a type of shock or awe, yet another factor that serves to weaken my emotional reserves. Other times, I am a giggling ball of hyperactive energy completely delighted with the fact someone or something is still there!

Sometimes I breakdown or have minor setbacks; simple requests for change or unexpected happenings pull me out of my comfort zone and can lead to anxiety attacks, panic attacks, nervousness, crying spells, or a variety of other emotional responses. With alterations in routine, I might incorporate negotiation tactics or enter a complete state of shutdown (isolating and not speaking). When faced with a daunting obstacle or challenge, a type of numbing denial occurs, in which I would rather not face the issue. I become overwhelmed thinking about the cognitive and physical energy involved in completing the task or finding a solution. In this case "autistic inertia" may set in, which can be perceived as a type of hiding (in the mind) to offset the anguish or act of confronting what seems to be an unapproachable challenge.

Sometimes I might exhibit behaviors that appear to be out of harmony with a given circumstance. If highly agitated (e.g., extremely hurt, confused, disappointed), I tend to act out without considering the outcome (e.g., screaming, blaming, saying things I don't mean). This doesn't happen often, but when it does it's astonishing—like someone else has body-snatched me. She can be rather blunt, bratty, bitchy, and appallingly sharp witted. She's the master of the intentional, evil-eye, resting-bitch face. When something challenging occurs that causes emotional upheave, I might retreat into a state of utter panic. I also get this annoying emotional gag reflex in which I overly focus on how I should respond to a given situation. This leads to a type of verbal self-punishment over my perceived lack of emotional know-how. Instead of focusing on the situation at hand, such as bad news or a crisis, and responding to what is happening in an expected manner, I might very well slip into a state of mental paralysis, unable to think of much more than my concluded "truth" that I am too self-focused and incapable of coping.

Strong emotions frighten and confuse me. I can handle more subtle emotions, such as a sense of ease, simple pleasure, or happy anticipation, but other more abrasive and overbearing states, not so much. Strong emotions—like anger, dread, disappointment, and fear—are hard for me to tolerate and digest. With strong emotions, I retreat into a small dark place, just as I did when I was a child. I have been known to cry in closets, bathrooms, and under tables. Sometimes I drive off in my van. My van is a nice means of escape because no one can hear me. Although, I am certain I have unnerved a few passing folks with my high-pitched wailing. If I have enough wits about me, I have trained myself to phone a friend. Though I cannot always do this, particularly, if I am in a state of extreme confusion or self-pity.

Concerning my reaction to an emotional event, first response does not typically indicate end response. There are times I feel emotionally numb when I have taken in too much too fast. In those moments I might become stoic, untouchable, and distant. In times of upset, it is also not uncommon for my nervous giggle to mask feelings of confusion and disappointment. I don't nervously laugh on purpose; it's an instinctual response—a protective mechanism; it feels safer to laugh than to face uncomfortable and disjointed feelings. Given time to process, I experience a delayed emotional response and find myself crying or distraught—sometimes days after an initial event.

In most instances, regarding strong emotions, I am unable to pinpoint the exact feelings I am experiencing. There are also situations where I don't realize I have been triggered until later. In that case, when the rush of emotions first enters and I don't know why, it's a double-whammy: I am confused by the emotions and I am also confused about what triggered me in the first place. When given space and time to process, I am typically able to identify the trigger, understand my feelings, and act accordingly.

It is always better that I don't try to "solve" my emotions and instead allow myself to go through the emotions. Even though I know this, I have a hard time remembering to follow through. During a triggering event, I have a clusterfu** of churned-up emotions. No matter how many times I am triggered emotionally, I am always, without fail, perplexed by the confusion. It's like my feelings all hide behind the couch at regular junctions and jump out, hollering, "Surprise!" Only they forget it's not my birthday. And likewise, I forget how much they confuse the heck out of me. I think to myself, in times of subtle tranquility, that the next time my feelings will get easier. That they'll just sprawl out casually on the couch and chill.

After the initial surprise of emotions, the party is over and the emotional overwhelm sets in. Emotional overwhelm is akin to a train ride, wherein I know I've been on the ride before but I do not recognize the train, terrain, or the destination. I'm kind of just zipping by, my head out the window, the wind in my hair, being slapped in the face by an onrush of bugs. Splat! Splat! Splat!

Most days I do okay with my emotions. Most days I'm not on the train and the party-animal feelings are at someone else's house behind their couch. Yet there are definitely times I don't know how to handle them. I have a type of emotional amnesia. That is to say I don't tend to learn much about my emotional response based on prior experience. I don't carry what I've learned about my emotions from one situation to the next, primarily because I haven't really learned anything except to ride the train and let it pass.

When an emotional event is behind me, I can kindly reason with myself that the way I reacted to a given situation is just the way I am and reassure myself that how I am is okay. But when I am in a state of emotional upheaval, all bets are off! I forget—I forget that emotions are hard. I forget they are party animals. Of course, I quickly remember as I am running and ducking for cover as the feelings chase me around the room.

When I am upset, I remind myself not to exaggerate and compound the angst with logic. (I remind the little voice inside my head to shut the fu** up.) Being in a state of emotional mess is not the ideal time to delve into self-analysis, particularly because all the good stuff is vaporized and all the shitty aspects about myself persist. It's just not astute to evaluate the way I handle emotions when the emotions already have a death grip on me. When inner turmoil comes a-calling, I remind myself that I am not thinking rationally because those jumping-from-out-of-nowhere emotions frighten me. I end my self-talk there. More self-talk does more harm than good.

If I don't heed my own advice and stick with the plan of just letting the feelings pass, and instead try to fix the situation with cyclic analysis and tedious dissection of self, I end up blaming myself for whatever transpired and my resulting inability to handle the situation. Old tapes resurface. Oftentimes statements people have said to me in the past, such as, "What makes you think he will like you after he gets to know you?" or "I've been telling my friends for years that you frighten me." (It doesn't help the situation that those statements were from close relatives.) With the bombardment of past messages, emotional confusion, and self-blame, I might not be able to stop myself from self-harming—such as banging my fist over and over against a door. I lose myself in these damaging moments. They aren't frequent, but they are memorable, and carry with them a haunting reminder that strong emotions and I don't mix.

136. VIGNETTE, THE MISSING HOURS, AGE 14

On a Sunday morning in mid-December, I awoke still dressed in yesterday's clothes and walked out onto our backyard deck. All the neighboring yards on our hilltop street were fenceless, so the frosted winter grasses each combined together into a continual line of speckled white—all except for one yard. There, a high wooden fence wrapped around the entire property, like a barrier to a prison. This yard belonged to him.

As I searched out into the fields, I attempted to reconstruct the previous day and recall when I'd arrived home. The events of the last hours of the previous night were so very blurred that it was difficult to distinguish between when I'd fallen asleep and when I'd been awake. I remembered standing on the curbside with a plastic bag, preparing to cross the parking lot and begin the long trek home. It had been cold. I could see my breath. I had wrapped my hands beneath my wool sweater. But it wasn't snowing. The evening sky was clear. It was the mildest winter in years for the East Coast, while in California they were experiencing the worst rainstorms in over a decade. My Sony Walkman was on and the headphones warmed my ears. John Cougar's cassette tape was playing "It Hurts So Good." I had five dollars in my pocket. Nana, Father's mother, had written again. She was sending money for Christmas and couldn't understand why I wasn't making any friends. I missed her. For a moment, standing there in the cold, I had thought I could smell her, a soapy floral scent like the baby-blue balls she kept in a dish on the edge of her pink bathroom sink.

There were dozens of cars in the store parking lot that late day, their tail pipes puffing smoke. A car honked. My heart had leapt, and then, after seeing the familiar burgundy car, I'd sighed.

"Come on in," the driver had said, pulling over and waving me inside. "It's too cold to walk home."

Without much thought, I had left the cold and accepted the warmth of his car, easing my way across the burgundy leather bench seat.

"I'm glad I ran into you," he had said, while turning the steering wheel and pulling his car out of the parking lot.

I stopped.

Found myself back in the present time, still standing on my outdoor deck, shaking in the winter breeze. I backtracked. That wasn't the way he had sounded. Things had been different.

Leaving the deck, I walked back into the house and down the stairs into the dark study, ignoring Ben's snoring from the couch. Downstairs in my room, beneath the covers, I remembered again. And as I did, it seemed I was rewinding a movie. I recalled he had fumbled for words.

He had said, "I'm glad I ran into you. Do you think you might be able to watch my son . . .? I mean, I understand and all if you've got plans . . . with your friends. It must be great to be in high school again. Well. Not *again*." He had stopped to chuckle, covering his beige mustache with the hand that housed his gold wedding ring. "I mean it must be fun to *be* in high school."

I responded with an insecure nod, unsure if he had even asked me a question.

Turning the car onto a quieter stretch of road, he asked, "So, you can babysit?"

I ran one finger down the moist glass of the side window, searching my eyes outward. "Yes, that should be fine." I had supposed then, as my thoughts wondered about, I could have offered more. Told him how school wasn't great at all; that the place was horrible, the people were horrible, and I would have been better off having never gone.

Further down the road, I sensed he was worried. He gave me those signals—fidgeting fingers, and the smile that could not find a home. "What's in the bag?" he asked.

"Just a blouse," I whispered.

"Can I see it? I bet it's pretty."

In the way his voice dipped, I felt as if he had called *me* pretty.

I reached into my bag and then held up my purple blouse.

"It's beautiful," he said, dragging out the last syllables.

There was a long pause. I was angry with myself. He must have informed me of our destination and I must have blacked out into my own fantasyland, thinking on someone else's husband's handsome green eyes, when I should have been counting the blocks home. I drew the warm air in through my nostrils and held it there, not wanting to breathe out. I wished to stop thinking, to get the drive over with. I forced myself to speak. "Where are we going, again?"

He put one hand on my shoulder. My spine quivered. "Oh, didn't I tell you? I'm sorry. I must have forgotten," he apologized, his voice speeding up with each word. "We're just headed up the road a bit. I forgot about this errand—a real quick thing for a friend. I think you met him. You know my buddy with the red beard?"

I did not remember, but nodded anyway.

"Sorry it's taking so long. It's right around this corner and down this alley."

The alley was absent of light. I could barely make out the shape of anything.

He stopped the car. "What was the name of your boyfriend again? You still have the same boyfriend? You're seeing him still. Aren't you?"

My ears burned red. I pulled strands of my hair across the side of my face. "Jeff is his name. Can we go home now?"

He repeated the name *Jeff.* I focused on the plastic bag between my knees. "Can we please go home?" He leaned into me, inching his pressed slacks across the seat, squeaking his bottom, like I had done earlier. Only he didn't care, didn't care at all about the noise he made. "Sweetheart," he said, softly, "Jeff is a lucky man."

That Sunday morning, I rolled over in the covers, swaddling myself like an infant. The stale water of the mattress rippled below me.

I had screamed. I remembered that much. But that's all I could remember. It was a loud scream. The type where the words take on a life of their own, as if magically stretching across from one mountain peak to another to form a bridge.

Ben's footsteps creaked above the study's ceiling. I pictured the layers between us—the ceiling plaster, the floorboard and padding, the dirty shag carpet—and I imagined firing a gun into his large ass. With a gush of cold air Mother entered my bedroom by way of the garage door, and with a kind smile she stuffed a stack of bills into her brown briefcase. "Hi, can I have a hug?" she asked.

Startled, I looked up at Mother, a part of me wishing she would leave and another part ready to cast myself into her arms and weep. Mother drew me near. The loneliness of the last days descended upon me. She released quickly. "I sure missed you. Did you get my postcard? Oh, what am I saying? You'll get it in a few days." Mother had a conversation with herself, answering and filling in the blanks. And the emptiness came again, the emptiness of not really being seen. Still smelling her stale breath, I whispered, "Mom?"

Mother opened her eyes wide and stopped looking for the lighter in her purse. "What?"

"I need a sick note for school tomorrow. I don't feel so good."

She flattened down the bottom corner of the old blue comforter. She could not keep still. I struggled to control my need to cry. I only wanted a simple *yes*. There was nothing more Mother could offer. Her voice sounded baffled and overly concerned. She tried to compensate in tone and mannerism for her absence the last couple of days. "Oh, Ben didn't tell me you were sick. Do you have a fever? Have you eaten anything? You look pale."

I did not answer, certain Mother was about to speak again. She moistened her lips. "Have you seen my cigarettes? I think I left my pack out in the car. Shit. It's cold. What were you saying?"

Again, the emptiness.

I rolled over in bed pressing my face into the pillow.

Mother shook her head. "You were sick?"

I coughed in my hand, feigning a cold, hoping for a break, for Mother to mount the stairs and rummage through the near-empty kitchen cupboards for some expired medicine. She wiped her wide forehead and tucked a strand of hair behind her ear. My breath was sinking. If Mother asked how I was, if she even looked at me with tenderness, I knew I would break apart.

Mother, finding her cigarettes, spilt out everything all at once: her trip, her new friends, and even her favorite airline stewardess. I cringed and breathed into the pillowcase. I felt her touch my arm. She was surveying. I remained motionless like an opossum playing dead. I was no longer competing with my feelings of emptiness. Mother had stepped up ahead of everything.

She sucked in air through her nostrils. I sensed her scowl. She could not help but spit her words out. "So, I think this was meant to be, this trip, the whole thing." Clearing her throat, Mom reloaded.

Even without her invitation, I would speak. I would open my mouth, if only to get her to shut her own. I swallowed, lifted my head, and blurted out, "I'm fine now. I just need a shower."

Mother huffed and lifted her eyes to the ceiling.

And that was the end of it. The last time I would contemplate the missing hours. The last time I would ever come close to telling Mother.

137. Mind the Mind

I am the puzzle seeker in all ways. In knowing this about myself, I am practicing the act of not exploding events in my mind. I recognize I take a flat, one-dimensional problem and I tilt it into multiple 3-D forms. I take what is simple and I complicate the matter. Not on purpose, and not with intention to add complexity, only as a byproduct of my innate ability to solve. I have asked myself why. The ultimate answer remains in the unease brought on by the thought of unknowns.

Even as a child, my childhood games were not games. They were preparation to conquer the unknown and unfamiliar. Everything, from playtime to alone time, was set in its place. Everything was organized and every move stemmed from a sense of needing order. As I grew older, that didn't change. My need for order and detail remained. The structured play transformed into thoughts fashioned into recognizable systems and order. I became that one that believed she must remain the leader of her thoughts, in attempt, to survive the turmoil that seemed *me*.

Everywhere was chaos and everywhere something that could be organized back to original form of order. I became, with every year, more a person who depended on her thoughts in hopes of discovering a neutral zone set outside the disorder. I am still here, doing this—seeking out in hopes of escaping the disorder. This is what it comes down to. This is the end point. And it is this observation that makes perfect sense now. I am the watchtower viewing my own cyclic hibernation. I am steering my way into self, thinking if I am the constant seeker then I shall hide enough from what is in front of me. For even the anguish of overthinking, even the painstaking ways in which I torture myself with thought upon thought, becomes reasonable when compared to the unknowns which remain out there. In some ways, I have made myself mad in the interior to avoid the fear of the exterior. I have made myself a prisoner of thought to escape the overbearing burden of life. But in so doing, I have made myself twice the captive. Piercing first myself with anxiety, and then again causing casualty by the intrepid thoughts that follow thoughts.

In knowing this recognition, I have concluded that the only way in which to save myself is to ironically *stop trying to save myself*! It is mind-blowing, that through the act of theorizing, I have concluded that in order to live more fully, I must stop the act of continual theorizing—to forbid myself to enter the labyrinth of thoughts disguised as false salve and salvation.

138. ANNIHILATED SELF

I once had a vision of a room full of people. In my imagination, each person took a turn standing up on a soapbox to speak. As they spoke, they pulled from random subjective memories. Memories and recollections based on gathered ideologies, belief systems, environments, and experiences. They were all present in a large hall. All assembled to give their opinions about me. As each of the individuals took their place on the raised platform, I recognized that I was merely a random interpretation. A flower being evaluated: Some loved me for my sweetness. Some adored my beauty. Some merely saw me as a weed to be plucked. Some thought I stunk. Others inhaled and couldn't get enough.

Through this pictorial image in my mind, I further theorized that the loose interpretations others had about who I was as a person were not only dependent on a number of obvious variables, but also on random points of time. People's outlooks were affected by the moment in time in which they existed. I also realized, soon following, that any subtle change in the way in which I currently lived could result in a person having an altered interpretation of who I was. If I divorced my husband, if I abandoned my children, if I joined a nunnery—how might my action affect the outcome of an audience member's interpretation of me? And, in addition, if they, the viewers, made any life changes, or faced any crisis, or shifted personal ideologies, how might their views of me change?

I then witnessed my past self and images of my life and saw how my perceptions have gradually shifted through the ages, and, as a result, the way in which I once viewed others also gradually shifted. From there, it was only logical to conclude that I, ever changing, would remain incapable of being stagnant in my individualized viewpoints that were based on unavoidable, continual transitioning. And that likewise, in parallel fashion, others remained incapable of being stagnant in their viewpoints, and thusly incapable of maintaining a stagnant view of whom I was.

In understanding I was nothing more than random gathered evidence, and that this evidence itself shifted based on the moment, circumstance, and the observer, I concluded that another's loose interpretation of who I was never remained idle in interpretation long enough to be deemed factual. With this, I saw that all opinions of who I was no longer could be perceived as complete truth—even the so-called "positive" interpretations. It did not make logical sense to attach myself to fleeting self-descriptors based on random observers with random transitioning viewpoints. Plus, if I was an information gatherer shifting my gatherings of what others thought of me to form a self-identity, then how could I ensure that what I gathered was substantiated by steadfast evidence and not merely self-serving, biased, selective proof? And beyond this, if I had latched onto the semipermanent, and what I thought to be most likely true and reasonable, interpretations of myself, then how could I be judge and jury? How was I to decide what was true and what wasn't true in considering others' interpretations of me? How was I to allow myself to collect so-called "positive" attributes about myself while disregarding and discarding the rest?

It seemed logical, at this juncture, to conclude that the only way out of the process of defining who I was based on others' viewpoints was to disrobe myself of all opinions obtained from others. From here, it followed suit that if I were to discount others' opinions in totality, then in equal measure it was essential that I discount my opinions about others in totality. In other words, if I believed others could not define me, then I reasonably could not define others without being a hypocrite.

Next, the process became a matter of what to see, what to believe, and what to qualify as truth. And the only natural conclusion that arose no further conflict or query within myself was to choose to see another being as another being and nothing more, and to overlook the illusion of what appeared to be "wrong" or "against" me.

In a sense, I annihilated self through logic and through the recognition that no stagnant representation of "me" existed. Without a true "self," I had no true or stagnant opinions. In reality, my opinion couldn't be trusted. My thoughts were just that: thoughts. Nothing more. Nothing less. Not bad, just not real. I reasoned further that the act of evaluating another is indirectly self-abusive. But that's another story.

139. VIGNETTE, NEVER EXISTED, AGE 14

The days after the note dredged on slowly like the days leading up to an important event, such as a wedding or the birth of a child—only without the joyful anticipation. The time was more of a long, drawn-out waiting, a gradual emptying of hope. Surely Mother was well prepared, having spent days packing moving boxes, marking down the numbers on the calendar, and concentrating an excess amount of energy and time on travel itinerary. Yet I was entrapped with my thoughts, completely unaware of how to be in tune with anything and how to think beyond moving my body.

"It's time to go," Ben said, softly.

I wished for the phone to ring one last time.

"Are you ready?" he asked.

Banked with a somber mind, I glanced up at his dark eyes and searched for a sense of regret, some indication of remorse, some sign to indicate he cared. And for an instant, a brief second, I thought I could see sadness. A glimmer of an apology. I held onto the glimmer and walked across the dark study that had served as my bedroom, past the sheet-draped window, past the cold ashes in the fireplace, and past the indentations in the carpet where Ben's waterbed had once been. I stepped one foot after the other, leaving no trail of my presence, feeling as if I'd never even lived in the space. Sensing I had never existed.

Some days earlier, on a dewy, damp day about a week after Easter, a holiday that had proven both basketless and without a single egg (save scrambled), I had found a note on the bottom of the stairs. Thinking Ben or Mother had dropped something, I unfolded the paper with unsuspecting casualness. Inside I found Ben's familiar scribbles. They were all crooked and capitalized. The first line contained the word "please" and the last line Ben's block-lettered signature, all in caps.

There are times life seemingly takes a giant highlighter and smears a moment in its bright mark. I can still see myself stooped on the bottom of our staircase, coarse-faced and gulping in disbelief, gnawing at the words, biting my way through the few sentences, halting at the exclamation marks to regroup and breathe. Standing there on the bottom step I had replayed the last months living in the house. It was true I had disputed with Ben over his ridiculous curfew. I'd also laughed mockingly at his idea of not dating until college. A few times I had silently cursed his lack of effort around the house. But in all honesty, I hadn't done anything worthy of his unabashed wrath. Even if I had, he was supposed to be the adult.

And then the cruel injustice of the situation hit me. It was just in the last month I had started making a few friends: nice girls, genuine girls with good morals, friends who accepted me for who I was. Friends who complimented me on my poetry, who invited me to slumber parties, and who happily sat by my side at lunch. The climate at school was less hostile and most of the name-calling had disappeared. I was no longer the new kid from California. I was finally just another girl at school. I'd even considered trying out for the next year's cheerleading squad. And above all, there was Jeff, the boy I was in love with, the boy I planned on marrying someday.

I thought with certainty this had to be some cruel test. I'd been ridiculed and shamed, beaten in spirit and then given a glimpse of hope, a splinter of success, only to be prematurely yanked back. It was some horrible, horrible test.

Refolding the note, I did the only thing I could do, and marched upstairs to find Mother. Once inside her bedroom I tossed the paper beside her. "Here," I said flatly.

Never one to handle confrontation well, Mother eyed me cautiously as she snatched up the note. Still as a stone, I waited. Mother's eyes tracked the full of Ben's words once and then she reread the note again. The first time with rueful eyes and the latter with a wry wince. Then she pulled herself into a high stance, sitting upright at the edge of her bed. Next, she gracefully folded the note closed, collected me with her eyes, and said, "It's no surprise. I knew this was coming."

Taken aback, I pressed my eyes sharply into Mother, burying my pain and replacing it with bitter disgust, "You've got to be kidding me!" I shouted. "You can't do this! Not after everything!"

Mother, enthroned on her bed, looked as if she intended to speak.

"I hate you!" I hollered.

She stiffened on my remark and her expression hardened. She then left the bed and scuffed her slippers across the carpet. "I can't deal with you when you're like this," she said, in an exasperated tone. "Don't you think I already have enough on my plate?"

I took in her words like pebbles ground into an open wound. "It's not always about you," I said.

"Well, of course it isn't. I understand it must be hard on you. I just hope I can get through the next two weeks." She walked toward the bedroom door. "You are the one who always wanted this. Think of how happy everyone will be. It's not as bad as it seems. Things could always be worse."

Standing at the outskirts of her bed, I felt the familiar tightening of my intestines. "But it hasn't even been a year," I announced. Only then did I realize that my path was already preordained.

Mother prattled on. And I did what I knew best—shut my ears and eyes, becoming a mute audience. Only I still heard her, muffled somewhere, underneath the layers I'd placed between us. She rambled more, speaking about what would unfold in the next few days, on airplanes and relatives, and on boxes—grocery boxes. We'd have to collect them again. And then there was phoning everyone, especially her mother and my father. She continued, until several sentences later her voice changed, and thinking she would nap, she kindly asked me to leave.

I drifted across the room. My eyes set on the stale carpet. I swiped the folded paper off of the bed. Stepping out I tottered, reopening the note and thinking the words felt heavy and wet, like sliced bread dipped in soup: soaked, soppy, and breaking apart piece by piece. "Please leave this house as soon as you can," came the pieces. "I cannot stand to have either one of you under this damn roof any longer," the words dripped. "Just pack up your belongings and get the hell out," the heaviness pounded. "BEN." The end hurt.

140. THE BARBS

I can sense fear well enough. It doesn't come in needle form. It isn't injected by an outside source. There is no fluid that enters through a prick or an invasive probing. Fear bypasses exterior layers, rooting from within, expanding and growing as seedlings do. And I am but host to the cyclic process.

For most of my days I wasn't aware of the fear inside. Even as I was always anxious and scared, I couldn't easily identify my emotions of fright, basically because I *was* fright. Even as new fear entered, there was no obvious change I noticed. There was no alarm system in place. Fear was my normal. If there were trespasses against me, there was no way to tell because I was already overcrowded inside. One more pair of prodding footsteps made no difference to a well-established colony of thousands. Ironically, in a state of fear-equilibrium, I felt perpetually balanced.

In regard to the fear I housed inside, I don't know when I started to shift. It was sometime between the start of my public writings and the times I had delved deeply into spiritual studies. I'd been searching for answers. And something had clicked. And in those moments the fear became recognizable. Wherein it had been invisible before, this fear now had a voice and had taken form. It arrived aware of itself, pushing up and growing in a making-room-for-more manner. The fear was real then. It always had been, but now it was set outside the shadows and staring down at me.

I could feel it everywhere, a monstrosity. I knew of it, as if an old familiar friend had reappeared for fellowship. Foe he was, true, but more so a companion in the way he meandered and made himself at home, opening and closing whatever compartment he fancied. Seeing him move this way, amongst the others, amongst the piles of pain, in the conglomeration of fear, baffled me. A visibility granted, where once there had only been utter blindness, seemed a miracle.

In this way fear itself, in its manifestation, became an element of transformation. In this way fear was part of my breaking and making. With my new awareness, my body was like a musical organ, each key being pounded by some unknown trigger and in response piping out this obnoxious vibration; the sounds penetrating my interior and leaching out of the exterior—a lost song let out into the open.

Where before I might have survived in a state of saturated fear, my stagnation birthed through a tangible blindness, here, in this new awareness of continual pounding, I could not live. In response to the discomfort my instinctual nature took over. And at a subconscious level I began the process of sorting through and categorizing the discomfort. Later, I established a way to eradicate the unwanted tenants. I'd rely on my own body. Recognizing that I was contaminated by fear, I would remove each and every cause for pain, my body an informant verbalizing through careful unspoken word.

It whispered its tellings:

"Listen," stomach would say, "I am tight."

"Listen," heart would say, "I am pounding."

"Listen," hands would say, "I am clenched."

And from here the *whys* came forth. Stomach was sad from the way the stranger had frowned. Heart was upset in the way the word "stupid" reminded him of the past. Hands were startled by the loud boom of the car.

And I listened. Day after day I listened. Until, with much patience and practice, I began to hear less and less. Now new spaces opened, where none had existed before. Now when a stranger named fear appeared, when he rooted himself in me, the fear was no longer cloaked by the masses. Now when the fear came, it came with a loud blow into an empty room. Now when fear arrived, I knew immediately. The tables had turned. Instead of housing the fears that had used me for room and board for decades, now I removed the newbies, the ones that had hitchhiked in hopes of permanent residency. Now I gathered the barbs and released them—their freedom, my freedom.

141. THE GIRL IN THE CHEER SKIRT

Mother and I moved back to the West Coast before my freshman year in high school on the East Coast was even over. With the move back across the states to a new school with my familiar childhood peers, for some reason—perhaps my East Coast metamorphism, e.g., new clothes, new hair, new makeup, and new figure—I went from an East Coast, ostracized, conceded slut to a West Coast, popular, sought-out friend. Needless to say, this was in every way confusing.

By the time my senior year in high school came along, through much trial and error, I'd developed skills for social survival. I'd learned how to blend in, how to keep a friend and how to not make waves. By age seventeen, I was the captain of the cheerleading squad, the homecoming princess, the spirit coordinator for school rallies (assemblies), and working part-time at a retirement home for senior citizens. I cannot say I was happy, though. In fact, I sought out a therapist convinced I was entirely wired wrong. Yet I can say, by all mainstream impressions, I was successful.

Since leaving the East Coast, I spent many an evening crying, primarily because I felt entirely alone and an outcast in the world, despite my best friend, boyfriend, and accomplishments. I was trapped in a deep lingering depression. I ended up intentionally missing so much school that the school counselor called Mother in for an emergency meeting to discuss the potentiality of me not graduating. There was that, and there were blessings—such as my English teacher who took a liking to my poetry and writings and became a type of advocate for my well-being and school survival, as well as the continual kindness and attention from my high school sweetheart and his family, and my loving Catholic confirmation teacher, Helen.

People, my peers mainly, would never have guessed then, looking at me, that I had any trouble whatsoever. Taken as a whole, I appeared to *have it all*—a reputation that only added to my sense of guilt in not being able to appreciate what I had. Profoundly, I had all the outer makings of that all-American girl. I even had a white picket fence.

Even with that, if anyone were to dig into the truth of me, if I were ever to have let anyone try, there would have been a whole other girl inside. Back then, I walked most days half-alive, just barely surviving; playing that role they (my classmates) had all cast me in. This new way of being on the West Coast truthfully didn't beat being ostracized for my oddities and called out for my imperfections on the East Coast. More so, the transition seemed as if I'd swung from one bad end of the pendulum to the next. In one place, I was pressed down so low I was suffocating at the bottom. In the other place, I was lifted up so high I lived in constant fear of falling. And in both places, no one ever saw me.

Had I known any different then, I suppose I would have disrobed every last inch of the dressings I was garbed in. But as it was, I did my best to survive, primarily through escaping in writing, daydreaming, sleeping, and cheerleading. I had poured my heart and soul into cheerleading. Cheering was my fixation, the place where I found a sense of normalcy, security, and stability. I liked that the cheers stayed the same, that each word or two had a movement that matched, and that those movements were predictable and ordered.

However, it was during the time period I was elected the captain of the cheer team that I was to receive one of the deepest emotional wounds of my life. Perhaps not as detrimental as the outcomes that resulted in my overtrusting of predators, but equal in measure in the way the event tore me to bits and further enforced that the world was unsafe and unmanageable.

My first two years of cheering were filled with good memories, as joyful as memories could be for a damaged dyslexic cheerleader with Aspergers. I greatly aspired to be the cheer captain from the get-go. I tried out each year. Leading and teaching had always come second nature to me; the structure and rigidness both suited and soothed me. Having finally earned the title of *captain* my senior year felt a dozen elevator levels better than grand, at least for the first week.

As fate would have it, although I was the same age as my new squad members, I was the opposite in many ways. Soon I realized the girls weren't going to listen to me. If I turned my back, they were poking fun at the way I stood. If I spoke, they were poking fun at the way I talked. All my hopes of being a *real* captain were lost in their ways. Despite the challenges and sense of pending doom, I didn't falter in my want to succeed. Perchance, I believed, I might pull these girls up from their place of dillydallying. Perhaps, I thought, they would grow out of their silliness and eventually listen. But of course they didn't change. And neither did I.

It wasn't long following my election to captain status that three of the squad members reported untruths about me to the cheer advisor. As a result of their false assumptions and cruel lies, I was instantly disqualified from my leadership role. In essence, demoted, shamed, and punished for something I never did. It was seconds after the announcement of my demotion that I had an emotional outburst and quit the squad altogether. I became entirely lost—my identity and special interest torn away for no logical reason, and certainly for no fair reason. This was another one of those devastating points in time that will forever rest in my memory banks. I can still see myself in my red and gold pleated skirt sprinting miles and miles down the city blocks, with the tears streaming down my face, and the thought, the very intense, terrifying thought, of no longer knowing who I was.

142. TRUTH TELLER

There are moments I want to tape my mouth shut. I can tell myself, even promise myself profusely, that I will not tell someone something. But it doesn't matter how I try to stop the train of words. For despite my best attempts, the charging locomotive comes. I don't want to be this way, but there is a driver beyond me. He is the one making the calls. Personally, this me, this person now that is consciously aware and writing, she would like to stop; she would like to remain silent; she would like to keep something to herself, but she cannot. She isn't allowed to house secrets. She is sworn to this all-encompassing law of "the truth shall set you free."

Only the truth is confusing. The truth can be convoluted and mixed up, and come with a whole bunch of strings attached. The truth can be buried under an avalanche of manipulation and selfish desire. The truth can be jaded by subjective perception and personal collected truths. Yet to be as authentic as possible, the truth itself must be unmasked, dug up, and examined. Herein lies more work. For all at once, I am dissecting the elements that classify true truth.

I can't even tell a partial truth without reflecting upon why I did such a (horrible) thing. I concentrate on the elements I left out—the *whys* of why I only told half a truth. I do the same if I leave out a small detail of a story.

Many times, after I speak, I partake in an elaborate, grand scale playback—some unseasoned director rewinding the film footage and noting flaws. I decipher if what I said was (1) true, (2) based on the best of my recollection, (3) reflected from a state of wanting nothing in return but to be heard, (4) lacking selfish motivation, manipulation, or covering up of any sort, (5) not said to win someone over or to gain sympathy, and (6) not missing parts that would take away from the true meaning or events.

While I am in review mode there is a background interpreter who is (1) reliving the past events through a pictorial overview, (2) rewriting a script of how I could have said something in a more authentic or kinder way, (3) watching myself go back in time and correcting what was said to better amplify truth, and (4) justifying said actions and suggestions through connecting back to previous learnings. Need I say this all gets rather exhausting?

143. CONTEMPLATING MUTISM

A loved one criticized me. And, in my all-too-common fashion, I stepped back and watched myself wade through the bullets of my rapid-firing brain. Or better yet, I observed the domino effect as one thought kicked another thought's ass. And one after the other, I collapsed.

Here is a very brief scenario:

"I complain a lot. I should kill myself. If I am that terrible of a person, I shouldn't be on earth. If I think in this type of martyrdom fashion, like the last two thoughts, I am surely not worthy of anyone's love. How could he say that? Do I really complain a lot? Is this his reality, my reality, or some other reality? Whose perspective is real? I should reread my Buddhist books for the third time. I have such a bad memory. He is cruel and unjust. I am never speaking to him again. Actually, I am going to be mute for the rest of my life. I will never speak to *anyone* again. If I still can't get things right after this many years, I am doomed. What is right? I hate that there are rights and wrongs. They don't make sense. I can do it. I will start with one day. If I am mute, no one will ever judge me. Well, at least not my spoken words. Should I still write? I will have to write. But to whom? And how much? I will be a saintly mute, like the older lady on the popular prison show. I kind of look like her anyway. I wonder how my children will react. Would my silence traumatize them? Maybe I should slowly become mute—little by little each day. I could write on a yellow legal notepad."

(Intermission: I looped into a fantasy of my life as a kind mute.)

And then, anger: "I will show that asshole. I shall never speak again! He complains, too. He is pessimistic. He is moody. He is . . . It's not fair he pointed this out to me. I hate him for doing this. I hate him. Doesn't he know how much goes on inside my head already? How hypersensitive I am to everything? That I am trying my best? I don't want to ever see him again. Ever! I miss being around people who aren't honest all the time. No, I don't. Yes, I do."

Tears (again).

"Well, I point out things to people, and I am sure it makes them uncomfortable, and they process what I said. Or they just ignore. I don't have the capacity to ignore. What would it be like to think everyone else is the problem and not look at self? Freeing, I suppose. I am still caught up in this perfectionism. Damn him. Damn me. I don't deserve to be here anymore. I just can't do it. I can't function in any type of relationship, friendship or romantic, not even casual. I don't know how to do it. I hate being alive. Do I really complain a lot? That's it. I am marching up to my bedroom and I shall stay there and sleep the day away. I am locking my door. I am not coming out."

(Toss and turn, replaying all past hurtful things *anyone* has *ever* said to me in my *entire* life . . . stab, stab, *stab*.)

"I can't sleep. I will run away. I will drive away. I will just leave. No one will miss me. They will be better off without me."

Marching downstairs. (I actually step lightly, but in my imagination I am stomping.)

"Hi Violet. You want to go outside to potty?" (Asked with baby-talk inflection to my wagging-tail shadow.)

"Shit!"

I can't be mute to my dog. Mute plan demolished, after thoughts of buying clickers, whistles, teaching my dog hand signals, and buying her extra treats, and after I'd already told her, "Good girl for going potty!" and her eyes lit up.

Driving away in my van . . . forever!

Logical me stepped back in, after one mile. Did errands. Paid bills. Texted a friend. Waded in self-pity. Analyzed self-pity. Analyzed myself analyzing self-pity. Analyzed my therapist's feasible thoughts of me having self-pity. Is it still self-pity if I am aware I am wallowing and analyzing the pity and making measures to eliminate the wallowing and admitting to martyrdom? Analyzed general truism at the time: never returning to my old life and ways. Like the victims in *Body Snatchers*, I shall arise reborn. Maybe half-dog. Wondered if I begged really loud, my home planet would beam me up.

Drove home. Pretended nothing was wrong but planned on never speaking again. Forgot I wasn't speaking ever again. Threw out that plan once and for all—though not before fantasizing about a commune where all mute Aspies lived together and developed telepathic abilities, so not one person had to open their eyes. Wondered if people would miss my voice. Wondered if other people get sick of hearing their own voice. Contemplated if life would be easier sensory-wise if I couldn't see. Yes, it would, I decided; but not before mourning the feasible loss of an azure sky honeycombed in powder-puff, morphing clouds above the evergreens. Sigh. I needed to see.

Continued to cry sporadically when no one was looking, punishing myself for yet another thing I did wrong, not right enough, and not good enough, and wondering how I could ever be enough for anyone, particularly my own self. Dead set settled on the fact that every person who was ever critical toward me in the past was right. Set about to analyze each and every person, and concluded they all have issues. We all have issues. But I suck the most. At least it's feasible I do. Wondering what the world would be like without me and if my death would affect and hurt people. Yes, it would. Not a good idea in general. Question: *Was I suicidal or just wallowing?* Wallowing was the outcome, blended in with self-persecution and lack of survival plan or skills for this round, mostly blue planet.

Held pain inside. Did not speak of it. Did not mention it to anyone. Stab. Stab. Stab. Decided to send emotional daggers out in every direction in attempt at self-preservation. Youngest son enters. He is miserable about something. Not him, too! He projects harmful statement toward me. I explode. I break down. I just can't hold on. Freak out. Freak out more. Rush to fix what is broken. Rush to fix family issue. Rush to redeem myself and help my son. Sink back into temporary reprieve. Distracted by other urgency, only to return to original funk of "I am not good enough," now accentuated by previous encounter with son. Sad. Very sad. Terribly sad. I obviously take things too personally. How can I dish out stuff but not be able to take it? That's hypocritical. I am a bad person.

Cycle back through these thoughts and multiple thoughts, over and over and over. Project into future what life will be like without certain people in my life. Become closed off and quiet. Nonrespondent. Function with normalcy, at least my normalcy, smile when expected, answer when expected. Nothing more.

Stuff. Stuff. Stuff. Occasional stab. Bleed out until dry.

Finally arrive, after days, at conclusion: everyone complains. At least, most people. But I can complain a bit less. It will be good for me. Having had uprooted my ego bits and experienced the pain of wounded self-image, I begin rebuilding.

Logic again: Yes, I complain more than some, but likely about average for my kind. I think? But compared to what is in my head, I only share one percent of what I hear inside. And I am so very grateful about so many things I think of constantly. Should I speak aloud all of those things to counterbalance what is perceived as negative? And how do I separate what is anxiety from what is considered complaining? Triggers from what is considered complaining? Truth telling from what is considered complaining? How do I know what to hold inside and what to tell? When does withholding thoughts or information become an untruth? When do I stay quiet? How much? For how long? How much can I share about what's inside before I sound like I am complaining? If it's to inform, and I don't feel like it's complaining, and it's just informational and logical, with no obvious emotion or intention, is it still complaining? When is sharing complaining? At what point?

Still contemplating mutism—after my dog dies.

144. COMMUNICATION IN REVIEW

1. **I understand the fact that a non-autistic person thinks differently than me, but I forget this fact in the heat of conversation**. Just as a typical person might understand that an autistic person thinks differently, but not thoroughly understand what it is like to have autism; likewise I can understand to a degree the way another person without autism thinks, but never quite grasp how this alternate thinking occurs.

2. **I have challenges with pragmatic language skills (a.k.a. social language skills)**. Sometimes I look away instead of looking someone in the eyes. I also take things literally. I am frequently candid and exhibit matter-of-fact mannerisms. I can be pedantic. Other people sometimes interpret my intonation and body language as angry, obstinate, or stuck-up. I have a nervous giggle that might come across as condescending. Due to my innate nature to see things outside of the box, I am a natural-born comedian. Even so I have a hard time distinguishing when it is acceptable to tell a joke and knowing the appropriate perimeters of a joke.

3. **There is a pronounced tendency for me to overexplain things**. Sometimes I elucidate beyond what might be deemed necessary because (a) I have difficulty differentiating between what is the least and greatest of importance to a given topic (e.g., thinking if I omit a piece of information that the omission might have been an essential part of the puzzle and/or that the omission would reflect a lack of honesty); (b) I think in complexities and at high speed, and perceive I am only ejecting a small percentage of my thoughts into the conversation, yet this so-perceived small percentage is often viewed as a large percentage; (c) I long to be heard and for my perception to be given consideration. It's not necessarily that I need validation or to prove a point; moreover, I wish to be allowed opportunity for expression without continual communication barriers and the resulting cross-countering; (d) I am partaking in a type of stimming (repeated, self-soothing behavior) in which the talking alleviates anxiety.

4. I have challenges censoring my spoken thoughts. This is primarily because I have an alternative thought-filtering system than most. I often do not have thoughts of another's reaction at heart as much as the desire to be honest, forthright, and transparent. As is such, I might appear to be lacking tact, when in actuality my act of not censoring my thoughts may be a mere result of my inability to instinctually employ people-pleasing techniques or other commonly used communication tactics. In theory, I am speaking without a filter. In other words: simply speaking without any other purpose than to speak.

5. **I interrupt.** There are several reasons I might interrupt: (a) I might cut someone short during a conversation in order to express my ideas before I cease to remember them. Because of my short-term memory challenges, I have difficulty retaining what is being spoken after a sentence or two. I feel anxiety related to the mental energy I will have to exert in order to remember what I was thinking because my thoughts come so fast; (b) I measure my thoughts as urgent and necessary to get out; it's like I have an interior aha sensation sparking my need to utter; (c) I am a visual thinker. I think in pictures. As a result I might interject in order to picture what is being said; (d) It is difficult for me to determine the end of a person's turn in conversation. Talking seems like a back-and-forth game.

6. **While conversing I am actively engaged in recalling and rehearsing the rules of communication.** I am juggling two conversations at once— what is being said in the two-way conversation with another and what is being said in the two-way conversation in my mind. I have to reteach myself the rules of conversation and then remind myself during the conversation how to act. My body language usually takes a back seat. I don't have enough energy reserves to consciously control my body all the time. Body language comes naturally and automatically to the typical person, like riding a familiar bike. Body language is not easy for me; it's more akin to riding a surfboard for the first time, over and over.

145. SMALL TALK

I coach myself. I truly do. Before and after discourse, however brief or so-perceived minor, I beseech the person within this person to be calm, to leave space in the conversation, to not be too logical, to not critique. And so it goes that each encounter is a great stretch of energy exertion: the coaching beforehand, the coaching afterwards, the coaching during. Always I am wondering what the other person thinks and what he or she is deciphering regarding my input and approach. And always I am that absent judge pulling apart the pieces and examining each on their own, in hopes of finding the missing part—the flaw, the inadequacy.

Case in point: Last night, I was in the local grocery store and the male checker locked eyes with me and asked, with a toothy grin, "So what have you been working on?"

What have I been working on? My face squished up in confusion. Number one thought barged in: *Glad I am wearing a winter hat to hide my burning red ears.* The bombardment of thoughts that followed went something like this:

What does this question mean? I am embarrassed. Can he tell I am beet red? I wonder if it bothers him he is balding. I wonder if he is single. What does he think of me? Why would he ask this? What am I supposed to say? He is staring at me. Can he tell I am embarrassed? What is he thinking? How should I respond? I am taking too long? Do I look autistic, shy, or stuck-up? I don't want to look at him. I don't want him to think I am in a bad mood. I am not. I thought I was better equipped than this. I thought I was prepared. I bet I look stuck-up. Just like in high school—always misinterpreted. The people in line are looking at me. I wonder if they are married? I wonder if they can tell I am so embarrassed. They are frowning. Are they tired or sad or mad at me? I look flustered. How much time has gone by? Why did I choose the shortest line and not the line with the female checker? (That's about half the thoughts, anyhow.)

Only seconds had past, but in my reality it seemed hours. I refocused. All I could think to say was, "What made you ask that question?" I realized immediately that I sounded evasive, suspicious, and even perhaps flirtatious. By this time, I wondered if he was psychic and could sense I was working on many projects. The checker responded quickly and easily, in a manner that screamed, "This is so easy for me!"

"Oh, I was just making small talk to pass the time."

Small talk? Small talk? Small talk! Should I explain there isn't such a thing in my mind?

He stared me down, and I knew, as the blood shot through my cheeks and up to the bridge of my nose, that in this communication game, it was my turn to speak. I stuttered some and then formed some shaky sentences about my new job and such, remembering of course, with screaming reminders in my head, to ask him about himself.

By the time the three minutes were over, and the checker had scanned and bagged my ten items, I felt I'd been to war and back.

146. VIGNETTE, FADED SUN, AGE 37

"Was it your voice or another voice that told you to kill yourself?" the stranger asked.

"My own voice," I whispered, from a mouth I could no longer feel.

I brought myself forward in a chair, a purposeful push, only to prove to myself I could move, that my brain synapses still fired, and then nodded solemnly in the direction of a blank white space. There was a stain in the high corner.

There, in that cramped room, I was unable to focus, unable for the first time to pretend. I had always been able to follow someone, to take cues from the people around me. Here I could not. Here, though I was clothed, I was stripped naked, paralyzed with the thought that there were no answers. From across the room my husband stirred his body, first to the left and then to the right, needing to get comfortable in a room with no comfort. Pen in hand, the serious woman with the questions balanced her clipboard on one leg. Once again my husband moved, taking the chair with him as he tilted and then rebalanced. I was long used to him, to his motions. I knew what they meant. I could read him like the time, like a sailor could read the wind. He was turning, shifting to the outer part of his thoughts, trying to unscramble what had been left. In the early years, I had expected my husband to change, for his patience to falter, for his colors to transform. But he hadn't. He'd remained steadfast, dedicated, concerned. And what was I but the quake bringing the waves?

Without wanting to, without deciding to, I whispered, "I'm sorry," taking in an ache tenfold. The stranger across the room, I imagined she was someone else. I turned her into a person I knew, someone with a face I could read.

"What did the voice say?" she asked.

I stared past her, washing her out like the old faded print of the pastel sunset hanging above her, led my eyes upward into the still glass frame, and stayed there, a witness to my own voice. "To end it all—to stop trying to hold it all together—to give up—to finally do it."

With narrowed eyes, the lady beneath the drab sunset moved her pen again. "What happened next?" she asked.

My husband's lips pressed together. He fingered the arm of his chair in a circular motion. I became still in thought, unable to think clearly. Something was slipping away—pride, pretense, normalcy. Everything inside me collided.

I responded, slowly, "I was on the freeway and had a strong desire to drive into oncoming traffic. I called my husband and I told him . . ." Here my voice cracked. Here my heart sped. "And I told him I wanted to die." A silence sat in the room, nodding for me to continue. Despite the claustrophobic heat, I shivered. Despite the encroaching numbness, I ached. I lowered my head and continued. This time the words came faster. Not high speed, but above normal, above where I wanted them to be. "I didn't know what to do, so I drove to our family doctor and fell apart. I fell onto my knees. Told him I couldn't go on like this anymore that I needed something to end the pain. Then I begged him to kill me. It was the endless voices, the wanting to be good enough, the needing to be accepted, the constant sense of failure. I couldn't do it anymore. Not one more day." A tear slithered down, and then another and another, until I could no longer count.

The silence in the room left; now there was only my heartbeat, and the knowing that I did not want to look up—not now, not ever. Curling my body inward was not possible. I was already turned. So instead I tucked my eyes into my lap. A cold shudder splintered down my spine. I remembered I held a tissue, remembered it was still there, and led my hand to my nose, pressing the pink to my skin, breathing in the scent of something that did not come from this place.

The woman addressed me gently. "I am going to ask you some more questions about your history. Can you do that?"

And here the room laughed, at least I thought it did, came alive like my distant haunted duplex: Her history? Her history? Ha!

"It's complicated," I heard myself say. I managed to curl my lip and attempt a smile, thinking the smile was the right thing to do. But I didn't want to *do* anymore. I just wanted to be without thinking about what to do.

The woman wrote down more in her loud ink. After a page of scribed sorrows, she looked up. "You know it is very unusual for a person with your history to not have become an addict or ended up in some type of serious trouble." Sniffling, I nodded. "What do you think made you strong?" she asked.

I twisted the tissue in my hand and looked out, searching into her blue-gray eyes. "God," I answered.

"You have a strong faith, then?" she asked.

I thought about the question, and then the tears came faster. "Not anymore," I whispered. "Not anymore."

An hour later, after two colored pills, I entered the last room at the end of the long blue hall. Muffled snores, bleach, staleness—each welcomed me. I found my bed. I pulled off my sweatshirt and spread it across the thin pillow. Darkness. I stared up at the shadowed ceiling. There was no sleeping.

As midnight approached, I stepped through the vacant corridor, light and clumsy, like a puppet pulled by a master puppeteer. "I can't sleep in there," I mumbled, looking at the nurse's wide forehead. "I can't sleep with a stranger in my room." I lowered my eyes to her white shoes with long laces and scuffed toes. The nurse looked me over with a cynical smile. "What are you afraid of?"

I felt a punch to my stomach. "I just can't sleep in there," I answered.

Huffing, the nurse pulled down her glasses. "Fine, come with me, then."

I padded down the hall thinking I might fall down, hoping I would wake up, knowing this was surely hell. The tall nurse stopped. She edged her eyes around me, trying to see inside. "You can stay in the Quiet Room for the night," she said. "But it's not where you are supposed to be."

Chastised, I didn't move. I knew this wasn't where I was supposed to be. None of this place was where I was supposed to be. She didn't know me.

"You'll have to return to your room in the morning. Do you understand?" she asked, marking something on her clipboard, something about me. My eyes swept the empty lobby. I glanced to the side where two nurses were chatting. I gave a slight nod. I smiled meekly. She had wanted me to smile.

The nurse spoke in a hushed whisper. "It's going to be loud. And it's not a very private place to sleep." I didn't have a voice. "Well, don't be surprised if we have to take you out in the middle of the night. If we get in a high-risk patient, we'll have to put them in here." I nodded.

Inside the Quiet Room, a space no bigger than a walk-in closet, my eyes searched out to the pale yellow walls. There were no pictures, no décor, nothing except for one narrow window that slid open to the nurse's station. The bed was made, the blanket thin. There were two doors—one that led to an attached bathroom and another door opening out to the lobby. On the other side of the wall was a large machine, perhaps a boiler or water heater, because every so often a rhythmic thump vibrated the room. Thump, thump— thump, thump—the room's heartbeat.

In reality, there was no bed, only a large wooden box with plywood set on the top. And there was no mattress, only a thick piece of yellow foam. My boots were on the floor, my socks rolled inside the boots. That was all of me that existed there—nothing more.

I sat hunched over on the foam, sinking in my thoughts, rewinding the day. I cried. I stopped, then cried again, stepping my eyes around the room. I cried up to God, "Why have you forsaken me? Why have you left me here? I did what you asked. I wrote every day. I did everything. I've always tried to be good and now you bring me here. This isn't right. This isn't how it's supposed to be. I'm tired of the pain. I'm tired of fighting. I can't do this anymore. I can't." I sank my head into the foam, taking in the unwanted smells. "I hate you!" I screamed. Jagged, scissoring despair. "I hate you," I sobbed.

Unable to escape, I thought back to a year prior. Drifted in my mind to another place and time. Only despite the turmoil, there was still hope then. It was the tail end of the spring of 2005, and, except for the light from the slivered moon, the road was black. My foot hit the pedal and I sped up faster and faster toward the tracks. Mangled is what I wanted. But I wouldn't have the nerve to stop, to wait for a train. There would have to be another way. Perhaps a motel off the interstate, perhaps some pills and a forever sleep. I shook away the thought and breathed a prayer. "Please, help me."

At that time, in my midthirties, the ache of the past had become my own Siamese twin. So much so, I didn't know where my pain stopped and my true self began. I was pain. I was the past. We shared the same blood. Everything and anyone could conjure up bitter memories, especially certain sounds and smells. Each day was yet another rerun of all the misery I'd viewed before. The scenery and characters might change, but the plot and outcome never altered. I knew all the psychological jargon, the self-talk, the imaging, meditation, and so on; and they served as my air, so to speak, the invisible space which kept me temporarily afloat as I waved back and forth in a stormy sea clinging to an inflatable raft filled with holes.

My minivan rattled across the wooden railroad tracks, whipping around a corner, a lone vehicle in a mostly sleeping town. I crossed half the city without much notice, flew by the clay-pottery yard and the Thompson's ranch, like they'd never existed, like all around me was just a blank-faced tunnel. I frowned in the mirror, scowled my brows so low that I quadrupled my age, let the wrinkles merrily line my forehead; let my eyes squint in disdain. "I hate you," I whispered. "I hate you," I cried.

Fear grew, thundering like the approaching storm. I nodded at my next thought, even smiled some. I would drive until there was nowhere else. And then, in the way of my old black cat, I would creep into a shadowed hovel, and cease to exist. Moving as a leaf in a crashing river, I went where the current took me, down the streets I'd barely touched before. The community pool, a palette of wavering violet hues, reflected the last glimpse of the lonely moon. The stars hid beneath a milky gray blanket. It was the end, the last cookie-cutter cluster of suburbia.

I mouthed, "I'm so scared." I shouted, lifting one hand off the steering wheel and forging through a fast-growing puddle. "Why me? Where is my shelter? Where is my reprieve?" The wind answered me, a mocking slap to the side window. "Who am I supposed to be?" I begged. "Please? I can't do this anymore." A burst of tears followed. "Please, please, help me."

From somewhere, perhaps inside, perhaps beyond, I was answered. In a whisper, a familiar voice directed: "Stop the car." There was a hush to the voice, like a mother hushing her babe to sleep. And then more words: "Pull over, right here and rest, rest here. My precious child."

"You're not real," I thought. "You've never been real." I cried, shaking in fear. I felt a failure, for holding on for so many years when I'd wanted to give up, wanted to collapse in someone's arms—let them take over, let them take the wheel. I'd longed to slip behind the curtain and rest . . . to just rest.

Then slowly something changed. I felt a smile, sensed a smile. Not in the way of man, but a smile just the same. I could see myself, a little girl with large brown eyes with a face creased in a generous grin—a trusting grin. All pains and misery erased. An enveloping trust surrounding an innocent.

Still, the older me, the one I considered rational and wise, was angry and doubtful. Tired of the games, the messages, all the confusion and mystery. I wanted to push the voice away like the debris on a driveway, let the garbage drift down the gutters into the brook. And then I remembered our greeting. The way through the years I'd made sure. The way I'd awake myself from my dreams—the nightmares that paralyzed and trapped me in another existence, another realm. "If this is not from the light, I rebuke you in the name of Jesus Christ!" I shouted.

The peace remained, more than steadfast, more than true. Remained and made a part of me into completion, repairing the fissured crack of my soul. As I sat still at the side of the road, there was a deafening silence. Even with the rain tumbling down and the wind whisking the trees, all around there was an insulating calm. A thousand twigs upon a thousand twigs crisscrossed and piled into an unbreakable peace. "Hush, child. Hush," I heard. "Just trust and believe. We are with you. We are always with you. Look out your window and see what is true."

I smudged my face with my sweatshirt and stopped my nose from draining. I turned, hesitating at first to even focus. I didn't know where I was. This side of town was unfamiliar. I expected to see nothing, at least nothing of meaning. But I looked, and looked again. Beside my van, outside the right passenger window, was the town's Catholic church, a structure battered in peeling white stucco and a forlorn tar rooftop. For a glimpse, I was back inside the tranquil walls of the church of my childhood, padding through the echoing corridors beneath the intricate archways and the steep, slanting balconies.

Looking further out my window through the pattering rain, my eyes beheld a new sight: a wooden cross, which stretched taller than a man, draped in a cloak of shimmering lights. And on this particular night, as the rain bled all around, the white bulbs, too numerous to count, illuminated the dark sky.

"We are with you. We are always with you," I heard.

This wasn't a vision. The cross was there. It was rooted into the ground, solid. What I beheld was plain as day to any other.

"Go home. Just believe. Just trust and believe, and go home."

I shook my head. I couldn't go home. I was still broken, and more than terrified to return. I looked up at the lit cross and cried louder. "I can't. I can't."

"Then drive."

I remembered to breathe, and without knowing what else to do, pulled out slowly onto the rain-slathered road. I drove a past a few streets, and then heard, "Turn here."

I felt crazy and delusional, but would try, if only once more. I turned into the narrow alleyway, an unfamiliar, dark road. Only a line of garbage cans and old garage doors greeted me.

"Stop here."

The van idled for a moment before I stopped the engine. The rain came louder.

"I don't want to go home. There is no reason. I'm useless," I cried, shrinking down into myself, wishing to be taken away. "Why should I go home? Why? Tell me why!"

"Look out your window and you will see why," the voice came again.

I turned to my left and raised my eyes. Beside where I'd parked was a tall street lamp. The lamp was shining down on a white, rectangular street sign. I was afraid. Afraid to know this was all just my twisted imaginings, a voice I had invented my entire life to stay afloat. I took in a sequence of breaths, each consecutively faster and harder, attempting to reassure myself. And then, after a labored intake, followed by one long, even release of air, I was ready. Here would be the truth of who I was, or at the very least a reckoning of the end, proof I should be done with it.

And there before my eyes, the truth stood clear, nailed to a wooden board, clear and bright beneath a flickering bulb. And effervescent light outlined the message. Aglow in the dark, a white street sign depicted two shadowed outlines of children playing in the street. Below the shadowed figures were the words "Think of the Children."

I knew then, knew beyond a doubt, that the children were why I should remain strong. Even as I bleed from the tattered past that shrouded me in misery, I knew I had to remain, if only for them. I had to keep fighting. I would have to find a way to pull myself out of the weight of physical and mental anguish. I had to win for my own children. I had to win for all of the children. All of this, these thoughts, fluttered inside like a rabble of monarchs bursting free from a net.

I thought again. Logically analyzed what had happened. I realized I had seen street signs before, usually yellow ones, and often around parks and schoolyards, but those signs typically displayed the words "Children at Play." Through all the years I had worked with children, first as a daycare employee, and later as an elementary and middle school teacher, I had never once seen a sign that read, "Think of the Children."

I whispered, "Think of the children." And the tears came again.

In the late hours of the night, I returned home and crept inside my boys' bedroom. Standing alone in the darkness, I looked down at my three small children—how sweet their faces, how tender their skin. I kissed them each, softly and purposefully, watched as their eyes fluttered. They hadn't known. None of them had known. To them I'd merely stepped out of the house. To them nothing had changed. My husband had had no indication of my true intentions either. Beyond what I had showed him, beyond my angry words and the act of leaving the house abruptly, all was well. To him, I'd appeared as an angry child, fed up. To him, I'd simply return when I'd cooled down. I'd return. I'd return, and then all would remain.

Inside my bedroom, my husband didn't stir. I found my nightclothes and slipped into bed. His snoring came in variants of alto and baritone, and sometimes in little rhythmic puffs. I rested on my back, staring up at the ceiling. "I'm home," I whispered. I closed my eyes. "Now what?"

"You will write. And your words will heal you and others," I heard.

My stomach turned nervously. My eyes opened. "What?" I questioned. "Not me."

"We are with you. We will be with you."

I protested with a deep sigh.

"You will write, and we will be with you."

I debated, momentarily, and then twisted under the covers and shut out the night.

In the early hours of morning, before the rooster crowed from the field beyond our property but long after the crickets and toads had stopped their serenading, I had a dream. In my vision a lone blue oak stood stalwartly on a towering hill in the shadows of the rising morning sun. The old tree's thick branches reached out in all directions, as high and as wide as the eyes could see. Purple and orange hues filled the sky. There was a sense of peace and serenity in the air, a feeling that all would turn out as planned. I was filled with a gentle peace and a knowing. I was filled with trust and understanding. I saw multitudes of people gather around the tree, hand-in-hand, their faces set in tears of recognition, their hearts smiling in joy. I was no longer alone, and neither were they.

I began writing that day.

The phone rang: one old, pale orange phone with a curled orange cord that hung on the light blue wall. A heavyset woman with a short-shaved haircut picked up. She looked like my mother's long-ago roommate, the heavy-boned woman who had taught me how to shower; the one I'd tried to forget. The one that reminded me of figs—how they can be split open with bare hands, and the insides all sucked out.

"Stew, it's for you!" The stout lady hollered across the lobby. Her eyes scanned the room like a mother surveying the clutter on a table. She hadn't wanted to truly look.

"Anybody seen Stew?" She scanned again, while yawning and then spoke. "Can't find him. Try again later."

I inhaled, taking in a breath to fill and shield me. Made no difference. I remained flat, non-dimensional, trapped in my own faded painting on a wall. The chair beneath me was hard plastic. Resembled the chairs in the classroom in which I taught. Where were my students now? Were they, too, all grown with their own pain? Could they see me here, by some type of magic? Peer inside this horror show.

The table, cafeteria style—cold, direct, nothing hidden—seemed a camcorder recording and displaying—shooting images of me across the universe. Captions of failure. Captions of stupid. Captions of unimportant.

A lanky nurse pushed a rolling cart with small white cups. "Here," she said flatly. Everything was flat here. Everything. I swallowed hard, the pills dropping down. I imagined them alive. From directly behind me a patient in stained pink pajamas squeaked open the fridge and brought out a cup of vanilla pudding. I thought about the haunted duplex, about the heavy-breathing ghost. The time of the storm, when I'd fled my house, running up the street to a stranger's door, pounding my fist, horrified, terrified to return to my own home for fear of the hauntings.

"Jack off! Jack off!" A man's voice called out.

"Jack off, here." He strutted by, some king of the forsaken castle, a comical stand-in for the real star. With an air of respect, he yanked at the tail of his striped hospital gown. Then he dug his eyes into me, real straight and narrow. They were sparkling, almost clear. "Jack Off. That's what they call me," he said, winking, his lashes thick beneath the flickering fluorescent light.

I tasted the soot in my mouth and suddenly wanted to weep over having not had a toothbrush to greet me in the morning. Just as I'd wanted to cry over yesterday's clothes.

"But you can just call me Jack," I heard. I lifted a brow. He was skinny like Mother's young boyfriend Lou from a time before, the guy that used to wear silver spikes up and down his leather pants. The lad only three years my senior, whose handsome dad had died in the tragic plane crash shortly after giving me that book, the book I had taken to the beach of France, the only book I had taken to Europe. My mind traveled and traveled.

"Is this your first time on these lovely premises?" Jack asked. He then paused, waiting for me to fill in the emptiness. I glanced up, twisting my fingers in my lap, and then wrapped my arms around my sweatshirt, and mumbled my name. My chair wobbled and the table shook. Nothing in this place seemed balanced.

A girl no older than twenty approached. She swept her arms across Jack's narrow shoulders. "Good morning," she whispered. "I missed you." She ran her finger playfully up and down his chest. Her hair was dark auburn, very straight and highlighted with grease. Jack turned around and gave her a tight squeeze, a lover's squeeze, their gowns joining together.

Jack looked to his side. "Hey there, Stew." A thin man walked past us and took his place on a black line on the floor. A silver-haired woman in a dressing gown filed in behind. Soon a middle-aged, red-bearded man joined the line. Jack leaned his arm on the table, the opulent green of his eyes half-masked by his tousled camel-blond hair.

"Stew doesn't look too good," Jack said. "They've been frying his brain with those electric *shock-o-matic* treatments." The girl standing next to Jack scratched her slender neck with overgrown fingernails. There were needle marks up her arms, dark circles under her eyes. I felt my hair. It was tangled. I tore the edging off a white napkin, thinking back to my friend's cousin, wondering if she'd ever seen the insides of a place like this, and if the hanger beatings had ever stopped.

"See that good-looking guy standing by the door? That's Freezer. If you're in here enough, you usually get a chance to see Old Freezer. Years back he tried to swallow antifreeze." Jack shook his head and streaked back his hair with both hands. His jaws and lips wiggled back and forth like he was rinsing with mouthwash, before he licked the top row of his yellow teeth and continued. "His parents signed some legal-type papers, can't afford to keep paying these hospital bills—disowning him. Now me, I don't have to worry about that none, seeing I don't have no parents."

"I'm sorry," I whispered. My eyes counted the crumbs on the cold gray table.

After yawning and cracking her neck to the side, Jack's lady friend stepped away into the line. "Looks like *caf-o-teria* time," Jack said, tipping his head to the left. "Sorry, sugar, you can't line up quite yet. Those hawk eyes aren't going to let you leave the premises," he laughed, "being you're a danger to society and all."

A nurse in a dark blue smock carrying a clipboard arrived and checked off the top box on her paper. "Jack? You coming to breakfast?"

"That's *Jack Off* to you." He spoke over his shoulder with a smirk and then turned around and leaned in real close. I could smell the cigarettes and mint. "Whatever you do, don't eat the eggs. And don't look them nurses in the eyes or they'll hypnotize you." He rolled his eyes around. I couldn't tell if he was humoring me or not. In the end, I figured it didn't really make a difference.

Someone from behind me approached and plopped a plastic tray down. I grimaced at a full plate of runny eggs. Jack made his eyes sparkle wide like half-dollars and ran his finger across his throat like a knife. "Watch out. Looks like death for you."

"Let's go, people. Time for breakfast," a nurse warned, and moved her hands in an ushering motion. I had flashbacks of elementary school lunchtime, of assemblies, of field trips, my mind searched for connections, to bring together the blurred past with the trapped present. Jack tipped an imaginary hat, and with a quick wink said, "Catch you later."

When most everyone had exited the room, I set my eyes on the Quiet Room where several nurses gathered. A woman was moaning inside.

"Sounds like she's having a hard time at it," a man, wearing bulky black headphones over a Red Sox baseball cap, said in a melodic baritone voice. His beard was grizzly thick and golden brown. He smiled and took a seat beside me at the small table. "I'm Zach," he offered, slightly adjusting his headphones back.

I said my name, with a struggling grin, and crossed my arms over my chest. He sat far back enough, I supposed. Freezer strode by in wide steps, barely balancing a food tray. Zach cleared his throat and tugged at his beard. "I'm in here getting sober." He looked to the left and then the right, letting out a slight chuckle. "Again," he added. "My boss—I work at the radio station—he said this was the last time. You heard of KWHIZ?"

"I'm not sure," I answered. I heard a high-pitched scream, and pulled my eyes away from the Quiet Room.

"That's where I work. I do the night selection. Doesn't pay much but can lead to other things. They call me Whiz. What are you in for?"

I grimaced and pushed aside my tray. I didn't answer.

"No problem. I get it. You met Jack, yet?"

I nodded.

"Quite the character. Has a good heart, though. He's my buddy. We're thinking about being roomies after this . . ." Whiz paused and gave a high wave to slender Stew. But Stew didn't seem to notice. He just ambled by staring straight ahead. "Poor Stew," Whiz said, shaking his head. "His wife comes down from the hills. He's been fighting this depression. They keep hoping those treatments will do something. I don't think frying him is helping at all. He can't be outside of these walls without someone watching him. I hate drinking. I hate what it does to me, but I'm sure glad I'm not him. See that lady over there, now don't go telling her I said this, but she's in here because of her daughter. Seems her daughter went and moved in with a known sex offender, a child molester, no less. And when she tried to pull her daughter out, the daughter said she didn't want anything to do with her anymore." Whiz fidgeted with a plastic fork on the table. "Can't get my finger on Freezer. You know about him?"

"Yes," I whispered.

"That's a tough way to go. I think I'd do the gas stove or car bit. You know, when you stick the hose in the exhaust pipe and sit in your car and fall asleep nice and easy. That's what I'd do. Not that I'd ever do it. But that's what I'd do, if I did."

I swallowed hard.

"How about you?"

I swallowed harder, and my eyes grew wide.

Alongside the north wall a frail elderly lady in a quilted robe strode across the floor calling out, "He should be here by now. He is coming. I shouldn't be here. He is coming. He promised he was coming." Her pale, thin arms lifted up into the air into a broad gesture. "I don't belong here. He is coming. He is coming!" She reached the wall, turned around, and started walking the other direction. She prattled on in Portuguese now.

Whiz nodded his head to the right. "It's not God she's calling. She doesn't belong here. Should be in an old folks' home. She needs to be in one of them places. She keeps thinking her nephew's going to come get her. But he ain't." He paused, stretched, scratched his chin, and then smiled lightly. "You can call me Whiz, if you'd like. But just for another day or two. I came in voluntarily. I can walk out any damn time I want to."

I sat up taller.

"That must be nice," I offered.

"Not really. Not really at all," Whiz said. His eyes lowered to the floor. His body collapsed. And his eyes grew sad. Then he looked straight into me, his voice cracking some. "You know, it's actually better when someone forces you to stay put. Makes you stay even though you don't want to. Makes you look at all those demons you've been thinking you could outrun."

147. BEHIND THE DOOR

There was a time of many tears, encompassing a thousand years,
To even glimpse a sense of joy seemed to me an endless void.
Where emptiness entrenched a whole, leaving still this shallow mold,
Of who I was supposed to be, of all the hopes drained out of me.
I searched for answers day and night. I prayed, I cried, I begged for light.
Still nothing ticked that I could hear. And all I am near disappeared.
What did remain, I did not know. But I continued, even so.
I stood and watched from way down low, that part of soul that yearned to grow.
Decades passed, and still I tried, to cease the pain that bled me dry.
No place to go, no one to ask. No way to understand my past;
I lived it all, the shadows gray, returning to the yesterdays;
Every smell, the sound, the face, could bring me back to fearful place.
And there was more than one or two, like the years a thousand grew.
The spots they shadowed up the sun, siphoning away the fun.
From pain to pain I hopped my path, never learning how to laugh.
Swirls of black and blue and red, stories that could not be said.
Time, he came; he watched, he left, taking with him all the best.
And where I looked through windowpane, the spinning world passed by again,
The rise, the fall, the nothingness, the dreaming more to not exist.
Until in faith one seed appeared and sprouted strong within the tears,
To something more than I could see, from something bright and bold and free.
This surfaced strong, a light to shine, a part no longer left behind.
The seed, it rose with every word; I shared and screamed, I scratched and blurred.
And in this way the mirror I shook, so I could take another look
Of what was done, and what was not, of what was lost, and what was sought,
Of all the little treasures blind, of all the nothings left behind.
I walked, I trekked, I even flew, passing by the girl I knew,
The way in which she smiled deep, the way in which she made me weep.
The precious one, heart pure as dew, I held her hand and one made two.
And thus in words I found a trail, to wave one last good-bye to fail.

The steps she made were never wrong; her heart was always ever strong.
Her wishes still she carried true, and in this way I grew anew.
In strength the mourning broke and quaked, and love was lastly made awake,
To forgive what was, to nod and rise, to finally claim the golden prize,
Of seeing where I'd been and gone, remembering the soft with strong.
And now when chance I cross and glance, another bled by circumstance,
In truth, I choose to sit and be, to hold the hand and place the key,
To understand that all that came, the hurt, the loss, engulfing shame,
Is nothing more than moving brook—a song, a dance, a storybook,
For what we are is so much more than what is locked behind the door.

148. A Beautiful Morning with a Beautiful Mind

My Aspie son and I have such deep and complex conversations that I swear he must be at least a thousand years old. He speaks philosophically, in a manner of viewing life that I have only discovered in the ancient wisdom of great scholars.

This morning, we spoke about truth, and the idea that when one threatens another's truth by confrontation through disagreement or differing opinion, how the other naturally instinctually responds with a fight-or-flight nature. We opted for the agreement that this human response is based on human nature, on the idea of wanting to protect singular intelligence and mentality. I scaffolded upon the initial points, mentioning the concepts of limited and isolated perception based on the singular collection of reality from a limited scope of an individualized sensory input. He understood entirely. I elaborated that I don't hold a singular truth, as my truths vary vastly compared to how I interpreted my world five years prior, and that I am continually changing. He concurred and expressed that I had made sense. Of course, most of this discussion was a dissertation on my son's part. His theories of human communication and outcomes are right up there with the geniuses of our time. It amazes me that he is Aspie and yet years ahead of his peers in understanding the complexities of human nature and societal responses to multiple environmental stimuli.

I suppose I have taught him some by example, and he has sought out his own form of awareness and truth through observation of others and the intake of literature and films; however, the intricate ways in which he pieces the found knowledge into linear, detailed outcomes and conclusions is awe-inspiring. If ever an old soul exists, I see this as my son.

When I offer a gentle reminder to him (at any time and in any genre of conversation) to please remember to keep in mind that he views the world a bit differently than others and that he and I have complex ways of interpreting events, he responds ever so humbly, consistently reminding me that he does not enjoy the comfort of setting himself above or beyond anyone else, and that all can see and comprehend as he does, but perhaps they do not understand what they are doing or in some way do not observe the connections.

He is insistent that his way is no better and that he is not superior by any means; to sit with the idea of being special is a great discomfort to him. And though my son may appear aloof, argumentative, and at the edge of his seat ready to engage in debate, he is a wise sage at heart, insistent upon remaining humble. A concept I did not set out to instruct upon him, but one he shares with me.

I am continually fascinated by his mind. He grows in spurts that are "unnaturally" fast, comprehending and taking in and retaining more than any student I have ever witnessed. He reworks ideas in his mind to match his view of reality, a view that is extremely open-minded whilst being seemingly narrow-minded. I mean to say that, to the typical observer, he comes across as strongly opinionated and limited in his viewpoints, but given the time for careful analysis, he is actually extremely open to reasonable and logical ideas that don't initially resonate as truth with him. And, in fact, he will easily dislodge a chosen truth for a new truth after taking in what another has shared. The barrier that exists between him and his peers (and some adults) appears to be that exact fight-or-flight mentality my son was theorizing upon. He speaks, and if another interprets him as threatening to any degree, then the other shuts my son down or out, no longer hearing what he is stating and instead closing off possible connection.

We were weaving out of conversation this morning, and I found myself going down an interesting course. I had started a sentence several times, never truly completing the string of words, as my son was interjecting (albeit while apologizing for doing so) with his rapid-fire thoughts and connections. I enjoy the way he is ignited with ideas and take no offense to his interruptions. I see a lot of myself in him, and him in me.

I was trying to explain something to my son. At first, I thought I was clear on my idea, but something inside of me self-corrected in the middle of my thought process. I was speaking aloud. I had thought of the isolating factor of Aspergers, how we are so often misunderstood and ostracized. And, on hearing my son talk so freely and blatantly, I imagined how this exact discourse might bring him further out of his collective circle of peers. I began to speak from fear, but didn't recognize what I was doing until most of the words were out of my mouth.

"As you get older, son, I think it would be beneficial if you monitored some of what . . ."

The words came through at last as one cohesive thread, and with that outpour, I had time to recollect what I had shared. I immediately backtracked.

"You know what? I have changed my mind," I shared. "I was originally thinking that you should be more careful around people who don't accept you unconditionally, so that you don't live an isolated life. But I disagree with this. I think you should be exactly you, and that people will love you for you."

We sidetracked for a bit to explore the concept of unconditional love. He didn't understand the idea of choosing not to have someone in your life but choosing to still love them unconditionally, e.g., to hold them in love and light, to pray or keep them in thought, to hold no ill will or resentment toward the individual and wish the person the very best.

He seemed to be taking in a lot more than I was saying.

My son looked at me and gave me a sheepishly wise grin. I knew that he knew. And we continued onward, back to the previous conversation.

I stated, "I mean, I tried the other way for years. To pretend and hold back myself, and I was miserable. Why would I want that for you? I just want you to be free to be you, and others to appreciate you for who you are."

He answered. "I know. I thought you might change your mind, once you said it. You realized you were contradicting yourself before you were finished. That is clear. I understand."

I smiled, still in disbelief at the level of this young man's ability to comprehend others' thought processes. I added, "I guess I just wish as you grow older that you can focus on being less injurious, if that makes sense. What I mean is there is a difference between choosing to say something that you are highly certain will hurt someone's feelings, and saying something that unintentionally hurts someone. If you are injurious, it will be harder to maintain friends. Does that make sense?"

"Yes," he said. "And I already do that, Mom. Don't worry. I understand."

We talked further about the complexities of human communication and the limitations based on others' interpretations and emotional responses. As we approached the school, he looked at me and responded, "Thank you for such intriguing conversation." He nodded, sounding much like the little professor I have grown to adore in astonishing amounts. "It was quite a good conversation."

I half expected him to add "indeed" to the end of his last statement.

His voice was monotone, without hints of rejoice; he made no eye contact, and he mostly huffed away as I said, "Enjoy your day, sweetie pie." But I knew how he felt. We'd connected at an intellectual level without judgment, without expectation, and with equally open minds and acceptance. It was another freeing moment, the way in which the two of us communicate, this unabashed arena in which anything said is okay and doesn't affect the other's equilibrium or sense of self or worth.

It was a beautiful morning, indeed.

149. Until the Rain Came

There once was a little girl named Sam. She spent her day in the wilderness amongst the walnut orchards and the towering oak trees, playing in the fields of tall grass. She was a friend to all creatures, grand and small. Every part of life was fascinating. Her own skin—soft and delightful. The pink of her dog's nose, poking through where the black had worn away— a wet treat. The ants she watched with fascination. The wind she breathed in to catch. And the sky, her endless dream.

This little girl, she loved to dance and be. She could sit for hours and play inside her imagination while amongst nature's gifts. Her bounty was the fallen twigs beneath her feet, the pebbles in her pockets, and the taste of nectar on her tongue. Nothing was missing or out of place. Everything moved as ordained in a perfect circle of give and take. Every part fit into place to make a glorious time, much like the intricate makings of a clock. All moved to produce one. All moved continually, and changed, and came back again. Returning to the eyes of the beholder what always was.

Love was all about this child, especially in the song of birds and the dipping of dragonflies as they danced, reflecting the light with their transparent wings. If colors were her world, then the spectrum was magnificent—a thousand rainbows intertwined to form hues uncommon to the adult eye, colors that danced their own symphony, producing brilliant songs from voices of angelic creatures. There wasn't a want or need, just the simplicity of moving as one with the rest that danced. She was as a caterpillar set free upon endless green, nibbling at the gifts before her.

Until the rain came.

With the rain, Caterpillar ceased and Butterfly was born. Butterfly was lovely, detailed and sketched in nature's beauty, and able to fly and reach heights previously unimaginable. However, now she could dance outside her realm and escape what she once knew as the only existence. From up above her angle changed. Her world became smaller and larger. Things she knew not of before appeared, and visions she once believed in vanished altogether. As she watched and flew higher, she began to see that where she'd been was nothing but a patch, a broken, shattered fragment that, given enough distance, simply disappeared from sight. When she returned and touched down everything was altered. As hard as she tried her new eyes could not see the same terrain. All was different. All tainted with logic and reason and this daunting inquiry.

That which was once simply existence was now struggle. That which was once simply peace turned to question after question. Her own beauty, which she had never doubted before or even considered, now faded with her thoughts. And those thoughts twisted within the others, creating a band so thick the toughest warrior could not break it. And now there were warriors. There were enemies and fighters. There were people who spoke untruths and hurt. There were diamonds that were stolen, treasures destroyed, and secrets kept. She knew then that the Butterfly World was not where she belonged. Though she had become Butterfly, she longed to return to the Land of Caterpillar. She longed for her old eyes.

As it was, she spent her days searching for kindness, for the place that once existed that was pure and innocent, the emerald of hope and faith that others now seemed to pierce and stab so often that she'd had to hide this essence out of fear of destruction. And thusly, she hid inside herself. When she was teased and admonished, she hid. When she was tortured with looks and words, she hid. When she tried to be as others wanted and she still was not enough, she hid. And all the time she hid she cried and wept for this land she knew before—where the birds sang and she heard only their music, where the wind blew and she felt only the air.

Now, everything came with explanation and reason. Now, everything came with doubt. And here in this Land of Butterflies, she wished for nothing but to pluck off her own wings and wither, if only to return to a part of her own self that could not fly above and see. She wished for death, like so many misplaced butterflies do. Not death from her own being but death from the world about her. To black out her surroundings and apply a fresh coat of white and paint again—a new picture, the one from before the rain came.

But still, she remained Butterfly. As Butterfly, she attempted to rebuild a cocoon, so she could crawl inside and wake up transformed to the time before. As Butterfly, she attempted to fly high so that she might leave behind all that was below. As Butterfly, she tried to protect herself in armor, to shield herself from the coming arrows. As Butterfly, she tried to smear herself in masks and makeup, to pretend. She tried and tried to no avail, and remained but a butterfly, broken and alone.

Until the time came and she heard an echo. And whispers poured in like dew quenching her unyielding thirst. She was shown then the way to Caterpillar Land. She was shown then how to bring peace to the butterfly. She was given the secret, the promise—a ray of hope so slender and tender that only this butterfly could keep safe. And she did, deep inside of her; she carried the precious ray through many years.

Until the time came again, and she knew what to do.

And thusly—with the coming season, with her heart knowing, as the light called—she set to spinning her ray, setting her thoughts to words in hopes that the world might know of the caterpillars and of the butterflies, and of how the journey of the broken was also a journey of hope. In her weaving the light shined and shined so bright that the other lost butterflies found a way to this little butterfly; and soon there were thousands of butterflies collected, their wings together fluttering to carry them onward. They moved and moved together. At last returning back home to the Land of Caterpillar, to the place of innocence and love they remembered, to the place of unreason and truth, to the place they could dance again in the spectrum of light, united in their beauty. In a place where everywhere they looked they saw a reflection of self and in so seeing realized the butterfly, though lost, had been found.

And so they danced, because of the promise of who they were, because of the place they kept inside all these years. And slowly, they let go. Slowly, the armor came off. And slowly, the light of the caterpillar shone through each of them so brilliantly that the world began to see that butterflies don't have to let go of the caterpillar to fly.

150. TURN, TURN, TURN

I'd like to end my writings on a *high* note, primarily because life is filled with enough dreariness and all that boggy jazz—and because I wish for you to want to be my forever friend. So rest assured, Silly Sam is still here! Right now I am playing and replaying the song "Dancing Queen" by Abba—after that I'll likely play the theme music from the movie *Flash Dance*, followed by the Byrds' "Turn, Turn, Turn."

I have a generous amount of peace of mind today when considered in comparison to what was on my proverbial plate the first four decades of my life. Which gives me further trust in the dark-haired psychic who not only predicted the meeting of my (former) husband and the birth of our first two children, but also foretold that during the second half of my lifespan, I would reach a wide audience of people, switch careers, and become significantly happier! Of course, silly me, I continue to spend an excess amount of time processing my expiration date (a.k.a. impending death) based on the coming to pass of the first half of my life.

Believe it or not, I no longer have the need to process as much, speak as much, or fret as much. I also worry about death, dying, and all things feasibly deadly about 95 percent less of the time. Now that's something! I continue to like the repetition of threes, though. The university experience (you know, the whole de-meaning "broken brain" incident), that has yet to come to full closure, but I think about mailing them these pages with a sweet pink Post-It note that reads, "By the way, the villains—that's you guys. Have a nice day (smiling-face emoticon)."

(Just a sec. I am turning to Google God for "Flash Dance: What a feeling." Okay. I am back now . . . *Take your passion and make it happen*! LV, dressed in blue chiffon, and Sir Brain, in his stately white briefs, are totally rocking out. Sir Brain just slid across the floor like Tom Cruise in *Risky Business*.)

As I steer away from my beloved story and venture into brand new territories (in all realms of my little life), and as this heck-of-a-long chapter of my days comes to a much-anticipated close, I thought you and I could pretend we are just now meeting for the first time! Wouldn't that be grand?

I mean, I am much more put together now (sarcasm). So how about it? How about you sit right down in this charming café with *moi* and order up your favorite beverage (my treat) and a side of mashed potatoes, please? Just for now, erase anything and *everything* you know about Sam (as I do daily) and pretend! Oh, instead of a café we can build a blanket fort and perch ourselves below my dining-room table, and wear violet and magenta floppy hats and oversized floral dresses (or striped '70s pants), and sip sweet tea from china cups (or guzzle down hard pear cider from long-necked bottles)!

Beginnings are so much better than endings, aren't they? I mean generally speaking. So here we are, and here I am . . . in repeat (erase-prior-knowledge) mode. You haven't spoken yet, but I have, of course. And this is what I am saying:

I make up words. I eat chocolate for breakfast. I take myself *far* too seriously. I have three wonderful teenage sons and don't know how I survived the earlier years, like when I came home to find the new babysitter pacing the room as my three-year-old son streaked naked with a broken bowl over his head and a stream of his second full roll of toilet paper in hand, trimming the hallways, while his two older brothers cheered him on. That, and the time my two youngest barricaded themselves in a bedroom to block their irate older brother with a fire poker from getting in and gouging them. Thousands know me by the name "Sam," and I actually answer to Sam, and turn around when I hear the name Sam, and refer to myself as Sam. And use Sam's Facebook page. But that's my pen name, and my real name is Marcelle. (I'm not French. I am actually named after my stunningly beautiful great-aunt who lives in Malta). I am psychic, empathic, and oftentimes a pain in the ass—not like a cyst or boil or hemorrhoids, not even a pimple, but more like a small tag in your underwear that irritates you to no end because you have sensory issues. I plan on returning to a happy-flappy state as soon as feasibly possible, and coffee mochas seem to be helping. Either that or a loony state, or perhaps a crazy, running-naked-in-the-street state—something to that degree. I am all pruned up from spending far too much time in a deep pool of self-analysis. I can write the most complex shit you've ever read and it all comes out in one sitting. In case you doubt it, I can provide proof. And here's a random picture of me when I was four. When I was four I liked to eat green apples and play in the gutter . . .

Your Turn!

ABOUT THE AUTHOR

Samantha Craft, EdM, is the author of the well-received blog *Everyday Aspergers*. She was featured as one of the twenty autistic mentors led by Dr. Temple Grandin in the best-selling *I Am AspienWoman*. Her works have been published in peer-reviewed journals and shared by thousands of individuals across the globe. Craft is best known for "Ten Traits," an article outlining the characteristics of a female Aspergerian. When she is not writing, she works as a community manager for a technology company that employs neurodiverse individuals. Craft lives in the beautiful Pacific Northwest with her three teenage boys, her partner, and a neurotic dog; there she enjoys walks in nature, quaint cafes, painting, poetry, and the performing arts. She offers her story as a testimony of the courage and love found in the heart of an autistic woman.

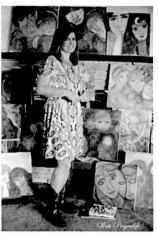

Photo credit by Wati Mixon Photography

Author Contact Information:

Email Sam at: info@myspectrumsuite.com

Twitter Sam at: @aspergersgirls

Join Everyday Aspergers Facebook Clan at: https://www.facebook.com/Everyday-Aspergers-387026824645012/

See Sam's company at: myspectrumsuite.com

Check out Sam's writings here:

everydayaspergers.com

everydayaspie.wordpress.com

bellyofastar.wordpress.com

UPCOMING BOOKS

Everyday Aspergers: Guided Journal

Everyday Aspergers: Poetry and Prose